Thieme
BRITISH MEDICAL ASSOCIATION

0832932

Neurosurgery Board Review

Questions and Answers for Self-Assessment

Third Edition

Cargill H. Alleyne Jr., MD
Professor and Marshall Allen Distinguished Chairman
Residency Program Director
Department of Neurosurgery
Medical College of Georgia at Georgia Regents University
Augusta, Georgia

M. Neil Woodall, MD
Chief Resident
Department of Neurosurgery
Medical College of Georgia at Georgia Regents University
Augusta, Georgia

Jonathan Stuart Citow, MD, FACS
Chief of Neurosurgery
Advocate Condell Medical Center
Libertyville, Illinois
Assistant Clinical Professor of Neurosurgery
Rosalind Franklin University Medical School
North Chicago, Illinois
and
President of the American Center for Spine and Neurosurgery
Libertyville, Illinois

268 illustrations

Thieme
New York · Stuttgart · Delhi · Rio de Janeiro

Executive Editor: Timothy Y. Hiscock
Associate Managing Editor: Kenneth Schubach
Managing Editor: Elizabeth Palumbo
Director, Editorial Services: Mary Jo Casey
Production Editor: Heidi Grauel
International Production Director: Andreas Schabert
Vice President, Editorial and E-Product Development:
    Vera Spillner
International Marketing Director: Fiona Henderson
International Sales Director: Louisa Turrell
Director of Sales, North America: Mike Roseman
Senior Vice President and Chief Operating Officer:
    Sarah Vanderbilt
President: Brian D. Scanlan

Library of Congress Cataloging-in-Publication Data

Alleyne, Cargill H., author.
    Neurosurgery board review : questions and answers
for self-assessment / Cargill Alleyne, M. Neil Woodall,
Jonathan Citow. — Third edition.
    p. ; cm.
    Includes bibliographical references and index.
    ISBN 978-1-62623-104-7 — ISBN 978-1-62623-105-4
I. Woodall, M. Neil, author. II. Citow, Jonathan Stuart,
    author. III. Title.
    [DNLM: 1. Neurosurgery—Examination Questions. WL 18.2]
RD593
617.4'80076—dc23   2015028124

Copyright © 2016 Thieme Medical Publishers, Inc.

Thieme Publishers New York
333 Seventh Avenue, New York, NY 10001 USA
1 800 782 3488, customerservice@thieme.com

Thieme Publishers Stuttgart
Rüdigerstrasse 14, 70469 Stuttgart, Germany
+49 [0]711 8931 421, customerservice@thieme.de

Thieme Publishers Delhi
A-12, Second Floor, Sector-2, Noida-201301
Uttar Pradesh, India
+91 120 45 566 00, customerservice@thieme.in

Thieme Publishers Rio de Janeiro, Thieme Publicações Ltda.
Edifício Rodolpho de Paoli, 25° andar
Av. Nilo Peçanha, 50 – Sala 2508
Rio de Janeiro 20020-906 Brasil
+55 21 3172 2297

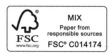

Cover design: Thieme Publishing Group
Typesetting by: Grauel Group
Printed in the United States by Sheridan Books, Inc. 5 4 3 2 1

ISBN 978-1-62623-104-7

Also available as an e-book:
eISBN 978-1-62623-105-4

This book is dedicated to my wife, Audrey, and children, Nathan and Nicole, whose love and support keep me grounded; my parents, Cargill Sr. and Linnette, and sister, Carlin, who taught me the meaning of family; and to the many residents with whom I have worked over the years.

Cargill H. Alleyne Jr., MD

To my wife, Anneliese, my son, Art, and my parents, James and Linda, for their unconditional love and support.

M. Neil Woodall, MD

This book is dedicated to my three most interesting children, Benjamin Joseph, Emma Caroline, and Harrison Atticus Chamberlain. Hopefully when you each join the clan of neurosurgeons (no pressure there...), you will correct any inaccuracies we have made here in this text, just as you are so wont to do with anything I touch at home.

Jonathan S. Citow, MD

Contents

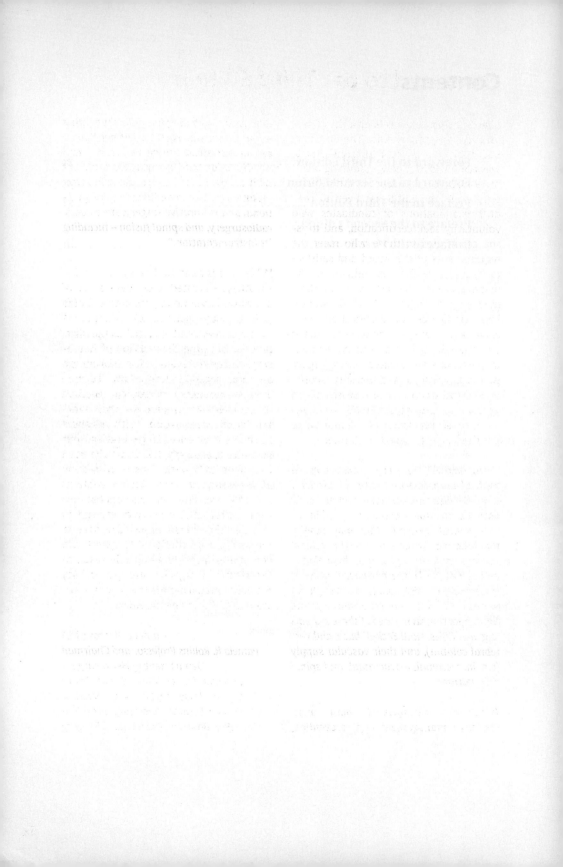

Foreword to the Third Edition

Board certification has been a rite of passage in our specialty since The American Board of Neurological Surgery (ABNS) was approved as a new examining board in 1940. Since its inception, the primary purpose of the ABNS has been to conduct examinations of candidates who voluntarily seek certification, and to issue certificates to those who meet the requirements of the Board and satisfactorily complete those examinations. The first official meeting of the ABNS was held in Chicago on October 17, 1940. Twenty-four candidates for certification were examined. Those 24 men were examined on a specialty that was relatively elementary by today's standards. Neurosurgery was simply defined as a specialty focused on surgical treatment of diseases of the nervous system. As the ABNS celebrates its 75th anniversary, that definition of our specialty has been transformed.

*"**Neurological surgery** constitutes a medical discipline and surgical specialty that provides care for adult and pediatric patients in the treatment of pain or pathological processes that may modify the function or activity of the central nervous system (e.g. brain, hypophysis, and spinal cord), the peripheral nervous system (e.g. cranial, spinal, and peripheral nerves), the autonomic nervous system, the supporting structures of these systems (e.g. meninges, skull & skull base, and vertebral column), and their vascular supply (e.g. intracranial, extracranial, and spinal vasculature).*

Treatment encompasses both non-operative management (e.g. prevention, *diagnosis – including image interpretation – and treatments such as, but not limited to neurocritical intensive care and rehabilitation) and operative management with its associated image use and interpretation (e.g. endovascular surgery, functional and restorative surgery, stereotactic radiosurgery, and spinal fusion – including its instrumentation."*

While a resident at Emory University, Dr. Alleyne created a prodigious list of questions based upon preparation for his written board examination. In an effort to assist other residents, that compilation later became the first edition of *Neurosurgery Board Review*. That monograph and the second edition have become a time-honored and popular method for residents to prepare for their written board examination. With advances in the neurosciences in general and our specialty specifically, has come the need to update this work. This third edition of *Neurosurgery Board Review* contains not only questions and answers but also explanations of those correct answers to enhance the overall knowledge base of the reader. I am confident this work will continue to provide a valuable resource for all neurosurgeons, but particularly residents preparing for the first step toward certification by the ABNS.

Daniel L. Barrow, MD
Pamela R. Rollins Professor and Chairman
Department of Neurosurgery
Director, Emory MBNA Stroke Center
Emory University School of Medicine
Former Director, Secretary, President
American Board of Neurological Surgery

Foreword to the Second Edition

Most learned professions require their membership to demonstrate aminimal level of competency to be fully accepted into that pursuit. Certification by the American Board of Neurological Surgeons (ABNS) is a rite of passage in the educational process of our chosen profession.

For the assiduous neurosurgical resident, assembly and organization of the material necessary to study for Part I of the ABNS examination can be an onerous task. Dr. Alleyne has compiled a set of questions he originally developed while studying for the oral boards during his residency at Emory University School of Medicine. Based in part on his outstanding performance on that examination, he was encouraged by his co-residents and colleagues to share his efforts and eventually publish them. In doing so, Dr. Alleyne has provided a valuable study guide for individuals preparing for the primary examination of the American Board of Neurological Surgeons. This effort also provides an outstanding resource for physicians involved in the neurosciences at any level of their career who may be motivated to assess their current knowledge. In addition to self-assessment this volume guides readers to appropriate resources to expand their knowledge in areas of deficiency.

Many factors influence a neurosurgeon's choice to pursue an academic career. A passion for teaching, however, is an essential feature of the successful academian. Dr. Alleyne has demonstrated his passion for teaching through the production of this valuable volume.

Daniel L. Barrow, MD
Atlanta, Georgia

Preface to the Third Edition

Dr. Alleyne wrote the first edition of his board review book while preparing to take the written portion of the ABNS exam as a resident. Seven years later, in 2004, he and Dr. Citow improved the book with additional questions and images. Much has changed in neurosurgery over the past 10 years, including the widespread use of endovascular techniques for the treatment of cerebral aneurysms, the availability of a new armamentarium of advanced imaging techniques, and major changes in the treatment of acute ischemic stroke.

Certainly every resident taking the ABNS primary exam wants to do his or her very best, but a high score on the exam is not the primary endpoint. Our goal as students and practitioners of neurosurgery is *understanding* of the material. The goals of this third iteration of Dr. Alleyne's classic book are threefold: (1) increase the number of questions and high-yield images to reflect the changing scope of neurosurgery; (2) correct any errors contained in the second edition; and (3) most importantly, provide detailed explanations for each question. We hope that the reader will be able to use this text for self-assessment, but also to enhance his or her understanding of the material. The format of the book has also been changed to make it more user-friendly.

Preparing for the ABNS primary exam is a substantial undertaking. We hope that this third edition will aid in your self-assessment, enhance your understanding of the material, and give you confidence when you get ready to sit for the boards.

M. Neil Woodall, MD
Augusta, Georgia

Preface to the Second Edition

In the 7 years since the publication of the first edition, there have been several other review texts published to aid in the review for the written portion of the Neurosurgery Board Examination. This second edition remains a text to be used for self-assessment and review to facilitate, not replace, primary study. The format remains the same, but the total number of questions has been increased to over 1,200. These include approximately 200 new questions, 100 of which were contributed by Jonathan Stuart Citow, MD. Several of the excellent anatomic dissections by Dr. Al Rhoton are included in the Neurosurgery section. I would again like to thank the editorial and production staff at Thieme for their excellent work. I also thank Andy Rekito, our illustrator in the Department of Neurosurgery at the Medical College of Georgia, for his superb artwork.

Cargill H. Alleyne Jr., MD

Preface to the First Edition

This work materialized as I was studying for the written portion of the Neurosurgery Board Examination; it is based largely on the question content areas revealed by the American Board of Neurological Surgery over the last several years. As the examination loomed closer, I was able to use the questions I had previously written to aid in the review process. The text should mainly benefit neurosurgery residents, but it may also appeal to residents in other neuroscience subspecialties. It is composed of over 1,000 multiple choice questions in seven sections: Neurosurgery (132 questions, including 3 photographs), Clinical Neurology (214 questions), Neuroanatomy (185 questions), Neurophysiology (146 questions), Neuropathology (134 questions, including 52 photographs), Neuroradiology (83 questions, including 51 photographs), and Clinical Skills/Critical Care (126 questions). The proportion of questions in each section approximately mirrors that of the Neurosurgery written Board examination. Each section is accompanied by answers that have been referenced to major texts in the respective subspecialty areas. Unless the questions are deemed self-explanatory, brief explanations are also provided. Every attempt was made to ensure the clarity of questions and the accuracy of answers, but the reader is urged to refer to the references listed or to other standard textbooks for further detail should the need arise. Sincere gratitude is expressed to the faculty on the editorial board for their critique of the manuscript. I would also like to thank the editorial and production staff at Thieme for their excellent work. It is hoped that the use of this text for self-assessment will facilitate the arduous task of review for the written portion of the Neurosurgery Board Examination.

Cargill H. Alleyne Jr., MD
Resident in Neurosurgery
Emory University School of Medicine
1997

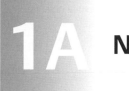

⇨ For questions **1** to **9**, identify the following structures. The figure illustrates a right transcallosal approach to the third ventricle.

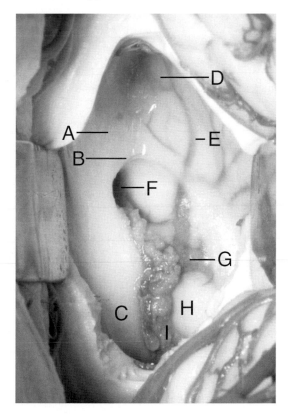

1. Caudate nucleus

2. Choroid plexus

3. Foramen of Monro

4. Columns of the fornix

5. Septum pellucidum

6. Thalamostriate vein

7. Thalamus

8. Body of the fornix

9. Anterior caudate vein

10. Surgical procedures utilized in the treatment of spasmodic torticollis include
     I.   Upper cervical ventral rhizotomies and spinal accessory neurectomy
     II.   Stereotactic thalamotomy
     III.   Microvascular decompression of the spinal accessory nerve
     IV.   Myotomy
  A.   I, II, III
  B.   I, III
  C.   II, IV
  D.   IV
  E.   All of the above

11. Which surgical approach for thoracic disk herniations is associated with the highest rate of neurologic injury?
  A.   Costotransversectomy
  B.   Lateral extracavitary
  C.   Midline laminectomy
  D.   Transpedicular
  E.   Transthoracic

12. Most patients with intrinsic brainstem gliomas initially present with
  A.   Cranial neuropathies
  B.   Headache
  C.   Hydrocephalus
  D.   Nausea and vomiting
  E.   Papilledema

13. Each of the following is characteristic of complex regional pain syndrome II (causalgia) *except*
  A.   Atrophic changes in the limb
  B.   Hypesthesia
  C.   Increased sweating
  D.   Lack of major motor deficit
  E.   Good relief with sympathetic block

⇨ For questions **14** to **18**, match the description with the structure.
  A.   Dermoid cyst
  B.   Epidermoid cyst
  C.   Both
  D.   Neither

14. Bacterial meningitis

15. Aseptic meningitis

16. Associated congenital malformations

17. Most often midline

18. Responsive to radiation therapy

19. Ventricular enlargement from choroid plexus papillomas can be secondary to
    I.   Entrapment of cerebrospinal fluid (CSF)
    II.   Decreased absorption of CSF from hemorrhage-induced arachnoiditis
    III. Tumor growth
    IV. Excessive production of CSF
  A. I, II, III
  B. I, III
  C. II, IV
  D. IV
  E. All of the above

20. Which approach is favored for a patient with an 8-mm acoustic neuroma in which hearing preservation is a goal?
  A. Middle fossa
  B. Suboccipital
  C. Translabyrinthine

21. Uncinate seizures typically produce
  A. Auditory hallucinations
  B. Gustatory hallucinations
  C. Olfactory hallucinations
  D. Vertiginous sensations
  E. Visual seizures

⇨ For questions **22** to **25**, match the description with the structure.
  A. Calcarine sulcus
  B. Lateral mesencephalic sulcus
  C. Posterior communicating artery
  D. Tectal plate

22. Separates the P1 and P2A segments of the posterior cerebral artery

23. Separates the P2A and P2P segments of the posterior cerebral artery

24. Separates the P2P and P3 segments of the posterior cerebral artery

25. Separates the P3 and P4 segments of the posterior cerebral artery

26. The radial nerve or one of its branches innervates each of the following *except* the
  A. Abductor pollicis longus
  B. Adductor pollicis
  C. Brachioradialis
  D. Extensor pollicis brevis
  E. Supinator

27. Each of the following is true of intraventricular hemorrhage (IVH) in the newborn *except*
    A. Periventricular hemorrhagic infarction is one sequela.
    B. Posthemorrhagic hydrocephalus can result in persistent bradycardia and apneic spells.
    C. The capillary bed of the germinal matrix is composed of large irregular vessels.
    D. The germinal matrix is the most common site of IVH in the full-term neonate.
    E. The risk of IVH is greater in the preterm than in the term infant.

28. The ossification centers of the odontoid consist of
    A. One primary and two secondary centers
    B. One secondary and three primary centers
    C. Three secondary and one primary center
    D. Two primary centers
    E. Two primary and one secondary center

29. The most common single-suture synostosis is
    A. Coronal
    B. Lambdoid
    C. Metopic
    D. Sagittal
    E. Sphenozygomatic

30. The most sensitive method for detecting carpal tunnel syndrome is
    A. Needle examination of the abductor pollicis brevis
    B. Needle examination of the first and second lumbricals
    C. Motor amplitude of the median nerve
    D. Motor distal latency of the median nerve
    E. Palmar sensory conduction time of the median nerve

31. Coup contusions most commonly occur at the
    A. Cerebral convexities
    B. Frontal and temporal poles
    C. Orbital surface of the frontal lobes
    D. Posterior fossa
    E. Ventral surface of the temporal lobe

⇨ For questions **32** to **36**, match the aneurysm with the sign or symptom it is most likely to produce. Each response may be used once, more than once, or not at all.
    A. Anterior communicating artery aneurysm
    B. Intracavernous carotid artery aneurysm
    C. Middle cerebral artery aneurysm
    D. Ophthalmic artery aneurysm
    E. Posterior communicating artery aneurysm

32. Pupil-involving third nerve palsy

33. Seizures

34. Diabetes insipidus

35. Inferior nasal quadrantanopia

36. Exophthalmos

37. The essential difference between a syringomyelic and a hydromyelic cavity is that the cavity in
    A. Hydromyelia is lined with ependymal cells, and in syringomyelia is not
    B. Hydromyelia is lined with choroid plexus, and in syringomyelia is not
    C. Syringomyelia contains CSF, and in hydromyelia contains serum
    D. Syringomyelia is focal, and in hydromyelia is more extensive
    E. Syringomyelia is an enlargement of the central canal, and in hydromyelia is an enlargement of the anterior median septum

⇨ For questions **38** to **45**, identify the following structures. The figure illustrates the structures exposed through the right opticocarotid triangle.

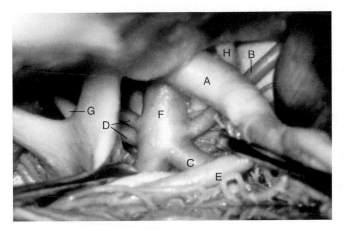

38. Basilar artery

39. Pituitary stalk

40. Right oculomotor nerve

41. Right posterior cerebral artery

42. Internal carotid artery

43. Left duplicated superior cerebellar artery

44. Right superior cerebellar artery

45. Right anterior cerebral artery (A1 segment)

46. Each of the following is true of basilar impression *except*
    A. Cerebellar and vestibular complaints typically overshadow motor and sensory complaints.
    B. McGregor's line is helpful in routine screening.
    C. McRae's line is helpful in clinical assessment.
    D. Short necks and torticollis are common.
    E. Vertebral artery anomalies are common.

47. Which of the following fractures has the poorest prognosis for healing without surgical intervention?
    A. Hangman's
    B. Jefferson's fracture with 4 mm displacement of lateral masses
    C. Type I odontoid
    D. Type II odontoid
    E. Type III odontoid

48. Sprengel's deformity refers to a(n)
    A. Congenital elevation of the scapula
    B. Congenital fusion of the upper cervical vertebrae
    C. Intravertebral disk herniation
    D. Postlaminectomy kyphosis
    E. Scoliosis resulting from tethering of the spinal cord

⇨ For questions **49** to **55**, match the fracture type with the mechanism. Each response may be used once, more than once, or not at all.

Force Neck Posture
    A. Flexing flexed
    B. Compressing flexed
    C. Compressing neutral
    D. Distracting extended
    E. Flexing axially rotated
    F. Compressing laterally bent

49. Hangman's fracture

50. Burst fracture

51. Unilateral facet dislocation

52. Teardrop fracture

53. Bilateral facet dislocation

54. Horizontal facet fracture

55. Jefferson's fracture

56. Lateral recess stenosis in spondylosis is most commonly caused by
    A. Disk herniation
    B. Hypertrophied pedicles
    C. Inferior articular facet hypertrophy
    D. Ligamentum flavum hypertrophy
    E. Superior articular facet hypertrophy

57. In the treatment of chronic pain, the undesirable effect(s) that is/are more common in stimulation of the periaqueductal gray than the periventricular gray region is/are
    I.   Diplopia
    II. Oscillopsia
    III. Reduction of upgaze
    IV. Sense of impending doom
    A.   I, II, III
    B.   I, III
    C.   II, IV
    D.   IV
    E.   All of the above

58. "Trilateral retinoblastoma" describes bilateral ocular retinoblastomas and a(n)
    A.   Astrocytoma
    B.   Medulloblastoma
    C.   Neurofibroma
    D.   Optic nerve sheath tumor
    E.   Pineoblastoma

59. Carotid artery ligation is absolutely contraindicated in patients with (a)
    A.   Bilateral intracavernous carotid aneurysms
    B.   Giant ophthalmic artery aneurysm and evidence of vasospasm on arteriogram
    C.   Giant ophthalmic artery aneurysm and extracranial atherosclerotic disease
    D.   Intracavernous carotid artery aneurysm and sudden loss of extraocular motility
    E.   Traumatic dissecting aneurysm of the petrous carotid artery

60. The syndrome of weakness in one upper extremity followed by lower extremity weakness on the same side, then contralateral lower extremity weakness, is most characteristic of a meningioma involving the
    A.   Clivus
    B.   Falx
    C.   Foramen magnum
    D.   Olfactory groove
    E.   Tuberculum sella

⇨ For questions **61** to **70**, the figure illustrates a lateral view of the left cavernous sinus. Match the following triangles with the descriptions/structures. Each response may be used once, more than once, or not at all.

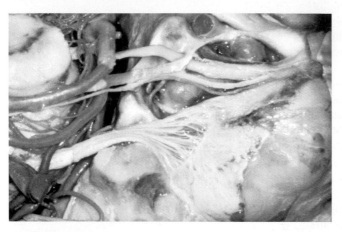

    A.   Clinoidal
    B.   Oculomotor
    C.   Supratrochlear
    D.   Infratrochlear or Parkinson's
    E.   Anteromedial
    F.   Anterolateral
    G.   Posterolateral or Glasscock's
    H.   Posteromedial or Kawase's

61. Clinoidal segment of the internal carotid artery

62. Intracavernous carotid artery

63. Intrapetrous carotid artery

64. Meningohypophyseal trunk origin

65. Optic strut

66. Sphenoid sinus and lower margin of V1

67. Two margins of this triangle are formed by the anterior and posterior petroclinoidal dural folds.

68. Located between V2 and V3

69. Contains the foramen spinosum

70. Contains the cochlea

71. Which of the following findings is most consistent with adherence of a posterior communicating artery aneurysm to the temporal lobe?
    A. Loss of consciousness
    B. Absence of third nerve palsy
    C. Projection of the aneurysm medial to the carotid on the anteroposterior (AP) angiogram
    D. Third nerve involvement
    E. Seizures

72. Weakness of the deltoid muscle is caused by injury to the
    A. Axillary nerve
    B. Dorsal scapular nerve
    C. Musculocutaneous nerve
    D. Suprascapular nerve
    E. Thoracodorsal nerve

73. Subdural empyema resulting after meningitis in an infant most commonly develops with
    A. *Escherichia coli*
    B. *Haemophilus influenzae*
    C. *Listeria*
    D. *Neisseria*
    E. *Staphylococcus*

74. Sudeck's atrophy, associated with reflex sympathetic dystrophy, refers to atrophic changes occurring in each of the following structures *except*
    A. Bone
    B. Joints
    C. Muscle
    D. Nerve
    E. Skin

⇨ For questions **75** to **79**, match the embryologic event with the postovulatory day. Each response may be used once, more than once, or not at all.

Postovulatory Day Number
    A. 13
    B. 17
    C. 22
    D. 24
    E. 26

75. Closure of the caudal neuropore

76. Closure of the cranial neuropore

77. Formation of the notochord

78. Formation of the primitive streak

79. Fusion of the neural folds to form the neural tube

80. Factors that predispose to the subclavian steal syndrome include
     I.   Occlusion of the left subclavian artery proximal to the origin of the left vertebral artery
     II.   Occlusion of the left subclavian artery distal to the origin of the left vertebral artery
     III. Active use of the left arm
     IV.   Occlusion of the left vertebral artery
     A. I, II, III
     B. I, III
     C. II, IV
     D. IV
     E. All of the above

81. The articular facet joint in the upper thoracic region is oriented
     A. Axially
     B. Coronally
     C. Obliquely
     D. Sagittally

82. The most common presenting symptom of a thoracic herniated disk is
     A. Back pain
     B. Leg numbness
     C. Leg weakness
     D. Thoracic numbness
     E. Urinary incontinence

83. Neurologic deficits thought to result from occlusion of the thalamostrate vein during the subchoroidal transvelum interpositum approach to the third ventricle include
     I.   Drowsiness
     II.   Hemiparesis
     III. Mutism
     IV.   Seizures
     A. I, II, III
     B. I, III
     C. II, IV
     D. IV
     E. All of the above

For questions **84** to **88**, the figure illustrates the right internal auditory canal through a middle fossa approach. Identify the following nerves.

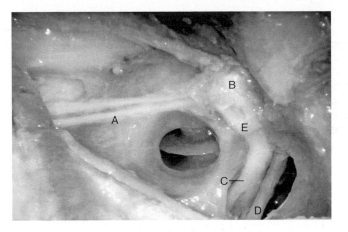

84. Labyrinthine segment of the facial nerve

85. Meatal segment of the facial nerve

86. Superior vestibular nerve

87. Greater superficial petrosal nerve

88. Geniculate ganglion

89. In the suboccipital transmeatal approach to an acoustic neuroma, the location of the facial nerve in relation to the tumor, in decreasing frequency of occurrence, is
 A. Anterior, posterior, inferior
 B. Anterior, superior, inferior
 C. Superior, anterior, posterior
 D. Posterior, superior, anterior
 E. Anterior, posterior, superior

90. Each of the following features is usually minimal or absent in patients with type 2 neurofibromatosis *except*
 A. Axillary freckles
 B. Café au lait spots
 C. Lisch nodules
 D. Multiple, typical skin neurofibromas
 E. Skin plaques

91. The single most important factor in the recurrence of meningiomas is
 A. Age of the patient
 B. Bone invasion
 C. Histologic type of benign meningioma
 D. Postoperative tumor residual
 E. Sex of the patient

⇨ For questions **92 to 98**, match the cistern with the structure it contains. Each response may be used once, more than once, or not at all.

    A.   Ambient cistern
    B.   Cerebellopontine angle cistern
    C.   Interpeduncular cistern
    D.   Lateral cerebellomedullary cistern
    E.   Prepontine cistern

92.   Contains the anteroinferior cerebellar artery (AICA)

93.   Contains the origin of the posteroinferior cerebellar artery (PICA)

94.   Contains the superior cerebellar artery

95.   Contains cranial nerve (CN) IV

96.   Contains CN V

97.   Contains the basal vein of Rosenthal

98.   Contains the choroid plexus at the foramen of Luschka

99.   The transverse crest separates the
    A.   Cochlear, facial, and superior vestibular nerves from the inferior vestibular nerve
    B.   Cochlear and inferior vestibular nerves from the facial and superior vestibular nerves
    C.   Facial and cochlear nerves from the superior and inferior vestibular nerves
    D.   Facial, cochlear, and inferior vestibular nerves from the superior vestibular nerve
    E.   Facial and inferior vestibular nerves from the cochlear and superior vestibular nerves

100.   Which of the following is true of hemifacial spasm?
    A.   Compression of the facial nerve by the superior cerebellar artery is the most common operative finding.
    B.   Deafness is more common than permanent facial weakness as a complication of microvascular decompression.
    C.   Men are more frequently affected than women.
    D.   Symptoms typically begin in the buccal muscles and move cranially.
    E.   The cure rate at 1 month after microvascular decompression is 95%.

101.   Each of the following surgical approaches may be considered for an aneurysm of the vertebrobasilar junction *except* the
    A.   Extended extreme lateral inferior transcondylar approach
    B.   Lateral suboccipital approach
    C.   Presigmoid transtentorial approach
    D.   Retrolabyrinthine transsigmoid approach
    E.   Subtemporal approach

102.   The most common presenting symptom in patients with colloid cysts is
    A.   Headache
    B.   Dementia
    C.   Seizures
    D.   Sudden attacks of leg weakness
    E.   Sudden death

For questions **103** to **106**, the figure illustrates the nerves occupying the right internal auditory canal through a middle fossa approach. Identify their relative positions.

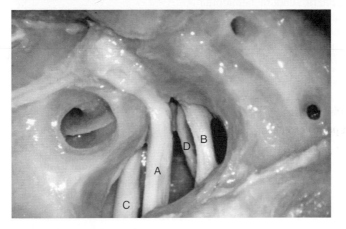

103. Inferior and anterior

104. Inferior and posterior

105. Superior and anterior

106. Superior and posterior

107. The most common presenting symptom of neonates with vein of Galen aneurysms is
  A. Congestive heart failure
  B. Hydrocephalus
  C. Intracerebral hemorrhage
  D. Seizures
  E. Subarachnoid hemorrhage

108. The most common upper thoracic spine injury is a
  A. Burst fracture
  B. Compression fracture
  C. Fracture-dislocation
  D. Seat belt injury

109. Which is true of thoracolumbar spine fractures?
  A. Burst fractures are the most common.
  B. Fracture-dislocations involve all three columns.
  C. Seat belt type injuries are generally stable.
  D. Wedge compression fractures are generally unstable.
  E. Wedge compression fractures involve the middle column.

110. Each of the following is true of diffuse brain swelling *except* that it is
  A. A result of cerebrovascular congestion
  B. A result of cytotoxic edema
  C. Associated with a 50% mortality rate in children with severe head injuries
  D. Manifested on computed tomography (CT) scan by a compression of the perimesencephalic cistern
  E. More common in children than in adults

111. Which of the following is *least* suggestive of child abuse?
    A. Acute and healing long bone fractures
    B. Interhemispheric subdural hematoma
    C. Parietal skull fracture
    D. Retinal hemorrhages
    E. Tentorial subdural hematoma

112. Trigonocephaly results from premature closure of the
    A. Coronal suture bilaterally
    B. Coronal suture unilaterally
    C. Frontosphenoidal suture
    D. Lambdoid suture
    E. Metopic suture

113. The cleft in the spinal cord associated with diastematomyelia is most commonly located in the
    A. Cervical region
    B. Lumbar region
    C. Sacral region
    D. Thoracic region

114. Up to what percentage of patients with bacterial arterial (mycotic) aneurysms carry an underlying diagnosis of subacute bacterial endocarditis?
    A. 10%
    B. 20%
    C. 40%
    D. 60%
    E. 80%

115. Each is true of bacterial intracranial aneurysms *except*
    A. Infected emboli lodge in the vasa vasorum.
    B. The middle cerebral artery is most commonly affected.
    C. The peripherally located branches are most commonly affected.
    D. Typical subarachnoid hemorrhage occurs in 18% of patients.
    E. *Staphylococcus aureus* and β-hemolytic streptococci are most commonly involved.

116. Each of the following is true of growing skull fractures *except* that they
    A. Can cross suture lines
    B. May be associated with underlying brain injury
    C. Occur if the edges of the initial fracture are separated by more than 3 mm
    D. Occur most commonly in the parietal bone
    E. Occur most commonly between the ages of 2 and 5 years

117. Approximately what percentage of infants with myelomeningocele have magnetic resonance imaging (MRI) evidence of a Chiari II malformation?
    A. 20%
    B. 40%
    C. 60%
    D. 80%
    E. 100%

118. Cardiovascular disease involving the heart and great vessels gives rise to which of the following types of emboli in the retina?

    I.   Cholesterol
    II.   Calcific
    III. Platelet-fibrin
    IV. Fat

A. I, II, III
B. I, III
C. II, IV
D. IV
E. All of the above

119. In the infratentorial supracerebellar approach to the pineal region, which of the following veins are usually sacrificed?

    I.   Superior vermian vein
    II.   Posterior pericallosal vein
    III. Precentral cerebellar vein
    IV. Basal vein of Rosenthal

A. I, II, III
B. I, III
C. II, IV
D. IV
E. All of the above

120. Each of the following is characteristic of an acoustic neuroma *except*
A. Békésy type III or IV audiogram
B. Loudness recruitment
C. Low short-increment sensitivity index
D. Poor speech discrimination
E. Pronounced tone decay

⇨ For questions **121** to **128**, the figure illustrates the right retrosigmoid approach. Identify the following structures.

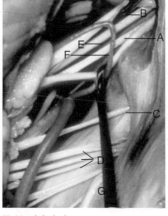

H–Not labeled

121. Subarcuate artery

122. Anteroinferior cerebellar artery

123. Cochlear nerve

124. Facial nerve

125. Glossopharyngeal nerve

126. Spinal accessory nerve

127. Posteroinferior cerebellar artery

128. Vagus nerve

129. Which of the following structures provides a marker for the most dorsal extent of the incision for anterolateral cordotomy for pain control?
A.   Dentate ligament
B.   Dorsal root entry zone
C.   Posterior intermediate sulcus
D.   Posterior median sulcus
E.   Zone of Lissauer

130. Occlusion of the anterior choroidal artery results in
  I.   Contralateral hemiplegia
  II.   Hemihypesthesia
  III. Homonymous hemianopsia
  IV.   Impaired cognition
A.   I, II, III
B.   I, III
C.   II, IV
D.   IV
E.   All of the above

131. Which of the following symptoms of Parkinson's disease is most likely to respond to a stereotactic lesion in the posterior ventral oval (VOP)/ventral intermediate (VIM) (ventrolateral) thalamus?
A.   Bradykinesia
B.   Gait disturbance
C.   Rigidity
D.   Speech disturbance
E.   Tremor

▷ For questions **132** to **136**, match the description with the syndrome or disease.
A.   Apert's syndrome
B.   Crouzon's disease
C.   Both
D.   Neither

132. Autosomal recessive inheritance

133. Exorbitism

134. Syndactyly

135. The majority of patients have preoperative intelligence quotients (IQs) greater than 90

136. Anterior open bite is common

▷ For questions **137** and **138**, match the description with the symptom.
A.   Primary empty sella syndrome
B.   Secondary empty sella syndrome
C.   Both
D.   Neither

137. Occurs primarily in women.

138. Visual disturbance may occur.

139. The most common etiology of os odontoideum is
   A. Congenital
   B. Iatrogenic
   C. Infectious
   D. Neoplastic
   E. Traumatic

140. The most common mechanism of translational C1–C2 subluxation is
   A. Axial loading
   B. Distraction
   C. Extension
   D. Flexion

141. The factor or substance with the *least* important role in the pathogenesis of cerebral vasospasm is probably
   A. Bilirubin
   B. Endothelin
   C. Intimal proliferation
   D. Lipid peroxides
   E. Oxyhemoglobin

⇨ For questions **142** to **148**, the figure illustrates the right presigmoid, retrolabyrinthine approach. Identify the following structures.

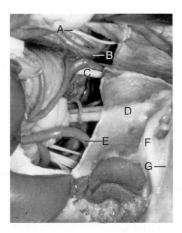

142. Internal acoustic meatus

143. Posterior inferior cerebellar artery

144. Chorda tympani nerve

145. Facial nerve

146. Superior cerebellar artery

147. Trigeminal nerve

148. Trochlear nerve

⇨ For questions **149** to **155**, match the descriptions with the type of arteriovenous malformation (AVM).
   A. Type I spinal AVMs
   B. Type II spinal AVMs
   C. Type III spinal AVMs
   D. Type IV spinal AVMs
   E. Types II and III spinal AVMs

149. Most common type of spinal AVM

150. Etiology believed to be acquired

151. Also known as juvenile malformations

152. Also known as glomus AVMs

153. Low flow and high pressure dynamics can be seen in type IV and this type

154. High flow and high pressure dynamics can be seen in type IV and this type

155. Type IV and this type typically present with progressively worsening symptoms without significant clinical improvement

156. Which of the following represents the correct sequence of removal of clamps from the arteries following carotid endarterectomy?
    A. Common carotid, external carotid, internal carotid
    B. Common carotid, internal carotid, external carotid
    C. External carotid, common carotid, internal carotid
    D. External carotid, internal carotid, common carotid
    E. Internal carotid, common carotid, external carotid

⇨ For questions **157** to **163**, the figure illustrates the subchoroidal transvelum interpositum approach to the third ventricle. Identify the following structures.

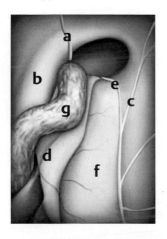

157. Anterior caudate vein

158. Column of the fornix

159. Internal cerebral vein

160. Septal vein

161. Tela choroidea

162. Thalamostriate vein

163. Thalamus

⇨ For questions **164** to **168**, the figure illustrates the right retrocondylar, far lateral approach. Identify the following structures.

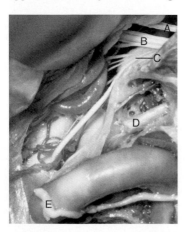

164. Dorsal ramus of C1

165. Glossopharyngeal nerve

166. Hypoglossal nerve

167. Spinal accessory nerve

168. Vagus nerve

➡ For questions **169** to **174**, the figure illustrates the pterional approach to aneurysm clipping. Identify the following structures.

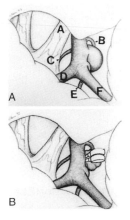

A

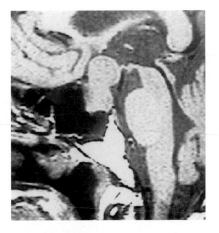

B

169. Anterior cerebral artery

170. Anterior choroidal artery

171. Middle cerebral artery

172. Optic nerve

173. Posterior communicating artery

174. Superior hypophyseal artery

175. Which of the following is most important in determining the propensity of a dural AVM to an aggressive clinical course?
A. Duration of symptoms
B. Leptomeningeal venous drainage
C. Location
D. Presentation
E. Size

➡ For questions **176** and **177**, refer to the image shown.

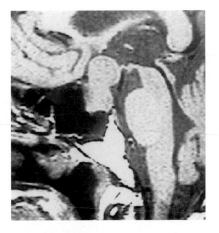

176. The MRI shown is that of a 40-year-old patient with bitemporal hemianopia and a prolactin level of 89. The best management of this lesion is
A. Bromocriptine
B. Bromocriptine, then surgery
C. Follow with serial MRIs
D. Radiation therapy
E. Surgery

177. If the prolactin level of the same patient in question **176** was found to be 650, the best management is
    A. Bromocriptine
    B. Follow with serial MRIs and prolactin levels
    C. Radiation therapy
    D. Surgery
    E. Surgery, then radiation therapy

178. Of the following, the *least* common location of intracranial meningiomas is (the)
    A. Intraventricular
    B. Olfactory groove
    C. Posterior fossa
    D. Sphenoid ridge
    E. Tuberculum sella

179. Each of the following statements is true of AVMs *except*
    A. Higher pressures have been measured in the feeding arteries of smaller as compared with larger AVMs.
    B. Smaller AVMs are more likely to bleed than larger AVMs.
    C. The annual risk of death from a ruptured AVM is 1%.
    D. The risk of bleeding from an unruptured AVM is 3 to 4% a year.
    E. The risk of rebleed in the first year after hemorrhage is highest in the first 2 weeks.

180. The most common complication of percutaneous radiofrequency trigeminal gangliolysis is
    A. Anesthesia dolorosa
    B. Decreased hearing
    C. Keratitis
    D. Masticatory weakness
    E. Paresthesias or dysesthesias

181. In the technique of percutaneous radiofrequency trigeminal gangliolysis, the needle is inserted into the
    I. Foramen rotundum
    II. Trigeminal cistern
    III. Foramen spinosum
    IV. Foramen ovale
    A. I, II, III
    B. I, III
    C. II, IV
    D. IV
    E. All of the above

⇨ For questions **182** to **189**, the figure illustrates a lateral view of the contents of the right orbit. The eyeball attachment of the lateral rectus muscle has been divided. Identify the following structures.

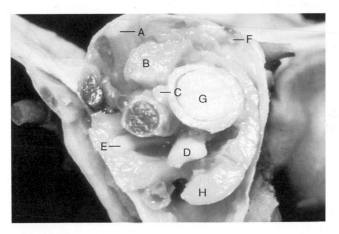

182. Inferior rectus muscle

183. Inferior division of the oculomotor nerve

184. Abducens nerve

185. Frontal nerve

186. Nasociliary nerve

187. Superior division of the oculomotor nerve

188. Optic nerve

189. Trochlear nerve

⇨ For questions **190** to **195**, match the condition with the most appropriate treatment option. Each treatment option may be used once, more than once, or not at all.

    A. Cingulotomy
    B. Dorsal root entry zone (DREZ) rhizotomy
    C. Morphine infusion
    D. Pallidotomy
    E. Sympathectomy
    F. Ventral rhizotomy

190. Brachial plexus avulsion

191. Causalgia

192. Obsessive-compulsive disorder

193. Nociceptive cancer pain above C5

194. Parkinson's disease

195. Spasmodic torticollis

196. Donor nerves that may be used for neurotization after brachial plexus avulsion include
     I.   Intercostal nerves
     II. Spinal accessory nerve
     III. Cervical plexus
     IV. Phrenic nerve
     A. I, II, III
     B. I, III
     C. II, IV
     D. IV
     E. All of the above

197. The pterion is formed by which of the following bones?
     A. Frontal, greater wing of the sphenoid, parietal, and squamous part of the temporal
     B. Frontal, lesser wing of the sphenoid, parietal, and squamous part of the temporal
     C. Frontal, greater wing of the sphenoid, parietal, and zygomatic arch
     D. Frontal, lesser wing of the sphenoid, parietal, and zygomatic arch
     E. Frontal, lesser wing of the sphenoid, squamous part of the temporal, and zygomatic arch

198. The most common external beam radiation therapy regimen for brain metastases is
     A. 30 Gy in 2 weeks
     B. 30 Gy in 4 weeks
     C. 60 Gy in 2 weeks
     D. 60 Gy in 4 weeks
     E. 45 Gy in 4 weeks

199. The most appropriate radiation treatment protocol for glioblastoma is
     A. 8,000 cGY in 400 cGY daily fractions
     B. 6,000 cGY in 200 cGy daily fractions
     C. 6,000 cGy in 100 cGy daily fractions
     D. 4,000 cGy in 400 cGy daily fractions
     E. 4,000 cGy in 200 cGy daily fractions

200. Cerebral salt wasting and syndrome of inappropriate antidiuretic hormone (SIADH) may best be distinguished by measuring
     A. Plasma arginine vasopressin (AVP)
     B. Serum osmolality
     C. Serum sodium
     D. Urine sodium
     E. Volume status

201. A patient presents status post a high speed motor vehicle collision with a cervical 5/6 fracture dislocation. Power in the deltoid, biceps, and wrist extensors is 5/5, and all other muscle groups are 2/5 including triceps, grips, and lower extremities. Rectal tone and perianal sensation are intact. What is the appropriate grade of this acute spinal cord injury?

A. ASIA A
B. ASIA B
C. ASIA C
D. ASIA D
E. ASIA E

202. What is the likelihood that the patient in the previous question (**201**) will be ambulatory at long-term follow-up?

A. < 3%
B. 50%
C. 75%
D. 95%
E. 100%

203. A patient presents with facial trichilemmomas, fibromas of the oral mucosa, hamartomas of the GI tract and breast, and a thyroid mass. Further workup reveals Lhermitte-Duclos disease in this patient, as well. What is the most likely genetic abnormality?

A. CAG trinucleotide repeat
B. mTOR amplification
C. p53 deletion
D. *PTEN* mutation
E. Trisomy 21

204. Which of the following best describes the standing radiograph seen here?

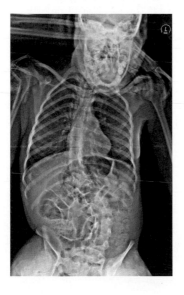

A. Major lumbar dextroscoliosis and minor thoracic levoscoliosis
B. Major lumbar levoscoliosis and major thoracic dextroscoliosis
C. Major lumbar levoscoliosis and minor thoracic dextroscoliosis
D. Minor lumbar dextroscoliosis and major thoracic levoscoliosis
E. Minor lumbar levoscoliosis and major thoracic dextroscoliosis

205. Which nerve(s) is (are) at risk during harvesting of iliac crest bone graft via an anterior approach?
A. Iliohypogastric nerve
B. Ilioinguinal nerve
C. Lateral femoral cutaneous nerve
D. All of the above
E. None of the above

206. Which of the following features is suggestive of ulnar nerve compression at the wrist (Guyon's canal)?
A. Aching along the medial proximal forearm
B. "Claw" hand
C. Paresthesias in an ulnar distribution
D. Sparing of dorsal hand sensation
E. Weakness of the third and fourth lumbricals

207. All of the following are true of SCIWORA *except*
A. Acronym for "spinal cord injury without radiographic abnormality"
B. More common in children
C. MRI is always unremarkable
D. No evidence of spinal fracture is seen
E. Thought to be due to ligamentous laxity

208. A patient presents status post fall with an acute type II odontoid fracture. Good spinal alignment is maintained. The patient has good bone quality, is otherwise healthy, and is neurologically intact. An MRI reveals disruption of the transverse ligament. Which of the following is the most appropriate treatment?
A. C-collar immobilization
B. No treatment
C. Occiput to C2 posterior fusion
D. Odontoid screw placement
E. Posterior C1–C2 instrumented fusion

1.	D	27.	D
2.	I	28.	E
3.	F	29.	D
4.	B	30.	E
5.	A	31.	A
6.	G	32.	E
7.	H	33.	C
8.	C	34.	A
9.	E	35.	D
10.	E	36.	B
11.	C	37.	A
12.	A	38.	F
13.	B	39.	G
14.	A	40.	H
15.	B	41.	C
16.	A	42.	A
17.	A	43.	D
18.	D	44.	B
19.	E	45.	E
20.	A	46.	A
21.	C	47.	D
22.	C	48.	A
23.	B	49.	D
24.	D	50.	C
25.	A	51.	E
26.	B	52.	B

53.	A	92.	B
54.	F	93.	D
55.	C	94.	A
56.	E	95.	A
57.	E	96.	B
58.	E	97.	C
59.	B	98.	D
60.	C	99.	B
61.	A	100.	B
62.	D	101.	E
63.	H	102.	A
64.	D	103.	C
65.	A	104.	D
66.	E	105.	A
67.	B	106.	B
68.	F	107.	A
69.	G	108.	B
70.	H	109.	B
71.	B	110.	B
72.	A	111.	C
73.	A	112.	E
74.	D	113.	B
75.	E	114.	E
76.	D	115.	A
77.	B	116.	E
78.	A	117.	E
79.	C	118.	A
80.	B	119.	B
81.	B	120.	B
82.	A	121.	B
83.	A	122.	F
84.	E	123.	A
85.	C	124.	E
86.	D	125.	C
87.	A	126.	G
88.	B	127.	H
89.	B	128.	D
90.	E	129.	A
91.	D	130.	A

131.	E	170.	E
132.	D	171.	F
133.	C	172.	A
134.	A	173.	B
135.	B	174.	C
136.	A	175.	B
137.	A	176.	E
138.	C	177.	A
139.	E	178.	A
140.	D	179.	E
141.	C	180.	E
142.	D	181.	C
143.	E	182.	H
144.	G	183.	D
145.	F	184.	E
146.	B	185.	A
147.	C	186.	C
148.	A	187.	B
149.	A	188.	G
150.	A	189.	F
151.	C	190.	B
152.	B	191.	E
153.	A	192.	A
154.	E	193.	C
155.	A	194.	D
156.	C	195.	F
157.	C	196.	E
158.	B	197.	A
159.	D	198.	A
160.	A	199.	B
161.	G	200.	E
162.	E	201.	C
163.	F	202.	C
164.	E	203.	D
165.	A	204.	C
166.	D	205.	D
167.	C	206.	D
168.	B	207.	C
169.	D	208.	E

1C Neurosurgery—Answers and Explanations

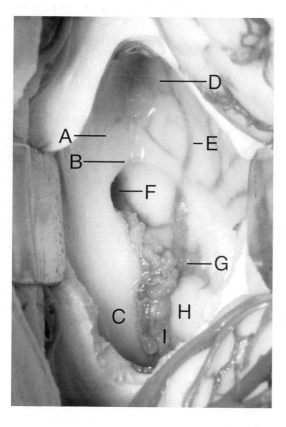

1. **D** – Caudate nucleus
2. **I** – Choroid plexus
3. **F** – Foramen of Monro
4. **B** – Columns of the fornix
5. **A** – Septum pellucidum
6. **G** – Thalamostriate vein
7. **H** – Thalamus
8. **C** – Body of the fornix
9. **E** – Anterior caudate vein

Figure 1.1 is a transcallosal view of the right lateral ventricle. The left side of the image is medial, the right side of the image is lateral, the top of the image is anterior, and the bottom of the image is posterior. The **septum pellucidum (A)** separates the right lateral ventricle from the left lateral ventricle in the midline. The **columns of the fornix (B)** make up the anterior aspect of the **foramen of Monro (F)**. Posteriorly, the **columns of the fornix (B)** turn into the **body of the fornix (C)**, which is separated from the laterally situated **thalamus (H)** by a tuft of **choroid plexus (I)** and the superior choroidal vein (not labeled). The **caudate nucleus (D)** can be appreciated in the anterolateral wall of the lateral ventricle. The **anterior caudate vein (E)** drains this area and ultimately joins the **thalamostriate vein (G)**. Understanding of these anatomical relationships is important for transchoroidal approaches to the third ventricle. For questions 1–9, figure used with permission of Dr. Al Rhoton.[1]

10. E –   All of the above

Myotomy was the earliest surgical procedure used to treat spasmodic torticollis. About 70% of patients improve after microvascular decompression of the spinal accessory nerve, and 81 to 97% of patients improve after upper cervical ventral rhizotomies and spinal accessory denervation procedures. Roughly two-thirds of patients undergoing stereotactic thalamotomy obtain a satisfactory result.[2]

11. C –   Midline laminectomy

Costotransversectomy (A), **lateral extracavitary (B)**, **transpedicular (D)**, and **transthoracic (E)** approaches all facilitate access to the thoracic disk space without the need for retraction on the thecal sac. Approaching a thoracic disk herniation through a simple **laminectomy (C)** would require thecal sac retraction and risk resultant neurologic injury. Posterior decompression alone (**laminectomy [C]** without diskectomy) is unlikely to improve symptoms as the pathologic process involves ventral compression across an already kyphotic spinal segment. The risk of either neurologic deterioration or no benefit with laminectomies for thoracic disk herniation is 45%.[3]

12. A –   Cranial neuropathies

The initial symptoms in most patients with brainstem gliomas are **cranial neuropathies (A)** followed by weakness or ataxia. **Headache (B)**, **nausea and vomiting (D)**, and **papilledema (E)** usually occur later in the course of the illness.[4]

13. B –   Hypesthesia

> Complex regional pain syndrome type II (CRPS II, formerly causalgia) is characterized by **atrophic changes in the affected limb (A)**, **increased sweating (C)**, **absence of a major motor deficit (D)**, **good response to sympathetic blockade (E)**, and hyperesthesia (increased sensitivity to stimulus). CRPS II is diagnosed in the setting of a known nerve injury. The diagnosis CRPS I (formerly reflex sympathetic dystrophy or Sudeck's atrophy) is made only in the absence of known nerve injury. Neither condition is associated with **hypesthesia (B)**, decreased sense of touch or sensation.[3]

14. A –   Bacterial meningitis → dermoid cyst
15. B –   Aseptic meningitis → epidermoid cyst
16. A –   Associated congenital malformations → dermoid cyst
17. A –   Most often midline → dermoid cyst
18. D –   Responsive to radiation therapy → neither

> Intracranial **dermoid cysts (A)** comprise 0.3% of brain tumors and usually present in the pediatric population. They occur when cell rests with dermal and epidermal components are included within neural ectoderm in the midline during neurulation. Communication of the dermoid cyst with the exterior via a sinus tract predisposes the patient to bacterial meningitis (question 14). Congenital malformations (question 16) may be associated with **dermoid cysts (A)**. Intracranial **epidermoid cysts (B)** comprise 0.5 to 1.8% of brain tumors and usually present in the adult. Spillage of the epidermoid cyst contents can lead to aseptic meningitis (question 15). **Epidermoid cysts (B)** result from epidermal cell rests and are most often located eccentrically (e.g., the cerebellopontine angle), whereas **dermoid cysts (A)** tend to be situated in the midline (question 17). Radiation (question 18) is not first-line therapy for either of these lesions.[2]

19. E –   All of the above

> Choroid plexus papillomas can cause ventricular enlargement by entrapment of cerebral spinal fluid (blocking CSF pathways at the foramen of Monro, cerebral aqueduct, or foramina of Luschka and Magendie), blocking CSF absorption at the arachnoid granulations due to hemorrhage-induced arachnoiditis, by tumor growth (causing ventricular expansion by the tumor itself), and by production of excessive cerebrospinal fluid.[2]

20. A –   Middle fossa

> This question is based on the assumption that an 8 mm acoustic neuroma would be an intracanalicular lesion. Small (<1 cm) intracanalicular acoustic neuromas can easily be approached via the middle fossa route. A **translabyrinthine (C)** approach would sacrifice hearing. The middle fossa approach is preferred to a **suboccipital (B)**, retrosigmoid approach for intracanalicular lesions.

21. C – Olfactory hallucinations

> Seizure foci in the mesial temporal lobe (uncinate seizures) tend to produce **olfactory hallucinations (C)**. **Auditory hallucinations (A)** intuitively would seem to be associated with a focus near Heschl's gyrus, but the data do not support that assumption. **Gustatory hallucinations (B)** are rare and can be brought about by stimulation of the posterior insula. **Vertiginous sensations (D)** are associated with foci in the superoposterior temporal lobe near the junction with the parietal lobe. **Visual seizures (E)** suggest a focus in the striate cortex of the occipital lobe.[4,5]

22. C – Posterior communicating artery (PComA)
23. B – Lateral mesencephalic sulcus
24. D – Tectal plate
25. A – Calcarine sulcus

> The posterior cerebral artery is divided into four segments. The P1 segment arises from the basilar bifurcation and extends through the interpeduncular cistern to the junction with the **posterior communicating artery (C)**. The P2A (anterior) segment runs in the crural cistern, extending from the **PComA (C)** to the **lateral mesencephalic sulcus (B)** where it becomes the P2P (posterior) segment. The P2P segment runs in the ambient cistern, lateral to the midbrain. The P2P and P3 segments are separated by the **tectal plate (D)**; the P3 segment runs in the quadrigeminal cistern. The P4 segment begins at the **calcarine sulcus (A)**. (Questions 22–25 from the microsurgical anatomy course; with permission of Dr. Al Rhoton.[1])

26. B – Adductor pollicis

> The **adductor pollicis (B)** is innervated by the ulnar nerve. The **abductor pollicis longus (A)**, **brachioradialis (C)**, **extensor pollicis brevis (D)**, and **supinator (E)** are innervated by the radial nerve or one of its branches.[6]

27. D – The germinal matrix is the most common site of IVH in the full-term neonate (false).

> The **germinal matrix** is the **most common site of IVH in the *preterm* infant**, not the *full-term* infant as presented in the question **(D)**. The most common site of IVH in the full-term neonate is the choroid plexus. The germinal matrix is characterized by a **capillary bed of large irregular vessels (C)** and begins to involute at 43 weeks. The **risk of IVH is greater in the preterm than the term infant (E)** and can lead to **periventricular hemorrhagic infarction (A)** as well as **posthemorrhagic hydrocephalus leading to persistent bradycardia and apneic spells (B)**.[7]

28. E – Two primary and one secondary center

> The odontoid consists of **two primary and one secondary ossification center**. The two primary centers lie inferiorly on either side of midline. The secondary ossification center is apical.[7]

29. D – Sagittal synostosis

Isolated **sagittal synostosis (D)** causes scaphocephaly and is the most common single-suture synostosis, accounting for up to 50% of craniosynostosis patients in some series. **Metopic synostosis (C)** causes trigonocephaly; **coronal synostosis (A)** causes anterior plagiocephaly and is less common than sagittal synostosis. **Lambdoid** and **sphenozygomatic synostosis (B, E)** are both less common than sagittal synostosis.[8]

30. E – Palmar sensory conduction time of the median nerve

Eighty-five to 90% of patients with carpal tunnel syndrome manifest abnormalities of the nerve conduction velocities. The palmar sensory conduction time is the most sensitive electrical test for carpal tunnel syndrome. The **abductor pollicis brevis (A)** and **the first and second lumbricals (B)** are innervated by the median nerve, but needle examination alone is not as sensitive as sensory conduction time for diagnosis. Decreased **motor amplitude (C)** is more sensitive and specific for axonal loss. **Motor latency (D)** of the median nerve is less sensitive than **palmar sensory conduction time (E)** of the median nerve for the diagnosis of carpal tunnel syndrome.[3]

31. A – Cerebral convexities

Contrecoup contusions, produced by rotational force, occur where the **frontal and temporal lobes** rub along bony prominences **(B, C, E)**. Coup contusions (the least common type) are located over the **cerebral convexities (A)**.[9]

32. E – Posterior communicating artery aneurysm
33. C – Middle cerebral artery aneurysm
34. A – Anterior communicating artery aneurysm
35. D – Ophthalmic artery aneurysm
36. B – Intracavernous carotid artery aneurysm

The close proximity of an **anterior communicating artery aneurysm (A)** to the hypothalamus can lead to endocrine abnormalities, including diabetes insipidus. A ruptured **intracavernous aneurysm (B)** produces a carotid-cavernous fistula, one of the hallmarks of which is exophthalmos. Compression of the medial temporal lobe by a **middle cerebral artery aneurysm (C)** may result in seizures. **Ophthalmic artery aneurysms (D)** may initially present with an inferior nasal field cut because of pressure on the optic nerve from the overlying falciform ligament (the dural fold between the anterior clinoid processes). A pupil-involving third nerve palsy is extremely suggestive of a **posterior communicating artery aneurysm (E)**.[2]

37. A – Hydromyelia is lined with ependymal cells, and syringomyelia is not

Hydromyelia represents a dilatation of the central canal of the spinal cord, which is lined by ependymal cells. Syringomyelia dissects through the spinal cord tissue outside of the central canal and is therefore not lined by ependyma (**A, E**). Neither lesion is lined with **choroid plexus (B)**. Both lesions contain **CSF (C)**. Both syringomyelia and hydromyelia may be either **focal or extensive (D)**, depending on the individual patient.[9]

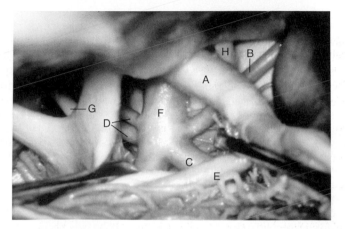

38. F – Basilar artery
39. G – Pituitary stalk
40. H – Right oculomotor nerve
41. C – Right posterior cerebral artery
42. A – Internal carotid artery
43. D – Left duplicated superior cerebellar artery
44. B – Right superior cerebellar artery
45. E – Right anterior cerebral artery (A1 segment)

In this figure the right opticocarotid triangle is exposed. On the left of the image, the optic chiasm (unlabeled) is being retracted with an instrument. The **pituitary stalk (G)** is noted between the paired optic nerves (unlabeled). The **basilar artery (F)** is noted in the center of the image, as is its bifurcation into the left and **right posterior cerebral arteries (C)**. A single **right superior cerebellar artery (B)** takes off proximal to the basilar bifurcation, and a **left duplicated superior cerebellar artery (D)** takes off on the contralateral side. The **right oculomotor nerve (H)** can be seen crossing underneath the **right SCA (B)** on its way to the superior orbital fissure. The **internal carotid artery (A)** is being retracted laterally at its bifurcation. The **right A1 segment (E)** is noted distal to the ICA bifurcation. (For questions 38–45, figure used with permission of Dr. Al Rhoton.)

46. A –   Cerebellar and vestibular complaints typically overshadow motor and sensory complaints (false).

In cases of basilar impression, motor and sensory complaints are seen more often than are cerebellar and vestibular symptoms. The lines of **McGregor (B)** and **McRae (C)** may be helpful in the radiographic assessment of patients with basilar invagination. **Short necks, torticollis (D)**, and **vertebral artery anomalies (E)** are common in patients with basilar invagination.[10]

47. D –   Type II odontoid fracture

Type II odontoid (D) fractures have the worst prognosis for healing of the choices presented. **Type I (C) and type III (E)** fractures generally heal well with immobilization. **The burst fracture of C1 (Jefferson's fracture) (B)** usually heals by rigid immobilization unless the transverse ligament is disrupted (lateral masses displaced more than 7 mm) or the patient is elderly.[10]

48. A –   Congenital elevation of the scapula

Sprengel's deformity refers to a congenital asymmetry of the scapula, with failure of one scapula to completely descend during development. Sprengel's deformity is often associated with the Klippel-Feil syndrome **(congenital fusion of the upper cervical vertebrae [B])**. **Intravertebral disk herniation (C)** is known as a Schmorl's node. **Postlaminectomy kyphosis (D)** and **scoliosis resulting from tethering of the spinal cord (E)** are incorrect responses.[11]

49. D –   Distracting extended
50. C –   Compression neutral
51. E –   Flexing axially rotated
52. B –   Compressing flexed
53. A –   Flexing flexed
54. F –   Compressing laterally bent
55. C –   Compressing neutral

Conditions of extreme flexion (e.g., **flexing in the flexed position [A]**) may result in bilateral facet dislocation. **Compression** (axial loading) **in the flexed position (B)** is the mechanism of the teardrop fracture. **Compression in the neutral position (C)** may lead to burst fractures of the subaxial spine as well as burst fractures of the C1 ring (Jefferson's fracture). **Distraction while in extension (D)** is the underlying mechanism of the Hangman's fracture. **Flexion with axial rotation (E)** may lead to unilateral facet dislocation. **Compression with lateral bending (F)** is the mechanism of horizontal facet fractures.[11]

56. E –   Superior articular facet hypertrophy

> This question tests the examinee's understanding of lumbar anatomy as well as the pathogenesis of lumbar stenosis. The superior articular facet is situated anterolaterally to the inferior articular facet of the level above, and makes up much of the posterior limit of the lateral recess of the lumbar spinal canal. Therefore, **superior articular facet hypertrophy (E)** is the most common cause of lateral recess stenosis in spondylosis. **Disk herniation (A)** and **ligamentum flavum hypertrophy (D)** may contribute to lateral recess stenosis but are less likely to cause lateral recess stenosis than **superior articular facet hypertrophy (E)**. **Inferior articular facet hypertrophy (C)** is incorrect because the **superior articular facet** is more closely associated with the lateral recess. **Hypertrophy of the pedicles (B)** does not contribute to lateral recess stenosis.[10]

57. E –   All of the above

> **Diplopia, oscillopsia, reduction of upgaze**, and **a sense of impending doom** are all more common with stimulation of the periaqueductal gray than with stimulation of the periventricular gray region.[2]

58. E –   Pineoblastoma

> The presence of bilateral ocular retinoblastomas along with the presence of a **pineoblastoma (E)** is known as "trilateral retinoblastoma." An understanding of this association is facilitated by the recognition that the pineal gland is a photoreceptor organ. **Astrocytoma (A)**, **medulloblastoma (B)**, **neurofibroma (C)**, and **optic nerve sheath tumor (D)** are incorrect responses.[2]

59. B –   Giant ophthalmic artery aneurysm and evidence of vasospasm on arteriogram

> **Evidence of vasospasm on arteriogram (B)** implies the potential for inadequate collateral flow, which would put the patient at risk for ischemic neurologic deficits following vessel sacrifice. While the presence of **bilateral intracavernous carotid aneurysms (A)** or **extracranial atherosclerotic disease (C)** may be relative contraindications to carotid sacrifice in this clinical scenario, they do not represent absolute contraindications. Carotid artery ligation is not contraindicated in the setting of **sudden loss of extraocular motility in the presence of an intracavernous carotid artery aneurysm (D)** or in the setting of **traumatic dissecting aneurysm of the petrous carotid artery (E)**.[2]

60. C –   Foramen magnum

> The "clockwise" progression of weakness described in the vignette is classically associated with lesions at the **foramen magnum (C)** such as a meningioma. Meningiomas of the **clivus (A)** may present with cranial nerve palsies. **Olfactory groove (D)** and **tuberculum sella (E)** meningiomas may present with visual symptoms, behavioral disturbances, or symptoms from increased intracranial pressure. **Parafalcine (B)** meningiomas are not associated with the "clockwise" pattern of quadriparesis described.[4]

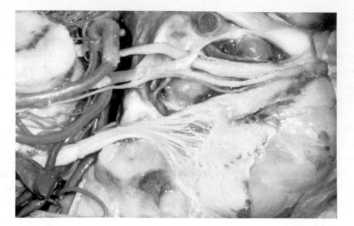

61. A – Clinoidal
62. D – Infratrochlear (Parkinson's)
63. H – Posteromedial (Kawase's)
64. D – Infratrochlear (Parkinson's)
65. A – Clinoidal
66. E – Anteromedial
67. B – Oculomotor
68. F – Anterolateral
69. G – Posterolateral (Glasscock's)
70. H – Posteromedial (Kawase's)

The clinoidal, oculomotor, supratrochlear, and infratrochlear triangles are the four triangles of the cavernous sinus. The **clinoidal (A)** triangle lies between the optic nerve and oculomotor nerve and can be exposed by removal of the anterior clinoid process to reveal the clinoidal segment of the internal carotid artery. The **oculomotor (B)** triangle is bordered by the anterior and posterior petroclinoidal dural folds and the intraclinoidal dural fold. The oculomotor nerve enters the cavernous sinus in the center of the **oculomotor (B)** triangle. The **supratrochlear (C)** triangle lies between the inferior margin of the oculomotor nerve and superior margin of the trochlear nerve—this triangle is very small. The **infratrochlear (D)** triangle, or **Parkinson's (D)** triangle, lies between the inferior margin of the trochlear nerve and superior margin of the ophthalmic nerve (V1) and contains the intracavernous carotid artery and the meningohypophyseal trunk. Parkinson described a surgical approach through the **infratrochlear (D)** triangle for the treatment of carotid-cavernous fistulas.

The anterolateral, anteromedial, posterolateral, and posteromedial triangles are the four triangles of the middle fossa. The **anteromedial (E)** triangle lies between the lower margin of the ophthalmic nerve (V1) and the upper margin of the maxillary nerve (V2). Drilling the bone in the **anteromedial (E)** triangle opens into the sphenoid sinus. The **anterolateral (F)** triangle lies between the inferior margin of the maxillary nerve (V2) and the upper margin of the mandibular nerve (V3). The **posterolateral (Glasscock's) (G)** triangle opens laterally to the mandibular nerve (V3), anterior to the point at which the greater superficial petrosal nerve crosses V3, and contains the middle meningeal artery in foramen spinosum. The **posteromedial triangle (Kawase's) (H)** contains the cochlea in its lateral apex, and also contains the petrous carotid artery. The medial portion of **Kawase's** triangle can be drilled in an anterior petrosectomy for approaches to the anterolateral brainstem and low-riding basilar bifurcations.[1] (For questions 61–70, figure used with permission of Dr. Al Rhoton.)

71. B –   Absence of third nerve palsy

Patients with posterior communication artery aneurysms who **do not have a third nerve palsy (B)** or whose angiogram reveals the aneurysm projecting *laterally* to the carotid are more likely to have aneurysm domes that are adherent to the temporal lobe. Choices **C** and **D** are incorrect because they contradict this statement. Neither **loss of consciousness (A)** nor **seizures (E)** predict aneurysm adherence to the temporal lobe.[5]

72. A –   Axillary nerve

Weakness of the deltoid muscle could be caused by injury to the **axillary nerve (A)**, which innervates the deltoid. The **dorsal scapular nerve (B)** innervates the rhomboid muscles as well as the levator scapulae. The **musculocutaneous nerve (C)** innervates the muscles of the anterior compartment of the arm including the biceps brachii and the coracobrachialis muscles. The **suprascapular nerve (D)** innervates the supraspinatus and infraspinatus muscles. An injury to the **thoracodorsal nerve (E)** would cause weakness of the latissimus dorsi muscle.[6]

73. A –   *Escherichia coli*

E. coli **(A)** is the most common cause of subdural empyema in the infant following meningitis. *Streptococcus pneumoniae* meningitis may also lead to subdural empyemas. *Listeria* **(C)**, *Neisseria* **(D)**, and *Staphylococcus* **(E)** are incorrect responses.[12]

74. D –   Nerve

The manifestations of Sudeck's atrophy are late changes of reflex sympathetic dystrophy (*CPRS I, RSD*). This condition may involve atrophic changes in the **bone (A), joints (B), muscle (C), and skin (E)**, but not the **nerve (D)**. The diagnosis of CRPS I, or reflex sympathetic dystrophy, is made only in the absence of a known nerve injury (in contrast with CRPS II, or causalgia, which requires a known nerve injury for diagnosis).[2]

75. E – Closure of the caudal neuropore: Day 26
76. D – Closure of the cranial neuropore: Day 24
77. B – Formation of the notochord: Day 17
78. A – Formation of the primitive streak: Day 13
79. C – Fusion of the neural folds to form the neural tube: Day 22

> Primary neurulation consists of the following events in this order: The primitive streak forms on **day 13 (A)**, notochord formation occurs on **day 17 (B)**, the neural folds fuse to form the neural tube on **day 22 (C)**, the cranial neuropore closes on **day 24 (D)**, and the caudal neuropore closes on **day 26 (E)**. Abnormalities during this stage of embryogenesis cause neural tube defects and Chiari malformations.[13,14]

80. B – I, III

> The subclavian steal syndrome is associated with symptoms of vertebrobasilar insufficiency. It occurs when increased **activity of the left arm (III)** results in shunting of blood into the left subclavian that is **occluded proximal to the origin of the left vertebral artery (I)**. The blood flow in the vertebral artery is reversed, resulting in partial brainstem ischemia exacerbated by use of the left arm. **Occlusion of the left subclavian artery distal to the origin of the left vertebral artery (II)** would not cause reversal of flow in the left vertebral artery, and therefore would not cause subclavian steal syndrome. **Occlusion of the left vertebral artery (IV)** might cause symptoms of vertebrobasilar insufficiency, but this would not be an example of subclavian steal.[3]

81. B – Coronally

> The coronal orientation of the facets in the upper thoracic spine leads to significant resistance to anterior translation but little resistance to rotation. In the lower thoracic spine, the facets become more sagittally oriented, and less resistance to anterior translation is offered.[3]

82. A – Back pain

> While it is possible for a thoracic disk herniation to cause either thoracic myelopathy, which may be characterized by **leg numbness (B)**, **leg weakness (C)**, **or urinary incontinence (E)**; or thoracic radiculopathy, which could cause **thoracic numbness (D)**; or thoracic pain in a dermatomal distribution, the most common presenting symptom of a herniated thoracic disk is **back pain (A)**. Back pain is the presenting complaint of 57 to 88% of patients with a thoracic herniated disk.[3]

83. A – I, II, III

> Occlusion of the thalamostriate vein during the subchoroidal transvelum interpositum approach to the third ventricle may result in **drowsiness (I)**, **hemiparesis (II)**, or **mutism (III)**. **Seizures (IV)** have not been reported after the ligation of the thalamostriate vein during this approach.[5]

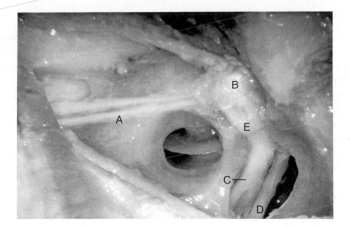

84. E – Labyrinthine segment of the facial nerve
85. C – Meatal segment of the facial nerve
86. D – Superior vestibular nerve
87. A – Greater superficial petrosal nerve
88. B – Geniculate ganglion

> This set of questions tests relevant anatomy for the middle fossa approach to the internal acoustic meatus. The **meatal segment of the facial nerve (C)** is noted in its superoanterior position in the internal acoustic meatus with the **superior vestibular nerve (D)** being located just lateral to it. The inferior vestibular nerve and cochlear nerve are obscured from view. The **labyrinthine segment of the facial nerve (E)** is noted just before the facial nerve enters the **geniculate ganglion (B)**. The **greater superficial petrosal nerve (A)** turns anteromedially to run along the middle fossa floor. The cochlea is noted in the angle formed by the facial nerve and greater superficial petrosal nerve.[1] (For questions 84–88, figure used with permission of Dr. Al Rhoton.)

89. B – Anterior, superior, inferior

> In the series of Sugita and Kobayashi, the facial nerve was anterior to the tumor in 50%, superior in 30%, and inferior in 15% of cases.[15]

90. E – Skin plaques (false)

> **Skin plaques (E)** are the most common skin lesions seen in neurofibromatosis type 2. They are well-circumscribed, raised, rough areas of skin that may be associated with excess hair. **Axillary freckles (A)**, **café au lait spots (B)**, **Lisch nodules (C)**, and **multiple typical skin neurofibromas (D)** are all characteristics of neurofibromatosis type 1.[6,12]

91. D – Postoperative tumor residual

Of the choices available, **postoperative tumor residual (D)** is the most important factor in meningioma recurrence. **Bone invasion (B)** could influence recurrence rates as it may limit the extent of tumor resection, particularly for lesions at the skull base. **Histologic type of benign meningioma (C)** is incorrect because this answer choice implies that the lesion is WHO grade I. Certainly WHO grade II (atypical) and WHO grade III (anaplastic) meningiomas have a higher recurrence rate than grade I (benign) lesions, but this is not an answer choice. **Patient age (A)** and **sex (E)** are incorrect responses.[3]

92. B – Cerebellopontine angle cistern
93. D – Lateral cerebellomedullary cistern
94. A – Ambient cistern
95. A – Ambient cistern
96. B – Cerebellopontine angle cistern
97. C – Interpeduncular cistern
98. D – Lateral cerebellomedullary cistern

The **ambient cistern (A)** contains portions of the superior cerebellar artery and the trochlear nerve as it courses around the lateral brainstem. The **cerebellopontine angle cistern (B)** contains the anteroinferior cerebellar artery and the trigeminal nerve. The **interpeduncular cistern (C)** contains the basal vein of Rosenthal. The **lateral cerebellomedullary cistern (D)** contains the choroid plexus at the foramen of Luschka and the origin of the posteroinferior cerebellar artery (PICA). None of the structures listed are located in the **prepontine cistern (E).**[16]

99. B – Cochlear and inferior vestibular nerves from the facial and superior vestibular nerves

This question tests the examinee's knowledge of the relationships of the nerves in the internal acoustic meatus. Anteriorly, the facial nerve is superior to the cochlear nerve ("7-up, coke down"). Posteriorly, the superior and inferior vestibular nerves are related to one another as their names imply. The transverse crest runs horizontally separating the two superior structures (facial nerve anteriorly and superior vestibular nerve posteriorly) from the two inferior structures (cochlear nerve anteriorly and inferior vestibular nerve posteriorly).[2]

100. B – Deafness is more common than permanent facial weakness as a complication of microvascular decompression.

Hemifacial spasm is more common in females (**C is incorrect**); it typically begins in the orbicularis muscles and progresses caudally (**D is incorrect**). At microvascular decompression the most common finding is compression by the posteroinferior cerebellar artery (PICA) (**A is incorrect**); the cure rate at 1 month is 86% (**E is incorrect**). Deafness occurs in 2.7% of patients, and permanent facial weakness occurs in 1.5% of patients after microvascular decompression (**B is correct**).[6]

101. E – Subtemporal approach

> Possible approaches to an aneurysm of the vertebrobasilar junction include the **extended extreme lateral inferior transcondylar approach (A)**, **the lateral suboccipital approach (B)**, **the presigmoid transtentorial approach (C)**, and **the retrolabyrinthine transsigmoid approach (D)**. The **subtemporal approach (E)** is best suited for aneurysms of the upper basilar trunk arising within 2 cm below the tip of the posterior clinoid.[3,5]

102. A – Headache

> **Headache (A)** is the initial symptom in more than 75% of patients with colloid cysts, and almost all patients with this lesion experience headache. "Drop attacks," possibly secondary to acute hydrocephalus that suddenly stretches corticospinal leg fibers **(sudden leg weakness [D])**, are associated with colloid cysts. **Dementia (B)** may be prominent, and **seizures (C)** occur in ~20% of patients. An association with **sudden death (E)** has been reported.[3]

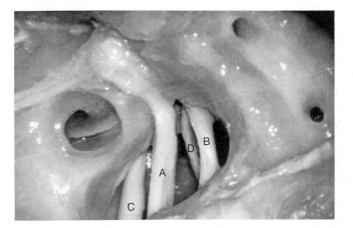

103. C – Inferior and anterior
104. D – Inferior and posterior
105. A – Superior and anterior
106. B – Superior and posterior

> This question tests the examinee's understanding of the anatomy of the internal acoustic meatus viewed through a middle fossa approach. The first step is getting oriented by identifying known structures. The cochlea has been exposed in the angle created by the facial nerve (A) and greater superficial petrosal nerve (not labeled), which we know is anteromedial to the internal acoustic meatus. A portion of the labyrinth has been exposed to reveal one of the semicircular canals posterolaterally (closest to B). As such, we know this is a view of the IAC from above (middle fossa approach) on the patient's right side. The facial nerve is noted **superior and anterior (A)** coursing toward the geniculate ganglion. The cochlear nerve is situated in an **inferior and anterior (C)** position on its way to the cochlea. The **superior** and **inferior** vestibular nerves are situated **posteriorly (B and D, respectively)** en route to the labyrinth. (For questions 103–106, figure used with permission of Dr. Al Rhoton.)

107. A – Congestive heart failure

Neonates with **congestive heart failure (A)** usually have multiple fistulas, and over 25% of their cardiac output is shunted. **Hydrocephalus (B)** and **seizures (D)** are more common in infants, whereas **subarachnoid hemorrhage (E)**, decreased cognition, and **intraparenchymal hemorrhage (C)** are more common in older children and adults.[3]

108. B – Compression fracture

This type of fracture is generally stable because the middle column is intact, by definition (utilizing the three-column spine model). Posterior column failure can still occur, however, if the anterior body height is reduced by more than half. The resulting kyphotic deformity can lead to neurologic deficit.[3]

109. B – Fracture-dislocations involve all three columns.

Compression fractures are the most common thoracolumbar spine fracture **(A is incorrect)**. Seat belt injuries refer to flexion-distraction type injuries that are often unstable **(C is incorrect)**. Wedge compression fractures generally involve the anterior column and are usually stable **(D and E are incorrect)**.[3]

110. B – A result of cytotoxic edema (false)

Diffuse brain swelling is a vasoactive posttraumatic phenomenon occurring within hours of head injury. It is thought to be a result of **cerebrovascular congestion (A)** and can be manifested on **CT scan by a compression of the perimesencephalic cistern (D)**. This pathologic process is **more common in children than adults (E)**, and may be **associated with a 50% mortality rate in severely head injured children (C)**. It is distinct from the vasogenic or **cytotoxic edema (B)** that occurs later.[7]

111. C – Parietal skull fracture

Of the choices listed, an isolated **parietal skull fracture (C)** is the least suggestive of child abuse, or nonaccidental trauma. **Acute and healing long bone fractures (A)**, **retinal hemorrhages (D)**, and **the presence of subdural hematomas (B and E)** should be treated as nonaccidental trauma until proven otherwise. When associated with abuse, skull fractures tend to be multiple or complex, depressed, and nonparietal.[7,9]

112. E – Metopic suture

Premature closure of the **metopic suture (E)** results in trigonocephaly. The incidence of trigonocephaly ranges from 10 to 16%.[7]

113. B – Lumbar region

The cleft is located in the **lumbar region (B)** in 47%, thoracolumbar region in 27%, **thoracic region (D)** in 23%, and **sacral (C)** or **cervical region (A)** in 1.5% of cases.[3]

114. E – 80%

> Up to 80% of patients with mycotic aneurysms carry an underlying diagnosis of subacute bacterial endocarditis.[3]

115. A – Infected emboli lodge in the vasa vasorum (false).

> Bacterial (mycotic) intracranial aneurysms are typically located in the **peripheral branches (C)** of the **middle cerebral artery territory (B)**. *Staphylococcus aureus* **and β-hemolytic streptococci species (E)** are the most common offending agents. The observation that vasa vasorum are found only on the first segment of the internal carotid artery (ICA), an unusual site of the development of bacterial aneurysms, has discredited the notion that **infected emboli lodge in the vasa vasorum (A)**. Although these aneurysms have a high tendency to bleed, typical **subarachnoid hemorrhage occurs in less than 20% of patients (D)**.[3]

116. E – Occur most commonly between the ages of 2 and 5 years (false)

> Growing skull fractures may **cross suture lines (A)**, may be **associated with an underlying brain injury (B)**, tend to occur if the **initial fracture is separated by more than 3 mm (C)**, and occur **most commonly in the parietal bone (D)**. Up to 75% of patients with growing skull fractures are < **1 year old (E is false, and therefore the correct answer choice)**.[7]

117. E – 100%

> **One hundred percent (E)** of infants with myelomeningocele have MRI evidence of a Chiari II malformation, the mechanism of which is thought to be due to CSF leaking through the myelomeningocele during development.[3]

118. A – I, II, III (cholesterol, calcific, and platelet-fibrin)

> **Cholesterol emboli (I)** (Hollenhorst plaques) are associated with ulcerated atheromatous plaques of the ICA. **Calcific emboli (II)** originate from the cardiac valves. **Platelet-fibrin emboli (III)** are thought to arise from large-vessel mural thrombi. **Fat emboli (IV)** result after trauma to marrow-containing bones and therefore are not due to cardiovascular disease of the heart and great vessels.[4]

119. B – I, III (superior vermian vein, precentral cerebellar vein)

> The **superior vermian vein (I)** and **precentral cerebellar vein (III)** are usually sacrificed during the infratentorial supracerebellar approach to the pineal region. The **basal vein of Rosenthal (IV)** and **posterior pericallosal vein (II)** are not sacrificed during this approach.[5]

120. B – Loudness recruitment (false)

> An absence of **loudness recruitment (B is incorrect)** is characteristic of a nerve trunk lesion, including an acoustic neuroma. Recruiting deafness occurs with a lesion in the organ of Corti (e.g., Ménière's disease). The other responses (**Békésy type III or IV audiogram [A], low short-increment sensitivity index [C], poor speech discrimination [D], and pronounced tone decay [E]**) are all characteristic of a retrocochlear (nerve) lesion such as an acoustic neuroma.[4]

121. B – Subarcuate artery
122. F – Anteroinferior cerebellar artery
123. A – Cochlear nerve
124. E – Facial nerve
125. C – Glossopharyngeal nerve
126. G – Spinal accessory nerve
127. H – Posteroinferior cerebellar artery
128. D – Vagus nerve

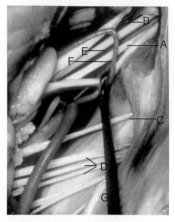

H–Not labeled

> This figure illustrates the structures of the right cerebellopontine angle as viewed through a retrosigmoid approach. A Rhoton dissector in the center of the image is retracting the inferior vestibular nerve inferiorly and is making contact with the **AICA (F)**. The **cochlear nerve (A)** is immediately anterior to the inferior vestibular nerve. The **subarcuate artery (B)** comes off of AICA and travels toward the subarcuate fossa. The superior vestibular nerve is being retracted superiorly in the upper right corner of the image to reveal the **facial nerve (E)**, which is immediately anterior to the superior vestibular nerve at the IAC. In the lower half of the image, the **glossopharyngeal nerve (C)**, the **vagus nerve (D)**, and the **spinal accessory nerves (G)** can be seen as they approach the jugular foramen to exit the cranial vault. The PICA vessel is not labeled but can be found in the lower left quadrant of the image crossing cranial nerves IX, X, and XI.[1] (For questions 121–128, figure used with permission of Dr. Al Rhoton.)

129. A – Dentate ligament

> The **dentate ligament (A)** is a paired structure that is an extension of pia that connects the lateral aspect of the spinal cord to the dura bilaterally—it marks the most dorsal extent of the incision for anterolateral cordotomy, a functional procedure for chronic pain. Lesioning at the **dorsal root entry zone (B)** is a useful technique particularly in cases of pain related to nerve root avulsion. The **posterior intermediate sulcus (C)** separates the fasciculus gracilis from the fasciculus cuneatus. The **posterior median sulcus (D)** runs in the dorsal midline separating the right and left dorsal columns. Afferent pain fibers enter the spinal cord and may ascend or descend up to three spinal levels in the **zone of Lissauer (E)** prior to terminating in the dorsal horn.[3,14]

130. A – I, II, III (contralateral hemiplegia, hemihypesthesia, homonymous hemianopia)

> The anterior choroidal artery is an intracranial branch of the internal carotid artery that comes off the ICA just distal to the origin of the posterior communicating artery. The anterior choroidal artery can be thought of as the most medial of the lateral lenticulostriate arteries, supplying the globus pallidus interna, the posterior limb of the internal capsule, and the optic tract. Occlusion of the anterior choroidal artery may lead to **contralateral hemiplegia (I)**, **hemihypesthesia (II)**, and a **homonymous hemianopsia (III)**. **Cognitive function (IV)** is unimpaired after occlusion of the anterior choroidal artery.[4]

131. E – Tremor

> The symptom of Parkinson's disease that is most likely to respond to a stereotactic lesion of the VIM of the thalamus is **tremor (E)**.[3]

132. D – Neither
133. C – Both
134. A – Apert's syndrome
135. B – Crouzon's disease
136. A – Apert's syndrome

> Both Apert's syndrome and Crouzon's disease are autosomal dominant conditions. Exorbitism and midface deficiency are seen in both. Anterior open bite and syndactyly are characteristic of Apert's syndrome. Although developmental delay is uncommon in patients with Crouzon's disease, mental retardation is seen in 50 to 85% of patients with Apert's syndrome.[3,7]

137. A – Primary empty sella syndrome
138. C – Secondary empty sella syndrome

> **Primary empty sella (A)** syndrome is an intrasellar herniation of the subarachnoid space occurring without previous pituitary surgery or radiation therapy. It typically occurs in middle-aged, obese women. Visual disturbance may occur in both the primary and secondary forms of the syndrome.[2]

139. E – Traumatic

Os odontoideum is a segment of odontoid that is well-corticated and is not fused with the body of the dens. The condition may be **congenital (A)** or **traumatic (E)**; trauma is the more common cause.[14]

140. D – Flexion

Translational C1–C2 subluxation is associated with **flexion (D)** injuries, rheumatoid arthritis, and tonsillitis (Grisel's syndrome).[14]

141. C – Intimal proliferation

While the mechanism of cerebral vasospasm has yet to be elucidated, studies indicate that **intimal proliferation (C)** is too mild and occurs too long after subarachnoid hemorrhage to play a significant role in vasospasm.[2]

142. D – Internal acoustic meatus
143. E – Posterior inferior cerebellar artery
144. G – Chorda tympani nerve
145. F – Facial nerve
146. B – Superior cerebellar artery
147. C – Trigeminal nerve
148. A – Trochlear nerve

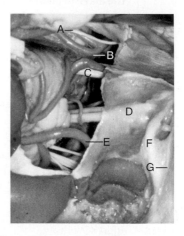

This figure illustrates the right presigmoid, retrolabyrinthine approach. The **trochlear nerve (A)** is noted at the rostral extent of the exposure, with the **superior cerebellar artery (B)** just below it. The **trigeminal nerve (C)** is closely associated with the superior petrosal vein in this image (not labeled). The VII–VIII complex is seen entering the **internal acoustic meatus (D)**. The temporal bone has been drilled to expose the course of the **facial (F)** and **chorda tympani nerves (G)**.[1] (For questions 142–148, figure used with permission of Dr. Al Rhoton.)

149. A – Type I spinal AVMs
150. A – Type I spinal AVMs
151. C – Type III spinal AVMs
152. B – Type II spinal AVMs
153. A – Type I spinal AVMs
154. E – Types II and III spinal AVMs

155. A – Type I spinal AVMs

> **Type I (A)**, or dural, spinal arteriovenous malformations (AVMs) are the most common type of spinal AVM, are believed to be acquired lesions, and manifest low flow but high pressure. They typically present with a slowly progressive course without significant clinical improvement. The etiology of types II, III, and IV spinal AVMs is believed to be congenital. **Type II (B)**, or glomus, AVMs are intramedullary. **Type III (C)**, or juvenile, AVMs are predominantly intradural. They are both true AVMs with rapid blood flow and are at risk for subarachnoid or intramedullary hemorrhage. **Type IV (D)** AVMs vary in size and in rapidity of blood flow. They are intradural, extramedullary, or perimedullary.[2]

156. C – External carotid, common carotid, internal carotid

> The correct sequence of removal of clamps from the arteries following carotid endarterectomy is the external carotid artery first, followed by the common carotid artery, with the removal of the clamp from the internal carotid artery last. This sequence ensures that any embolic material will be flushed into the external carotid circulation.[2]

157. C – Anterior caudate vein
158. B – Column of the fornix
159. D – Internal cerebral vein
160. A – Septal vein
161. G – Tela choroidea
162. E – Thalamostriate vein
163. F – Thalamus

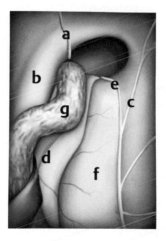

> The above figure represents a view of the contents of the right lateral ventricle that are relevant for the subchoroidal transvelum interpositum approach to the third ventricle.[5]

164. E – Dorsal ramus of C1
165. A – Glossopharyngeal nerve
166. D – Hypoglossal nerve
167. C – Spinal accessory nerve
168. B – Vagus nerve

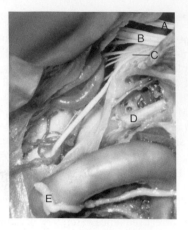

Questions 164–168 test the examinee's knowledge of the relevant anatomy exposed through the far lateral approach. A right-sided exposure is pictured here. The **glossopharyngeal (A)**, **vagus (B)**, and **spinal accessory nerves (C)** can be seen in transit to the jugular foramen in the upper right portion of the image. The **hypoglossal nerve (D)** has been exposed in its canal. The **dorsal ramus of C1 (E)** is adjacent to the vertebral artery at the lower margin of the figure. (For questions 164–168, figure used with permission of Dr. Al Rhoton.)

169. D – Anterior cerebral artery
170. E – Anterior choroidal artery
171. F – Middle cerebral artery
172. A – Optic nerve
173. B – Posterior communicating artery
174. C – Superior hypophyseal artery

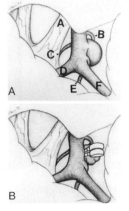

The above figures show the surgeon's view of the optic nerve, carotid artery, and its branches as seen through a right-sided pterional craniotomy. The ipsilateral **optic nerve** is labeled **A**. The internal carotid artery (ICA) bifurcates into the laterally projecting **middle cerebral artery (F)** and medially projecting **anterior cerebral artery (D)**. The most proximal ICA branch in this image is the **posterior communicating artery (B)**. The **superior hypophyseal artery (C)** can be seen projecting medially underneath the optic chiasm. The **anterior choroidal artery (E)** takeoff is just proximal to the internal carotid artery bifurcation.[2]

175. B – Leptomeningeal venous drainage

The risk of hemorrhage of dural AVMs seems related to the presence of tortuous and aneurysmal leptomeningeal arterialized veins.[2]

176. E – Surgery
177. A – Bromocriptine

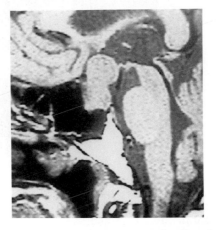

A prolactin level of 89 probably represents the "stalk effect" from this large pituitary tumor with suprasellar extension. A preoperative ophthalmologic examination should be documented, and surgery probably should be performed because chiasmal compression is evident. A prolactin level of 650 suggests a prolactinoma that should be bromocriptine responsive.[2,14]

178. A – Intraventricular

Lateral ventricular meningiomas account for 1 to 2% of intracranial meningiomas. **Olfactory groove (B)**, **posterior fossa (C)**, **sphenoid ridge (D)**, and **tuberculum sella (E)** are all more common locations.[2]

179. E – The risk of rebleed in the first year after hemorrhage is highest in the first 2 weeks (false).

The risk of rebleed from an AVM in the first year after hemorrhage is as high as 6 to 18%, but this risk is evenly distributed throughout the first year.[2]

180. E – Paresthesias or dysesthesias

Paresthesias (E) occur in 20% of postoperative patients; **dysesthesias (E)** occur in 5.2 to 24.2%.[2]

181. C – II, IV (trigeminal cistern and foramen ovale)

In the technique of percutaneous radiofrequency trigeminal gangliolysis, the needle is inserted into the **trigeminal cistern (II)** via the **foramen ovale (IV)**. The **foramen rotundum (I)** does transmit the maxillary division of the trigeminal nerve, but is not used in this procedure. The **foramen spinosum (III)** transmits the middle meningeal artery and is not used in percutaneous trigeminal gangliolysis.[2]

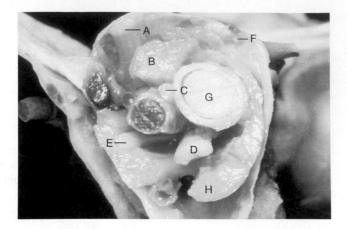

182. H – Inferior rectus muscle
183. D – Inferior division of the oculomotor nerve
184. E – Abducens nerve
185. A – Frontal nerve
186. C – Nasociliary nerve
187. B – Superior division of the oculomotor nerve
188. G – Optic nerve
189. F – Trochlear nerve

> The above figure represents a cross section through the right orbit (anterior view). The **frontal nerve (A)** and **superior division of the oculomotor nerve (B)** are noted superolaterally. The small **trochlear nerve (F)** is noted superomedially. The **optic nerve (G)** is seen in its sheath with the **nasociliary nerve (C)** just lateral to it. Inferior to the optic nerve lies the **inferior division of the oculomotor nerve (D)** and the **inferior rectus muscle (H)**. The **abducens nerve (E)** is seen inferolateral to the ophthalmic artery (unlabeled).[1] (For questions 182–189, figure used with permission of Dr. Al Rhoton.)

190. B – DREZ rhizotomy
191. E – Sympathectomy
192. A – Cingulotomy
193. C – Morphine infusion
194. D – Pallidotomy
195. F – Ventral rhizotomy

> **Cingulotomy (A)** procedures are used in the treatment of obsessive-compulsive disorder. For patients with nociceptive cancer pain above C5, **morphine infusion (C)** and periventricular gray matter stimulation are options. If chronic stimulation fails in brachial plexus avulsion pain, a **dorsal root entry zone (DREZ) procedure (B)** should be considered. The **pallidotomy (D)** is very effective in Parkinson's disease, whereas causalgia responds to **sympathectomy (E)**. Good results are obtained when spasmodic torticollis is treated with ventral **rhizotomy (F)** combined with spinal accessory denervation procedures.[2]

196. E – All of the above

These options (intercostal nerves, spinal accessory nerves, cervical plexus, and phrenic nerve) have all been used with varying degrees of success. Intercostal nerves are most commonly used for neurotization procedures involving the upper extremity.[2]

197. A – Frontal, greater wing of the sphenoid, parietal, and squamous part of the temporal

B is incorrect; the lesser wing of the sphenoid does not contribute to the pterion. **C** is incorrect; the zygomatic arch does not contribute to the pterion. **D and E** are incorrect because neither the lesser wing of the sphenoid nor the zygomatic arch contributes to the pterion.[17]

198. A – 30 Gy in 2 weeks

The most common external beam radiation therapy regimen for brain metastasis is **30 Gy given over 2 weeks (A).**[14]

199. B – 6,000 cGy in 200 cGy daily fractions

The most appropriate radiation protocol for glioblastoma is **6,000 cGy in 200 cGy daily fractions (B).**[14]

200. E – Volume status

Patients with cerebral salt wasting are volume depleted, whereas those with syndrome of inappropriate antidiuretic hormone (SIADH) are euvolemic or volume expanded.[2]

201. C – ASIA C

The ASIA impairment scale is used for the grading of acute spinal cord injuries. **ASIA A (A)** represents a complete spinal cord injury with no sensory or motor sparing in the sacral dermatomes. **ASIA B (B)** corresponds to a sensory incomplete spinal cord injury, with sparing of sensation but not motor function distal to the level of injury—this may include sensation in the sacral dermatomes only (perianal sensation or deep anal pressure). **ASIA C (C)** represents motor incomplete injuries where > 50% of the muscles below the level of injury have < grade 3 power—such as the patient in the vignette. **ASIA D (D)** is ascribed to patients with ≥ grade 3 power in > 50% of the muscle groups below the neurologic level. **ASIA E (E)** corresponds to patients who have sustained a documented spinal cord injury, but are now neurologically intact.[14]

202. C – 75%

> The ASIA impairment scale can help to predict ambulatory outcomes. The patient in the question stem has an ASIA C spinal cord injury. Please see the table below.[14]
>
> | Grade | % Ambulatory |
> |:-----:|:------------:|
> | A | < 3 |
> | B | 50 |
> | C | 75 |
> | D | 95 |
> | E | 100 |

203. D – *PTEN* mutation

> The diagnosis for the patient in the question stem is Cowden's syndrome, which is characterized by facial trichilemmomas, fibromas of the oral mucosa, hamartomas of the GI tract and breast, and thyroid tumors. There is also an association with Lhermitte-Duclos disease, a hamartomatous lesion of the cerebellum. Cowden's disease is due to mutations of the **PTEN gene on chromosome 10q (D)**. **CAG trinucleotide repeats (A)** are associated with Huntington's disease. The **mTOR pathway (B)** has been implicated in the pathogenesis of tuberous sclerosis. Germline **mutations of p53 (C)** are seen in the Li-Fraumeni syndrome. **Trisomy 21 (E)** is seen in Down's syndrome.[14]

204. C – Major lumbar levoscoliosis and minor thoracic dextroscoliosis

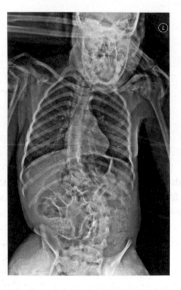

The curve is named based on the direction of the convexity of the curve. If the convexity of the curve is to the right, it is labeled dextroscoliosis. If the convexity of the curve is to the left, it is labeled levoscoliosis (**A and D are incorrect**). The major and minor curves are determined by the Cobb angles; the curve with the larger Cobb angle is the major curve. Conversely, the curve with the smaller Cobb angle is the minor curve (**E is incorrect**). In this case, the thoracic curve has its convexity pointed to the right with a Cobb angle of 33 degrees. The lumbar curve has its convexity pointed to the left and has a Cobb angle of 48 degrees. Therefore, the best description is choice **C, major lumbar levoscoliosis and minor thoracic dextroscoliosis.**[18]

205. D – All of the above

Iliac crest bone graft is harvested from a point at least 3 cm behind the anterior superior iliac spine to avoid ilioinguinal ligament disruption. Nerves at risk during this procedure (from lateral to medial) include the **iliohypogastric (A)**, **ilioinguinal (B)**, and **lateral femoral cutaneous nerves (C)**. The correct answer is **D, all of the above.**[18]

206. D – Sparing of dorsal hand sensation

A sensory deficit over the dorsoulnar aspect of the hand is seen in ulnar nerve compression at the elbow. With ulnar nerve compression at the wrist in Guyon's canal, this dorsal sensation is spared as the dorsal sensory branch of the ulnar nerve branches off proximal to the wrist. Therefore, **D** is the correct response. The other features can be seen in ulnar nerve compression at the elbow or the wrist.[8]

207. C – MRI is always unremarkable (false)

SCIWORA refers to **spinal cord injury without radiographic abnormality (A)** and is **more often seen in the pediatric population (B)**. Patients will present with signs and symptoms of spinal cord injury without **radiographic (X-ray or CT) evidence of a fracture (D)**. SCIWORA was first described before MRI was routinely used in the evaluation of spine trauma, and the mechanism is thought to be related to **ligamentous laxity in children (E)**. MRI scans in children with SCIWORA may reveal disruption of the discoligamentous complex and injury to the cord itself **(C is false).**[19]

208. E – Posterior C1–C2 instrumented fusion

Type II odontoid fractures have a high rate of nonunion, and therefore, surgical intervention is usually recommended **(A and B are incorrect)**. Generally, **odontoid screw placement (D)** and **posterior C1– C2 fusion (E)** either with transarticular screws or a screw/rod construct are acceptable options. In this case, the transverse ligament is disrupted, which is a contraindication to **odontoid screw placement** (the patient would have ongoing atlantoaxial instability even if the odontoid was stabilized due to ligamentous disruption between the dens and C1). Therefore, a **posterior C1– C2 fusion (E)** is the most appropriate treatment for this patient. Inclusion of the occiput would be unnecessary and introduces additional complexity and morbidity to the procedure **(C is incorrect).**[18]

References

1. Rhoton AL. Cranial Anatomy and Surgical Approaches. Schaumburg, IL: Lippincott Williams & Wilkins; 2003

2. Tindall GT, Cooper PR, Barrow DL, eds. The Practice of Neurosurgery. Baltimore, MD: Williams & Wilkins; 1995

3. Winn HR, ed-in-chief. Neurological Surgery, 5th ed. Philadelphia, PA: W.B. Saunders; 2003

4. Ropper AH, Brown RH. Principles of Neurology, 8th ed. New York: McGraw-Hill; 2005

5. Apuzzo MLJ. Brain Surgery. Complication Avoidance and Management. New York: Churchill Livingstone; 1993

6. Greenberg MS. Handbook of Neurosurgery, 5th ed. New York: Thieme Medical Publishers; 2001

7. Cheek WR, ed. Pediatric Neurosurgery: Surgery of the Developing Nervous System, 3rd ed. Philadelphia, PA: W.B. Saunders; 1994

8. Quinones-Hinojosa A, ed. Schmidek & Sweet Operative Neurosurgical Techniques, 6th ed. Philadelphia, PA: Elsevier; 2012

9. Nelson JS, Mena H, Parisi JE, Schochet SS, eds. Principles and Practice of Neuropathology, 2nd ed. New York: Oxford University Press; 2003

10. Rothman RH, Simeone FA, eds. The Spine, 3rd ed. Philadelphia, PA: WB Saunders; 1992

11. Frymoyer JW, ed. The Adult Spine, Principles and Practice. Philadelphia, PA: Lippincott-Raven; 1997

12. Rowland LP, ed. Merritt's Textbook of Neurology, 9th ed. Baltimore, MD: Williams & Wilkins; 1995

13. Cheek WR, ed. Pediatric Neurosurgery: Surgery of the Developing Nervous System, 3rd ed. Philadelphia, PA: W.B. Saunders; 1994

14. Citow JS, Macdonald RL, Refai D, eds. Comprehensive Neurosurgery Board Review. New York: Thieme Medical Publishers; 2009

15. Youmans JR, ed-in-chief. Neurological Surgery, 4th ed. Philadelphia, PA: W.B. Saunders; 1992

16. Yasargil MG, Kasdaglis K, Jain KK. Anatomic Observations of the Subarachnoid Cisterns of the Brain during Surgery. In: Selected papers of Professor Gazi Yasargil. Congress of Neurological Surgery. New York: Waverly Press; 1986

17. Moore KL, Dalley AF. Clinically Oriented Anatomy, 5th ed. Baltimore, MD: Lippincott Williams and Williams; 2006

18. Kim DH, ed. Surgical Anatomy and Techniques to the Spine, 2nd ed. Philadelphia, PA: Elsevier; 2013

19. Borden NM, Forseen SE. Pattern Recognition Neuroradiology. New York: Cambridge University Press; 2011

2A Clinical Neurology— Questions

For questions **1** to **7**, match the eye movement with the description. Each response may be used once, more than once, or not at all.

    A. Convergence nystagmus
    B. Dissociated nystagmus (internuclear ophthalmoplegia)
    C. Downbeat nystagmus
    D. Impairment of optokinetic nystagmus
    E. Ocular bobbing
    F. Seesaw nystagmus
    G. Spasmus mutans

1. A common sign of multiple sclerosis

2. Most often associated with large destructive lesions of the pons

3. Seen exclusively in infants

4. Associated with lesions of the cervicomedullary junction

5. Associated with lesions of the parasellar region

6. Associated with lesions of the parietal lobe

7. Associated with lesions of the pineal region

8. Which of the following is *false* of seizure foci?
    A. Epileptic foci are slower in binding and removing acetylcholine than normal cortex.
    B. Firing of neurons in the focus is reflected by periodic spike discharges in the electroencephalogram (EEG).
    C. If unchecked, cortical excitation may spread to the subcortical nuclei.
    D. Neurons surrounding the focus are initially hyperpolarized and are GABAergic.
    E. The change in seizure discharge from the tonic phase to the clonic phase results from inhibition from the neurons surrounding the focus.

9. An abnormal optokinetic response is more likely to be obtained by rotating the optokinetic nystagmus drum
    A. Away from an occipital lobe lesion
    B. Away from a parietal lobe lesion
    C. Toward an occipital lobe lesion
    D. Toward a parietal lobe lesion
    E. Toward a temporal lobe lesion

⇨ For questions **10** to **14**, match the EEG wave with the description. Each response may be used once, more than once, or not at all.
    A. Alpha
    B. Beta
    C. Delta
    D. Theta
    E. 3-per-second spike and wave

10. 4 to 7 Hz

11. Normally may be present over the temporal lobes of the elderly

12. Recorded from the frontal lobes symmetrically

13. Associated with absence seizures

14. Attenuated or abolished with eye opening or mental activity

15. Which of the following drugs is *least* effective in the treatment of trigeminal neuralgia?
    A. Baclofen
    B. Carbamazepine
    C. Clonazepam
    D. Phenytoin
    E. Ketorolac tromethamine (Toradol)

16. Which of the following is *true* of papilledema?
    A. Absence of venous pulsations is a reliable indicator of papilledema.
    B. Pupillary light reflexes remain normal.
    C. The congested capillaries derive from the central retinal vein.
    D. Unilateral edema of the optic disk is never seen.
    E. Visual acuity usually decreases.

17. Which of the following can occur in glossopharyngeal neuralgia?
    I.   Pain in the throat
    II.   Syncope
    III. Pain in the ear
    IV.   Bradycardia
    A. I, II, III
    B. I, III
    C. II, IV
    D. IV
    E. All of the above

18. Features of trisomy 13 (Patau's syndrome) include
- I.   Microcephaly
- II. Hypertonia
- III. Cleft lip and palate
- IV. Dextrocardia
- **A.** I, II, III
- **B.** I, III
- **C.** II, IV
- **D.** IV
- **E.** All of the above

19. Which of the following is *not* a feature of Parinaud's syndrome?
- **A.** Dissociated light–near response
- **B.** Lid retraction
- **C.** Nystagmus retractorius
- **D.** Paralysis of upgaze
- **E.** Third nerve palsy

20. Which of the following is *true* of tuberculous meningitis?
- **A.** Headache is usually absent.
- **B.** If untreated, the clinical course is self-limited.
- **C.** The inflammatory exudate is confined to the subarachnoid space.
- **D.** The inflammatory exudate is found mainly at the convexities.
- **E.** The protein content of the cerebrospinal fluid (CSF) is almost always elevated.

21. Which of the following CSF findings is *least* suggestive of acute multiple sclerosis?
- **A.** An IgG index greater than 1.7
- **B.** Increased myelin basic protein
- **C.** Increased protein to 200 mg/dL
- **D.** Presence of oligoclonal bands
- **E.** Slight to moderate monocytic pleocytosis

22. Each of the following is true of myasthenia gravis *except*
- **A.** A decrementing response to peripheral nerve stimulation is typical.
- **B.** Aminoglycoside antibiotics may worsen the symptoms.
- **C.** Females are more frequently affected in the < 40 age group.
- **D.** Females predominate in the subset of patients with a thymoma.
- **E.** Ten to 15% of patients have no antibodies to the acetylcholine receptor.

23. A defect in mitochondrial DNA is found in each of the following disorders *except*
- **A.** Kearns-Sayre syndrome
- **B.** Leber's hereditary optic atrophy
- **C.** Leigh's subacute necrotizing encephalopathy
- **D.** Mitochondrial myopathy, encephalopathy, lactic acidosis, and stroke (MELAS)
- **E.** Menkes' syndrome

24. Symptoms of spontaneous carotid artery dissection include
    I.   Dysgeusia
    II.   Eye pain
    III. Tongue weakness
    IV. Horner's syndrome
A. I, II, III
B. I, III
C. II, IV
D. IV
E. All of the above

25. Memory impairment is caused by discrete bilateral lesions of which of the following structures?
    I.   Amygdala
    II.   Hippocampal formation
    III. Mammillary bodies
    IV. Dorsomedial nuclei of the thalamus
A. I, II, III
B. I, III
C. II, IV
D. IV
E. All of the above

26. Genes responsible for cavernous malformations have been mapped to chromosomes
A. 1 and 3
B. 3 and 5
C. 3 and 7
D. 4 and 5
E. 5 and 7

27. Each of the following is characteristic of a diabetic third nerve palsy *except*
A. It develops over a few hours
B. It spares the pupil
C. It is usually painless
D. The lesion involves the center of the nerve
E. The prognosis for recovery is good

▷ For questions **28** to **36**, provide the best match of the toxicities with the description. Each response may be used once, more than once, or not at all.
A. Arsenic poisoning
B. Lead poisoning
C. Manganese poisoning
D. Mercury poisoning
E. Phosphorus poisoning

28. Transverse white lines in the fingernails

29. Black lines at the gingival margins

30. Later symptoms resemble those of Parkinson's disease

31. Treated with atropine

32. Penicillamine is the treatment of choice in the chronic form

33. Characterized by mood changes, tremors, and a cerebellar syndrome

34. Treated with ethylenediaminetetraacetic acid (EDTA) and dimercaprol (BAL)

35. Increased excretion of urinary coproporphyrin

36. Diagnosis can be made by the examination of hair samples

37. Which of the following is *not* a characteristic of Adie's syndrome?
- **A.** Degeneration of the ciliary ganglia and postganglionic parasympathetics
- **B.** More common in women than in men
- **C.** No reaction to 0.1% pilocarpine solution
- **D.** Paralysis of segments of the pupillary sphincter
- **E.** Pupil responds better to near than to light

38. Characteristics of infantile seizures include
- I. Lip smacking
- II. Hypsarrhythmia
- III. Generalized tonic-clonic activity
- IV. Myoclonic head jerks
- **A.** I, II, III
- **B.** I, III
- **C.** II, IV
- **D.** IV
- **E.** All of the above

⇨ For questions **39** to **42**, match the disease with the description. Each response may be used once, more than once, or not at all.
- **A.** Myasthenia gravis
- **B.** Eaton-Lambert myasthenic syndrome
- **C.** Both
- **D.** Neither

39. Muscles of the trunk and lower extremities are more frequently involved than the extraocular muscles

40. Poor response to anticholinesterase drugs

41. An incrementing response (marked increase in the amplitude of the action potential with fast rates of nerve stimulation) is typical

42. Associated with antibodies to the presynaptic voltage-dependent calcium channel

43. The dorsal scapular nerve innervates the
- I. Supraspinatus
- II. Rhomboids
- III. Subscapularis
- IV. Levator scapulae
- **A.** I, II, III
- **B.** I, III
- **C.** II, IV
- **D.** IV
- **E.** All of the above

⇨ For questions **44** to **50**, match the peripheral nerve with the muscle it innervates. Each response may be used once, more than once, or not at all.

    A.   Axillary nerve
    B.   Dorsal scapular nerve
    C.   Subscapular nerve
    D.   Suprascapular nerve
    E.   None of the above

44.   Teres major

45.   Teres minor

46.   Subscapularis

47.   Levator scapulae

48.   Supraspinatus

49.   Infraspinatus

50.   Rhomboids

51.   The motor unit potential in myopathy is of
    A.   Decreased voltage and decreased duration
    B.   Decreased voltage and increased duration
    C.   Decreased voltage and normal duration
    D.   Normal voltage and decreased duration
    E.   Normal voltage and increased duration

52.   Which is *true* of myotonic dystrophy?
    A.   Frontal balding occurs only in men.
    B.   Lens abnormalities are rare.
    C.   The congenital form is inherited only from the maternal line.
    D.   The inheritance is autosomal recessive.
    E.   Weakness always predates the myotonia.

53.   Subacute combined degeneration of the spinal cord is caused by a deficiency of
    A.   Cobalamin
    B.   Folic acid
    C.   Nicotinic acid
    D.   Pyridoxine
    E.   Thiamine

54.   The marker linked to the Huntington gene is localized to the short arm of chromosome
    A.   4
    B.   11
    C.   17
    D.   22
    E.   None of the above

55. Alexia without agraphia is most likely to occur with a lesion involving the
   A. Left geniculocalcarine tract and corpus callosum
   B. Left geniculocalcarine tract and Wernicke's area
   C. Left geniculocalcarine tract, corpus callosum, and Wernicke's area
   D. Right geniculocalcarine tract and corpus callosum
   E. Right geniculocalcarine tract and Wernicke's area

56. Deviation of the eyes to the right is most likely to occur with occlusion of the
   A. Calcarine artery bilaterally
   B. Calcarine artery on the contralateral side
   C. Contralateral paramedian branch of the basilar artery
   D. Ipsilateral superior cerebellar artery
   E. Superior division of the contralateral middle cerebral artery

57. Which of the following antiepileptic drugs has the shortest half-life?
   A. Carbamazepine
   B. Ethosuximide
   C. Phenobarbital
   D. Phenytoin
   E. Valproate

⇨ For questions **58** to **60**, match the description with the disease.
   A. Amyotrophic lateral sclerosis
   B. Syringomyelia
   C. Both
   D. Neither

58. Weakness and atrophy of the hands

59. Hypo- or areflexia

60. Absence of sensory changes

61. Biochemical studies of neurons from a seizure focus have shown all of the following *except*
   A. Increased levels of extracellular potassium in glial scars near seizure foci
   B. Decreased rate of binding and removing acetylcholine in the foci
   C. Deficiency of γ-aminobutyric acid (GABA)
   D. Decreased glycine levels
   E. Decreased taurine levels

62. The most reliable indicator of an *intracellular* cobalamin (vitamin B_{12}) deficiency is
   A. Low vitamin B_{12} on a microbiologic assay
   B. Low vitamin B_{12} on a radioisotope dilution assay
   C. Low vitamin B_{12} on a Schilling test
   D. The finding of hypersegmented polymorphonuclear neutrophil leukocytes (PMN) in bone marrow smears
   E. The finding of increased serum concentration of methylmalonic acid and homocysteine

63. Each of the following is true of radiation myelopathy (delayed progressive type) *except*
    A. Absence of pain is typical early in the course
    B. It occurs 12 to 15 months after radiation
    C. Magnetic resonance imaging (MRI) shows abnormal signal intensity; decreased on T1 and increased on T2
    D. Sensory changes usually develop after motor changes
    E. The most severe parenchymal changes are typical of infarction

64. Fasciculation potentials indicate
    A. Motor nerve fiber irritability
    B. Motor nerve fiber destruction
    C. Motor unit denervation
    D. Muscle atrophy
    E. Reinnervation of muscle units

⇨ For questions **65** to **70**, match the description with the potential.
    A. Fasciculation potential
    B. Fibrillation potential
    C. Both
    D. Neither

65. Di- or triphasic pattern

66. 5 to 15 milliseconds in duration

67. May take the form of positive sharp waves

68. Seen in poliomyelitis

69. Usually develops 24 to 36 hours after the death of an axon

70. May be visible through the skin

71. What characteristics of motor unit potentials are typical soon after reinnervation?
    A. Prolonged, high amplitude, and polyphasic
    B. Prolonged, low amplitude, and polyphasic
    C. Shortened, high amplitude, and polyphasic
    D. Shortened, low amplitude, and polyphasic
    E. None of the above

72. Which of the following ocular findings is *not* seen in myasthenia gravis?
    A. Abnormal pupillary response to accommodation
    B. Normal pupillary response to light
    C. Weakness of extraocular muscles
    D. Weakness of eye closure
    E. Weakness of eye opening

73. Risk factors for carpal tunnel syndrome include
    I.   Acromegaly
    II. Amyloidosis
    III. Hypothyroidism
    IV. Pregnancy
    A. I, II, III
    B. I, III
    C. II, IV
    D. IV
    E. All of the above

74. Which of the following is *true* of neurologic findings in sarcoidosis?
    A. Cranial nerve VI is most frequently involved.
    B. Sarcoidosis occurs in 25% of cases of sarcoid.
    C. Polydipsia, polyuria, somnolence, and obesity are common features.
    D. The granulomatous infiltration is most prominent over the hemispheres.
    E. Visual disturbances are usually secondary to lesions in the occipital cortex.

75. All of the following are associated with narcolepsy *except*
    A. Increased total number of hours per day spent sleeping
    B. Cataplexy
    C. Hypnagogic hallucinations
    D. Sleep paralysis
    E. Sleep patterns beginning with the rapid eye movements (REM) stage

76. Which of the following signs or symptoms occurring in a young person is the most suggestive of multiple sclerosis?
    A. Bilateral internuclear ophthalmoplegia
    B. Gait ataxia
    C. Lhermitte's sign
    D. Optic neuritis
    E. Vertigo

77. The muscles most often involved in thyroid ophthalmopathy are the
    A. Inferior, superior, and medial recti
    B. Inferior rectus and superior oblique
    C. Lateral and superior recti
    D. Lateral rectus and superior oblique
    E. Medial rectus and inferior oblique

78. Most cases of "idiopathic" hemifacial spasm are thought to result from
    A. Ephaptic transmission
    B. Hypersensitivity of facial muscles
    C. Hypocalcemia
    D. Psychiatric disorders
    E. Recurrence of latent viral infection

79. The diagnosis of neurosarcoidosis is based on
    A. Biopsy evidence of sarcoid granulomas in non–central nervous system (CNS) tissue and neurologic findings
    B. Computed tomography (CT) scan showing meningeal involvement
    C. Increased sedimentation rate and hyperglobulinemia
    D. Increased serum levels of angiotensin-converting enzyme
    E. MRI findings of periventricular and white matter changes

⇨ For questions **80** to **84**, match the paraneoplastic syndrome with the description. Each response may be used once, more than once, or not at all.
    A. Limbic encephalitis
    B. Eaton-Lambert syndrome
    C. Moersch-Woltman (stiff-man) syndrome
    D. Opsoclonus-myoclonus
    E. Sensory neuropathy

80. Seen most often in children with neuroblastoma

81. Anti-Hu antibodies

82. Anti-Ri antibodies

83. Autoantibodies to voltage-gated calcium channels

84. Autoantibodies to glutamic acid decarboxylase

⇨ For questions **85** to **88**, match the vascular syndrome with the description. Each response may be used once, more than once, or not at all.
    A. Basilar syndrome
    B. Lateral medullary syndrome (vertebral artery [VA] or posteroinferior cerebellar artery [PICA] occlusion)
    C. Lateral superior pontine syndrome (superior cerebellar artery [SCA] occlusion)
    D. Medial medullary occlusion
    E. None of the above

85. Contralateral hemiparesis sparing the face, contralateral loss of position and vibration sense, ipsilateral paralysis, and atrophy of the tongue

86. Contralateral pain and temperature loss in the body, ipsilateral Horner's syndrome, ipsilateral ataxia, ipsilateral paralysis of the palate and vocal cords, and ipsilateral pain and numbness in the face

87. Ipsilateral cerebellar ataxia, contralateral loss of pain and temperature in the body, partial deafness, and nausea and vomiting

88. Bilateral motor weakness in all extremities, bilateral cerebellar ataxia, and diplopia

89. The lesion in hemiballismus is localized to the contralateral
    A. Brachium conjunctivum
    B. Caudate nucleus
    C. Dorsomedial nucleus of the thalamus
    D. Substantia nigra
    E. Subthalamic nucleus

90. The long thoracic nerve innervates the
    A. Latissimus dorsi
    B. Levator scapulae
    C. Rhomboids
    D. Serratus anterior
    E. Teres minor

91. Which of the following is most consistent with Eaton-Lambert syndrome?
    A. Abnormal presynaptic vesicles
    B. Antibodies to the acetylcholine receptor
    C. Decreased numbers of acetylcholine receptors
    D. Defect in release of acetylcholine quanta
    E. None of the above

92. Von Hippel-Lindau disease has been associated with all of the following *except*
    A. A defect on chromosome 3
    B. Dominant inheritance
    C. Iris hamartomas
    D. Pancreatic cysts
    E. Renal cell carcinoma

93. Gerstmann's syndrome classically involves a lesion in the
    A. Dominant frontal lobe
    B. Dominant parietal lobe
    C. Dominant temporal lobe
    D. Nondominant parietal lobe
    E. Nondominant temporal lobe

94. Each of the following is true of dopamine pharmacology *except*
    A. Homovanillic acid is a metabolite.
    B. It is derived from phenylalanine.
    C. It is metabolized by monoamine oxidase (MAO).
    D. The activation of the D2 receptor decreases the release of transmitter at synaptic terminals.
    E. The rate-limiting step in its synthesis is dopa decarboxylase.

⇨ For questions **95** to **99**, match the antiparkinsonian drug with the description. Each response may be used once, more than once, or not at all.
    A. Amantadine
    B. Artane (trihexyphenidyl)
    C. Bromocriptine
    D. Eldepryl (selegiline)
    E. Sinemet (carbidopa-levodopa)

95. Contains a dopa decarboxylase inhibitor

96. Slows progression of the disease in its early stages

97. Stimulates D2 receptors

98. Dryness of the mouth and blurred vision are some of the side effects

99. Inhibits intracerebral metabolic degradation of dopamine

100. Wernicke's area corresponds most closely to Brodmann's area(s)
   A. 17
   B. 19
   C. 22
   D. 41 and 42
   E. 44

101. Complications of diabetes generally thought to be vascular in origin include
   I.   Ophthalmoplegia
   II. Acute mononeuropathy
   III. Mononeuritis multiplex
   IV. Distal sensorimotor polyneuropathy
   A. I, II, III
   B. I, III
   C. II, IV
   D. IV
   E. All of the above

102. Each of the following is consistent with a cholinergic crisis in a patient with myasthenia gravis being treated with pyridostigmine (Mestinon) *except*
   A. Bradycardia
   B. Diarrhea
   C. Increased strength after the Tensilon test
   D. Miosis
   E. Sweating

103. The genetic transmission of the MELAS syndrome is
   A. Autosomal dominant
   B. Autosomal recessive
   C. Maternal inheritance
   D. Sporadic
   E. X-linked recessive

⇨ For questions **104** to **107**, match the cord syndrome with the description. Each response may be used once, more than once, or not at all.
   A. Anterior cord syndrome
   B. Brown-Séquard syndrome
   C. Central cord syndrome
   D. A and B
   E. None of the above

104. Acute hyperextension

105. Flexion injury

106. Dissociated sensory loss

107. Among the incomplete syndromes, this has the best prognosis

⇨ For questions **108** to **113**, match the description with the sleep stage.
   A. REM sleep
   B. Non–rapid eye movement (NREM) sleep
   C. Both
   D. Neither

108. Dreaming

109. Adult somnambulism

110. Desynchronization of the EEG

111. K complexes

112. Sleep spindles

113. Glucose metabolism in the brain is increased in comparison to the waking state

⇨ For questions **114** to **117**, match the description with the disease.
   A. Glycogen storage disease type II (acid maltase deficiency)
   B. Glycogen storage disease type V (McArdle's disease)
   C. Both
   D. Neither

114. Myophosphorylase deficiency

115. Large amounts of glycogen are deposited in various organs

116. Three clinical forms are noted

117. X-linked recessive inheritance

118. Wilson's disease is characterized by
   I.   High urinary copper excretion
   II. High serum copper
   III. Low ceruloplasmin levels
   IV. Hyperdensity of the globus pallidus and putamen on CT
   A. I, II, III
   B. I, III
   C. II, IV
   D. IV
   E. All of the above

119. Each of the following is true of central pontine myelinolysis *except*
   A. A marked inflammatory response with destruction of nerve cells in the pons is seen.
   B. It is associated with rapid correction of hyponatremia.
   C. It is associated with chronic alcoholism.
   D. Quadriplegia, pseudobulbar palsy, and a locked-in syndrome can occur.
   E. Some patients have no signs or symptoms referable to the pontine lesion.

⇨ For questions **120** to **122**, match the description with the disease.
- **A.** Homocystinuria
- **B.** Marfan's syndrome
- **C.** Both
- **D.** Neither

120. Arachnodactyly

121. Mental retardation

122. Brain infarcts

123. Dressing apraxia is associated with a lesion in the
- **A.** Dominant frontal lobe
- **B.** Dominant parietal lobe
- **C.** Nondominant frontal lobe
- **D.** Nondominant parietal lobe
- **E.** Nondominant temporal lobe

124. The axillary nerve innervates the
- **A.** Coracobrachialis
- **B.** Rhomboids
- **C.** Supraspinatus
- **D.** Teres major
- **E.** Teres minor

125. All of the following are seen in Sturge-Weber syndrome *except*
- **A.** Calcified cortical vessels
- **B.** Facial nevus contralateral to seizure activity
- **C.** Hemisensory deficit contralateral to facial nevus
- **D.** Meningeal venous angiomas
- **E.** Tramline calcifications outlining the convolution of the parieto-occipital cortex

126. The normal sensory nerve conduction velocity in the median and ulnar nerves is approximately
- **A.** 10 meters per second (m/s)
- **B.** 25 m/s
- **C.** 50 m/s
- **D.** 100 m/s
- **E.** 150 m/s

127. Each of these statements is true of Charcot-Marie-Tooth disease *except*
- **A.** Autosomal dominance is the usual mode of inheritance.
- **B.** Distal muscle atrophy is prominent.
- **C.** It can affect the upper extremities.
- **D.** Steroids have no effect on disease progression.
- **E.** The autonomic nervous system is usually involved.

128. Cranial nerves that may be affected by a clival chordoma include
  I.   Cranial nerve XII
  II. Cranial nerve V
  III. Cranial nerve X
  IV. Cranial nerve II
  A. I, II, III
  B. I, III
  C. II, IV
  D. IV
  E. All of the above

129. Which of the following CSF findings is *least* consistent with tuberculous meningitis?
  A. Glucose of 30 mg/dL
  B. Lymphocytic predomination after 1 week of illness
  C. Opening pressure of 200 mm CSF
  D. Protein of 35 mg/dL
  E. White blood cell count (WBC) of 200 cells/mm³

130. The syndrome of PICA occlusion results in all of the following *except*
  A. Contralateral Horner's syndrome
  B. Contralateral loss of pain and temperature over the body
  C. Ipsilateral ataxia
  D. Ipsilateral numbness of the limbs
  E. Ipsilateral paralysis of the palate

131. Stage 2 sleep is characterized by
  A. K complexes
  B. Delta waves
  C. Desynchronization of the EEG
  D. REM sleep
  E. Somnambulism

⇒ For questions **132** to **141**, match the muscular dystrophy with the description. Each response may be used once, more than once, or not at all.
  A. Becker's muscular dystrophy
  B. Duchenne's muscular dystrophy
  C. Emery-Dreifuss muscular dystrophy
  D. Landouzy-Dejerine (facioscapulohumeral) dystrophy
  E. Myotonic dystrophy

132. The protein dystrophin is absent

133. The protein dystrophin is structurally abnormal

134. The most common adult form of muscular dystrophy

135. Prominent pseudohypertrophy of the calves is seen in Becker's and in this type

136. Contractures of the elbow flexors and neck extensors occur early

137. Abnormal gene is on chromosome 4

138. Lens opacities are found in 90% of patients

139. Occasionally associated with congenital absence of an involved muscle

140. Masseter atrophy, ptosis, and frontal baldness are characteristic

141. Abnormal gene is on chromosome 19

142. Monoplegia without muscular atrophy is most often secondary to a lesion in the
   A. Brainstem
   B. Cortex
   C. Internal capsule
   D. Peripheral nerve
   E. Spinal cord

143. The transmissible agent of Creutzfeldt-Jakob disease is inactivated by
   I.   Formalin
   II. Autoclaving at 132°C under pressure for 1 hour
   III. Alcohol
   IV. Immersion for 1 hour in bleach
   A. I, II, III
   B. I, III
   C. II, IV
   D. IV
   E. All of the above

144. The most common finding on audiography in patients with acoustic neuromas is
   A. Flat loss
   B. High-frequency loss
   C. Low-tone loss
   D. Normal audiogram
   E. Trough-shaped loss

⇨ For questions **145** to **149**, match the brachial plexus lesion with the description. Each response may be used once, more than once, or not at all.
   A. Lateral cord lesion
   B. Lower trunk lesion
   C. Medial cord lesion
   D. Middle trunk lesion
   E. Upper trunk lesion

145. Median sensory responses from the index and middle finger are low in amplitude, but motor conduction velocities of the hand muscles are normal.

146. Ulnar sensory response from the little finger is abnormal; electromyographic exam of the extensor indicis proprius and abductor pollicis longus is abnormal.

147. Ulnar sensory response from the little finger is abnormal; normal responses are seen from the extensor indicis proprius.

148. Action potentials from the deltoid and biceps are of low amplitude.

149. Abnormal median sensory responses and denervation are seen in the biceps and flexor carpi radialis; normal response is seen from the abductor pollicis brevis.

150. Persons migrating from a zone with high risk of multiple sclerosis (MS) to one of low risk after age 15 show a risk of developing MS that is
    A. Equal to that of the high-risk zone
    B. Equal to that of the low-risk zone
    C. Intermediate between the two zones
    D. Lower than that of the low-risk zone
    E. Unpredictable

151. Eye findings in botulism include
    I. Ptosis
    II. Strabismus
    III. Diplopia
    IV. Unreactive pupils
    A. I, II, III
    B. I, III
    C. II, IV
    D. IV
    E. All of the above

152. Repetition is least likely to be affected by a
    A. Broca's aphasia
    B. Conduction aphasia
    C. Global aphasia
    D. Transcortical sensory aphasia
    E. Wernicke's aphasia

153. Which stage of sleep is prominent on EEG at the onset of narcoleptic sleep attacks?
    A. Stage 1
    B. Stage 2
    C. Stage 3
    D. Stage 4
    E. REM

154. The most common cause of viral meningitis is
    A. Enterovirus
    B. Human immunodeficiency virus (HIV)
    C. Leptospirosis
    D. Lymphocytic choriomeningitis
    E. Mumps

155. Successive involvement of all cranial nerves on one side has been reported in
    A. Meningitis
    B. Sarcoidosis
    C. Tumors of the brainstem
    D. Tumors of the cavernous sinus
    E. Tumors of the clivus

156. Each of the following is true of Ménière's disease *except*
    A. Distention of the endolymphatic duct occurs
    B. Hearing loss is usually unilateral
    C. High-tone loss occurs early in the disease
    D. Horizontal nystagmus occurs during an acute attack
    E. Low-pitched tinnitus is typical

157. Each of the following is true of Eaton-Lambert syndrome *except*
    A. Autonomic disturbances are seen
    B. Fasciculations are not seen
    C. It has been associated with carcinoma of the stomach and colon
    D. Temporary increase in muscle power may occur during the first few contractions
    E. Women are more frequently affected than men

158. Type I (red) muscle fibers differ from type II (white) fibers in all of the following ways *except* that they
    A. Are more fatigable
    B. Fire more tonically
    C. Have slower contraction and relaxation rates
    D. Have more mitochondria
    E. Have more oxidative enzymes

159. Historically, one of the treatment modalities of Parkinson's disease was surgical ligation of the
    A. Anterior cerebral artery
    B. Anterior choroidal artery
    C. Middle cerebral artery
    D. Posterior communicating artery
    E. Recurrent artery of Huebner

160. Which of the following is *not* characteristic of diabetic mononeuritis multiplex?
    A. Lower extremities are more commonly affected than upper extremities
    B. Painful neuropathy
    C. Proximal extremities are more commonly affected than distal extremities
    D. Recovery is usual
    E. Symmetric neuropathy

For questions **161** to **165**, provide the best match of each antiepileptic drug with the seizure type. Each response may be used once, more than once, or not at all.
    A. Adrenocorticotropic hormone (ACTH)
    B. Ethosuximide
    C. Lorazepam
    D. Tegretol
    E. Valproic acid
    F. D or E

161. Status epilepticus

162. Absence seizures

163. Complex partial seizures

164. Infantile seizures

165. Atypical petit mal syndrome of Lennox-Gastaut

166. Each of the following is true of polymyositis associated with carcinoma *except*
    A. Carcinoma affects 9% of patients with polymyositis.
    B. It is most commonly associated with lung and prostate cancer in men.
    C. It is usually painful.
    D. Muscle biopsies show no evidence of tumor cells.
    E. Proximal muscles are initially affected more than distal ones.

167. Which of the following is *least* suggestive of cluster headaches?
    A. Associated with lacrimation and rhinorrhea
    B. Bilateral location
    C. Daily occurrence for 2 months
    D. Male predominance
    E. Orbital location

168. Organophosphate poisoning is characterized by all of the following *except*
    A. Bronchial spasms
    B. Dry mouth
    C. Miosis
    D. Sweating
    E. Vomiting

169. One of the cerebral biochemical defects in Huntington's disease is
    A. Decreased dopamine
    B. Decreased GABA
    C. Decreased norepinephrine
    D. Decreased somatostatin
    E. Increased acetylcholine

170. Prosopagnosia is associated with lesions of the
    A. Anterior corpus callosum
    B. Bilateral anteroinferior temporal lobes
    C. Bilateral medial temporo-occipital lobes
    D. Occipital poles
    E. Posterior corpus callosum

171. A lesion of the supplementary motor cortex produces
    A. Echolalia
    B. Palilalia
    C. Poverty of spontaneous speech
    D. Receptive aphasia
    E. No speech abnormalities

172. Lesions of the peroneal nerve produce weakness of the
    A. Abductor hallucis and gastrocnemius
    B. Extensor digitorum longus and brevis and abductor hallucis
    C. Gastrocnemius and flexor hallucis longus
    D. Tibialis anterior and extensor digitorum longus and brevis
    E. Tibialis anterior and flexor digitorum brevis

173. Which of the following is *not* characteristic of Tay-Sachs disease?
    A. Abnormal startle response
    B. Autosomal recessive inheritance
    C. Cherry red spots in the retina
    D. Deficiency of sphingomyelinase
    E. Macrocephaly

174. Which of the following deficits is *least* characteristic of Alzheimer's disease?
    A. Corticospinal tract dysfunction
    B. Dysnomia
    C. Korsakoff's amnesic state
    D. Personality change
    E. Spatial disorientation

175. Each of the following is true of Guillain-Barré syndrome *except*
    A. Disturbances of autonomic function are common
    B. High-dose steroids form the mainstay of therapy
    C. Hypo- or areflexia is characteristic
    D. The mortality rate is 3%
    E. The peak severity is 10 to 14 days after onset in 80% of cases

176. The second-order neuron in the sympathetic pathway to the pupil arises from the
    A. Ciliary ganglion to the iris
    B. Edinger-Westphal nucleus to the ciliary ganglion
    C. Hypothalamus to the lateral horn cells at C8 to T3
    D. Lateral horn cells at C8 to T3 to the superior cervical ganglion
    E. Superior cervical ganglion to the iris

177. The treatment of choice for toxoplasmosis is
    A. Penicillin
    B. Praziquantel
    C. Pyrimethamine and sulfadiazine
    D. Rifampin and nafcillin
    E. Thiabendazole

178. Which of the following is *true* of subacute sclerosing panencephalitis (SSPE)?
    A. Intracytoplasmic but not intranuclear inclusions are found.
    B. It is more common in patients > 18 years of age.
    C. Lesions are confined to the white matter.
    D. The EEG shows characteristic periodic waves that occur every 2 to 3 seconds.
    E. The CSF protein is normal.

179. The treatment of choice for optic neuritis is
    A. Intrathecal prednisolone
    B. Intravenous methylprednisolone followed by oral prednisone
    C. Oral prednisone only
    D. Oral prednisone followed by intravenous methylprednisolone
    E. Plasmapheresis

180. Schilder's disease most closely resembles
- **A.** Duchenne's muscular dystrophy
- **B.** Krabbe's disease
- **C.** Multiple sclerosis
- **D.** Trisomy 13
- **E.** Tuberous sclerosis

181. The cricothyroid muscle is innervated by the
- **A.** External branch of the superior laryngeal nerve
- **B.** Internal laryngeal branch of the superior laryngeal nerve
- **C.** Ninth cranial nerve
- **D.** Recurrent laryngeal nerve
- **E.** Seventh cranial nerve

182. Korsakoff's syndrome is best characterized by (a)
- **A.** Defect in learning and loss of past memories
- **B.** Global confusional state
- **C.** Manic-depressive state
- **D.** Paranoid ideation
- **E.** Stupor or coma

183. Werdnig-Hoffmann disease is notable for all of the following *except*
- **A.** Areflexia
- **B.** Autosomal recessive inheritance
- **C.** Hypotonia
- **D.** Involvement of chromosome 5q
- **E.** Mental retardation

184. Tricyclic antidepressants
- I.   Block norepinephrine uptake
- II. Block oxidative deamination of monoamines
- III. Block serotonin uptake
- IV. Bind to GABA receptors
- **A.** I, II, III
- **B.** I, III
- **C.** II, IV
- **D.** IV
- **E.** All of the above

⇨ For questions **185** to **189**, match the description with the disease.
- **A.** Amyotrophic lateral sclerosis (ALS)
- **B.** Cervical spondylosis
- **C.** Both
- **D.** Neither

185. Lower extremity spasticity

186. Hyporeflexia

187. Hyperreflexia

188. Absence or paucity of sensory symptoms

189. Atrophy of the hand muscles

⇨ For questions **190** to **195**, match the vasculitis with the description. Each response may be used once, more than once, or not at all.

    A. Cogan's syndrome
    B. Polyarteritis nodosa
    C. Systemic lupus erythematosus
    D. Takayasu's syndrome
    E. Temporal arteritis
    F. Wegener's granulomatosis

190. Antineutrophil cytoplasmic antibodies

191. Antinuclear antibodies and malar rash

192. Visual loss and claudication with chewing

193. Visual loss and loss of peripheral pulses

194. Mononeuritis multiplex, kidney involvement, and skin purpura

195. Deafness and keratitis

196. Wernicke's encephalopathy consists of all of the following *except*
    A. Defect in retentive memory out of proportion to other cognitive functions
    B. Gait ataxia
    C. Gaze palsy
    D. Mental confusion
    E. Nystagmus

197. Which of the following is *least* suggestive of a parietal lobe lesion?
    A. Astereognosis
    B. Loss of position sense
    C. Loss of temperature sensation
    D. Loss of two-point discrimination
    E. Atopognosia

198. The purest form of achromatopsia is caused by a lesion involving the
    A. Left calcarine cortex
    B. Left superior occipitotemporal region
    C. Right inferior occipitotemporal region
    D. Right occipital cortex and angular gyrus
    E. Right superior calcarine cortex

199. Failure of a miotic pupil to dilate after instilling 2 to 10% cocaine followed by 1% hydroxyamphetamine indicates a
    A. First-order Horner's syndrome
    B. Second-order Horner's syndrome
    C. Third-order Horner's syndrome
    D. First- or second-order Horner's syndrome
    E. Second- or third-order Horner's syndrome

200. Somnambulism occurs in which stage of sleep?
  A. Stage 1
  B. Stage 2
  C. Stage 4
  D. REM
  E. All of the above

201. The most effective treatment of enuresis is
  A. Klonopin
  B. Clonidine
  C. Haloperidol (Haldol)
  D. Imipramine (Tofranil)
  E. Methylphenidate (Ritalin)

202. In most cases, section of the corpus callosum causes
  A. Apraxia of both hands to command
  B. Apraxia of the left hand to command
  C. Apraxia of the right hand to command
  D. Object agnosia
  E. No deficit

⇨ For questions **203** to **208**, match the aphasia with the description. Each response may be used once, more than once, or not at all.
  A. Good comprehension, fluent speech, poor repetition
  B. Good comprehension, nonfluent speech, good repetition
  C. Good comprehension, nonfluent speech, poor repetition
  D. Poor comprehension, fluent speech, good repetition
  E. Poor comprehension, fluent speech, poor repetition
  F. Poor comprehension, nonfluent speech, poor repetition

203. Broca's aphasia

204. Conduction aphasia

205. Global aphasia

206. Transcortical motor aphasia

207. Transcortical sensory aphasia

208. Wernicke's aphasia

⇨ For questions **209** to **215**, match the description with the disease.
  A. Dermatomyositis
  B. Polymyositis
  C. Both
  D. Neither

209. May be associated with carcinoma

210. Men are more frequently affected than women

211. Necrosis and phagocytosis of individual muscle fibers are the principal changes

212. Perifascicular muscle degeneration and atrophy are found

213. Large numbers of T cells are found in the intramuscular inflammatory exudates

214. Immune complexes are deposited in the walls of arterioles and venules

215. Corticosteroids have no effect on symptoms

216. Which of the following anticonvulsants is associated with hyponatremia?
    A. Carbamazepine
    B. Gabapentin
    C. Levetiracetam
    D. Phenytoin
    E. Topiramate

217. All of the following statements regarding the use of single-photon emission computed tomography (SPECT) and positron emission tomography (PET) in epilepsy are true *except*
    A. Both ictal and interictal SPECT studies can be acquired and compared for seizure localization
    B. Ictal SPECT scans are generally easier to acquire than ictal PET scans
    C. Ictal SPECT scans show decreased tracer signal in the seizure focus
    D. Perfusion follows changes in metabolism during seizures
    E. Tracer needs to be injected within 1–2 minutes of seizure onset for an ictal SPECT study

218. All of the following are associated with mononeuritis multiplex *except*
    A. Diabetes
    B. HIV
    C. Neurocysticercosis
    D. Polyarteritis nodosa
    E. Sarcoidosis

219. The U.S. Food and Drug Administration (FDA) initially approved intravenous rtPA (recombinant tissue plasminogen activator) for use in acute ischemic stroke up to ___ hour(s) since symptom onset, but in 2009 extended the window to ___ hours since symptom onset.
    A. 1, 3
    B. 3, 4.5
    C. 4.5, 6
    D. 6, 8
    E. 8, 10

220. Based on the PROACT study, intra-arterial thrombolytic therapy is appropriate for patients with middle cerebral artery occlusions within ___ hours of symptom onset.
    A. 3
    B. 4.5
    C. 6
    D. 8
    E. 12

221. Based on the MERCI study, mechanical thrombectomy is appropriate for patients with middle cerebral artery occlusions within ___ hours of symptom onset.
    A. 3
    B. 4.5
    C. 6
    D. 8
    E. 12

222. All of the following are possible indications for endovascular therapy in the setting of acute ischemic stroke *except*
    A. Contraindication to intravenous tPA
    B. Diffusion-perfusion mismatch
    C. Failure to improve with intravenous tPA
    D. NIH stroke score of > 20
    E. Patient presents outside the therapeutic window for intravenous tPA

2B Clinical Neurology— Answer Key

1.	B	27.	C
2.	E	28.	A
3.	G	29.	B
4.	C	30.	C
5.	F	31.	E
6.	D	32.	D
7.	A	33.	D
8.	E	34.	B
9.	D	35.	B
10.	D	36.	A
11.	D	37.	C
12.	B	38.	C
13.	E	39.	B
14.	A	40.	B
15.	E	41.	B
16.	B	42.	B
17.	E	43.	C
18.	E	44.	C
19.	E	45.	A
20.	E	46.	C
21.	C	47.	B
22.	D	48.	D
23.	E	49.	D
24.	E	50.	B
25.	C	51.	A
26.	C	52.	C

53.	A	92.	C
54.	A	93.	B
55.	A	94.	E
56.	C	95.	E
57.	E	96.	D
58.	C	97.	C
59.	B	98.	B
60.	A	99.	D
61.	D	100.	C
62.	E	101.	A
63.	D	102.	C
64.	A	103.	C
65.	B	104.	C
66.	A	105.	A
67.	B	106.	A
68.	C	107.	B
69.	D	108.	C
70.	A	109.	B
71.	B	110.	A
72.	A	111.	B
73.	E	112.	B
74.	C	113.	A
75.	A	114.	B
76.	A	115.	A
77.	A	116.	A
78.	A	117.	D
79.	A	118.	B
80.	D	119.	A
81.	E	120.	C
82.	D	121.	A
83.	B	122.	A
84.	C	123.	D
85.	D	124.	E
86.	B	125.	A
87.	C	126.	C
88.	A	127.	E
89.	E	128.	E
90.	D	129.	D
91.	D	130.	A

131.	A	170.	C
132.	B	171.	C
133.	A	172.	D
134.	E	173.	D
135.	B	174.	A
136.	C	175.	B
137.	D	176.	D
138.	E	177.	C
139.	D	178.	D
140.	E	179.	B
141.	E	180.	C
142.	B	181.	A
143.	C	182.	A
144.	B	183.	E
145.	D	184.	B
146.	B	185.	C
147.	C	186.	D
148.	E	187.	C
149.	A	188.	A
150.	A	189.	C
151.	E	190.	F
152.	D	191.	C
153.	E	192.	E
154.	A	193.	D
155.	E	194.	B
156.	C	195.	A
157.	E	196.	A
158.	A	197.	C
159.	B	198.	C
160.	E	199.	C
161.	C	200.	C
162.	B	201.	D
163.	F	202.	B
164.	A	203.	C
165.	E	204.	A
166.	C	205.	F
167.	B	206.	B
168.	B	207.	D
169.	B	208.	E

209. C
210. D
211. B
212. A
213. B
214. A
215. D

216. A
217. C
218. C
219. B
220. C
221. D
222. D

2C Clinical Neurology— Answers and Explanations

1. B – Dissociated nystagmus (internuclear ophthalmoplegia)

2. E – Ocular bobbing

3. G – Spasmus mutans

4. C – Downbeat nystagmus

5. F – Seesaw nystagmus

6. D – Impairment of optokinetic nystagmus

7. A – Convergence nystagmus

Convergence nystagmus (A) is a "rhythmic oscillation in which a slow abduction of the eyes with respect to each other is followed by a quick movement of adduction," and may be accompanied by other signs of Parinaud's phenomenon, suggesting a lesion of the pineal region or midbrain tegmentum. **Dissociated nystagmus (B)** is horizontal nystagmus that occurs only in the abducting eye—this is a sign of internuclear ophthalmoplegia and is associated with multiple sclerosis. **Downbeat nystagmus (C)** has been associated with lesions of the cervicomedullary junction including Chiari malformation, syrinx, and basilar invagination. **Impairment of optokinetic nystagmus (D)** is associated with lesions to the parietal lobe—"the slow pursuit phase of the OKN may be lost . . . when a moving stimulus . . . is rotated toward the side of the lesion." **Ocular bobbing (E)** involves a "spontaneous fast downward jerk of the eyes followed by a slow upward drift to midposition," and has been associated with large destructive lesions of the pons. **Seesaw nystagmus (F)** is a "torsional-vertical oscillation in which the intorting eye moves up and the opposite (extorting) eye moves down, then both move in the reverse direction." **Seesaw nystagmus (F)** has been associated with chiasmatic bitemporal hemianopsia due to lesions of the parasellar region. **Spasmus mutans (G)** is a pendular nystagmus of infancy that is typically idiopathic and self-limited.[1]

8. E – The change in seizure discharge from the tonic phase to the clonic phase results from inhibition from the neurons surrounding the focus (false).

The change from the tonic to the clonic phase results from diencephalic inhibition of the firing cortex, not from inhibition of the neurons surrounding the focus as described in **(E)**. The other statements are true: Epileptic foci are slower in binding and removing acetylcholine than normal cortex **(A)**; firing of neurons in the focus is reflected by periodic spike discharges in the electroencephalogram **(B)**; if unchecked, cortical excitation may spread to the subcortical nuclei **(C)**; and neurons surrounding the focus are initially hyperpolarized and are GABAergic **(D)**.[1]

9. D – Toward a parietal lobe lesion

An abnormal optokinetic response (loss of the slow pursuit phase) is more likely to be obtained by rotating the optokinetic nystagmus drum **toward a parietal lobe lesion (D)**.[1]

10. D – Theta
11. D – Theta
12. B – Beta
13. E – 3-per-second spike and wave

14. A – Alpha

Alpha waves (A) are 8–12 Hz waves that are present in the occipital and parietal region and are attenuated or abolished with eye opening or mental activity. **Beta waves (B)** are of faster frequency (> 12 Hz) and lower amplitude than α waves and are recorded from the frontal areas symmetrically. **Theta waves (D)** are 4–7 Hz, and may be present over the temporal regions—especially in the elderly. **Delta waves (C)** are 1–3 Hz and are not present in the normal waking adult. A **3-per-second spike and wave (E)** EEG pattern is associated with absence seizures.[1]

15. E – Ketorolac tromethamine (Toradol)

Of the options listed, **ketorolac (Toradol [E])**, a nonsteroidal anti-inflammatory drug (NSAID), is the least effective in relieving the pain of trigeminal neuralgia. Anticonvulsants such as **carbamazepine (B), clonazepam (C), and phenytoin (D)** are often useful. **Baclofen (A)** is most helpful as an adjunct to one of the anticonvulsant drugs.[1]

16. B – Pupillary light reflexes remain normal

Venous pulsations are absent in 10 to 15% of normal individuals (**A is incorrect**). The congested capillaries are derived from the short ciliary arteries (**C is incorrect**). Unilateral edema can occur with optic nerve tumors (**D is incorrect**). Visual acuity is usually normal in papilledema (**E is incorrect**). Pupillary light reflexes typically remain normal in papilledema (**B**).[1]

17. E – All of the above

Glossopharyngeal neuralgia is less common than trigeminal neuralgia and is characterized by **pain in the throat (I)** that is often exacerbated by swallowing, talking, or yawning. Pain may also **radiate to the ear (III)**. Abnormal afferent inputs to cardioregulatory centers may trigger **syncope (II)** or **bradycardia (IV)**, which are not associated with trigeminal neuralgia or hemifacial spasm.[1]

18. E – All of the above

Trisomy 13, or Patau's syndrome, is characterized by **microcephaly (I), hypertonia (II), cleft lip and palate (III), and dextrocardia (IV)**. Other features of this dysgenetic syndrome include corneal opacities, polydactyly, impaired hearing, and severe mental retardation. Death usually occurs in early childhood. Trisomy 18, Edwards' syndrome, is characterized by low-set ears, micrognathia, mental retardation, and rocker-bottom feet.[1]

19. E – Third nerve palsy

Parinaud's syndrome (dorsal midbrain syndrome) is a constellation of symptoms that include **paralysis of upgaze (D)**, mydriasis and **lid retraction (B)**, **nystagmus retractorius (C)**, and a **dissociated light-near response (A)**. **Third nerve palsy (E)** is not associated with Parinaud's syndrome.[1]

20. E – The protein content of CSF is almost always elevated.

Headache occurs in more than half of cases (**A is incorrect**). Confusion, coma, and death usually result if the patient is untreated (**B is incorrect**). The inflammatory exudate occurs mainly in the basal meninges and frequently invades the underlying brain by spreading via pial vessels (**C is incorrect**). The CSF protein is always elevated to 100 to 200 mg/dL or higher (**E**).[1]

21. C – Increased protein to 200 mg/dL

The CSF protein is slightly increased in ~40% of patients with multiple sclerosis (MS). A concentration of > 100 mg/dL is rare (**C**). If the ratio of CSF IgG/serum IgG to CSF albumin/serum albumin is more than 1.7, the diagnosis of MS is probable (**A**). This ratio is known as the IgG index. Testing for **oligoclonal bands** (**D**) in CSF is the most widely used test for MS. Increased CSF **myelin basic protein** (**B**) can be present in acute MS exacerbations and is therefore consistent with a diagnosis of MS; however, increased MBP may be present in any process where myelin is destroyed. **A slight to moderate monocytic pleocytosis** (**E**) is present in approximately one-third of MS patients.[1]

22. D – Females predominate in the subset of patients with a thymoma (false)

The majority of patients with myasthenia gravis harboring a thymoma are older (50–60 years) and male (**D is false**). The disease is two to three times more common in women than men in patients < 40 years of age (**C is true**). A decrease in muscle action potential with nerve stimulation at 3 Hz (a decrementing response) is seen (**A is true**). Certain aminoglycoside antibiotics can impair transmitter release by inhibiting calcium ion fluxes at the neuromuscular junction (**B is true**). Ten to 15% of patients have no antibodies to the acetylcholine receptor (**E is true**).[1]

23. E – Menkes' syndrome (false)

Menkes' (kinky hair) syndrome (E) is a rare sex-linked recessive disease characterized by severe copper deficiency due to failure of intestinal absorption of copper. The other disorders (**Kearns-Sayre syndrome [A], Leber's hereditary optic atrophy [B], Leigh's subacute necrotizing encephalopathy [C], and mitochondrial myopathy, encephalopathy, lactic acidosis, and stroke [MELAS; D]**) have point mutations or deletions of mitochondrial DNA as part of their pathogenesis.[1]

24. E – All of the above

Symptoms of spontaneous carotid artery dissection may include **eye pain (II)** or unilateral headache as well as the presence of a **Horner's syndrome (IV)** that is due to the disruption of sympathetic nerves running along the carotid artery. Signs of ischemia in the territory of the affected internal carotid artery may be present. Small branches off of the carotid artery may supply the cranial nerves extracranially; ischemia to these branches may lead to cranial nerve dysfunction such as **dysgeusia (impaired taste, I)** or **tongue weakness (III).**[1]

25. C – II, IV (hippocampal formation and dorsomedial nuclei of the thalamus)

> Discrete, bilateral lesions in the **hippocampus (II)** and **dorsomedial thalamus (IV)** impair memory and learning out of proportion to other cognitive functions. Stereotactic lesions of the **amygdala (I)** and **mammillary bodies (III)** have failed to produce these symptoms.[1]

26. C – 3 and 7

> The gene (*CCM1*) responsible for familial cavernous malformations has been mapped to 7q11.2–q21. In addition, *CCM2* (7p13–15) and *CCM3* (3q25.2–27) have been identified in patients with cavernous malformations.[2]

27. C – It is usually painless (false)

> Diabetic third nerve palsy **develops over a few hours (A)**, and tends to be **pupil-sparing (B)** because it involves infarction of the **center of the nerve (D)**. **Recovery is typical (E)** but may take months. Diabetic third nerve palsy is usually **painful (C is false)**.[1]

28. A – Arsenic poisoning
29. B – Lead poisoning
30. C – Manganese poisoning
31. E – Phosphorus poisoning
32. D – Mercury poisoning
33. D – Mercury poisoning
34. B – Lead poisoning
35. B – Lead poisoning
36. A – Arsenic poisoning

> **Arsenic poisoning (A)** may be due to pesticide exposure, may cause **transverse white lines in the fingernails,** and may be diagnosed based on **examination of the hair** or urine. **Lead poisoning (B)** is less common in adults than in children and may present with anemia or peripheral neuropathy. **Lead poisoning (B)** may cause **black lines at the gingival margins, increased urinary excretion of coproporphyrin**, and may be **treated with ethylenediaminetetraacetic acid (EDTA) and dimercaprol (BAL)**. Chronic **manganese poisoning (C)** may result in extrapyramidal symptoms reminiscent of dystonia or **parkinsonism**. **Mercury poisoning (D)** may present with **mood changes, tremors, and a cerebellar syndrome** and is treated with **penicillamine**. **Phosphorous poisoning (E)** is typically due to exposure to organophosphate insecticides and is manifested by anti cholinesterase effects in the acute setting. Symptoms of **phosphorous poisoning (E)** can be treated with atropine and pralidoxime.[1]

37. C – No reaction to 0.1% pilocarpine solution

Adie's syndrome or Adie's tonic pupil results from **degeneration of the ciliary ganglia and postganglionic parasympathetics (A)** that are responsible for pupillary constriction. Adie's pupil **responds better to near (accommodation) than to light (E)**. The condition is **more common in women (B)** and involves **paralysis of segments of the pupillary sphincter (D)**. An **Adie's pupil will respond to 0.1% pilocarpine**, whereas a normal pupil would not (denervation hypersensitivity). **C is false.**[1]

38. C – II, IV (hypsarrhythmia, myoclonic head jerks)

Infantile seizures or spasms (West's syndrome) usually begin before 6 months of age and are characterized by sudden flexor or extensor **spasms of the head**, trunk, and limbs and an electroencephalogram (EEG) picture of bilateral high-voltage, slow-wave activity (**hypsarrhythmia**). **Lip smacking** and **generalized tonic-clonic activity** are not features.[1]

39. B – Eaton-Lambert myasthenic syndrome
40. B – Eaton-Lambert myasthenic syndrome
41. B – Eaton-Lambert myasthenic syndrome
42. B – Eaton-Lambert myasthenic syndrome

In **Eaton-Lambert myasthenic syndrome (B)**, muscles of the trunk and lower extremities are most frequently involved, there is an incrementing response to stimuli, and there is a poor response to anticholinesterase drugs. **Eaton-Lambert syndrome (B)** is associated with antibodies to the presynaptic voltage-dependent calcium channel. These are all features of **Eaton-Lambert syndrome (B)** and stand in contrast to the features of classic **myasthenia gravis (A)**.[1]

43. C – II, IV (rhomboids, levator scapulae)

The dorsal scapular nerve arises from the anterior ramus of C5 and pierces the middle scalene to innervate the **rhomboid muscles (II)** and **levator scapulae muscle (IV)**. The **supraspinatus muscle (I)** is innervated by the suprascapular nerve, which arises from the superior trunk of the brachial plexus and receives contributions from C5, C6, and C4. The **subscapularis muscle (III)** is innervated by the upper and lower subscapular nerves that are branches of the posterior cord receiving fibers from C5 and C6, respectively.[3]

44. C – Subscapular nerve
45. A – Axillary nerve
46. C – Subscapular nerve
47. B – Dorsal scapular nerve
48. D – Suprascapular nerve
49. D – Suprascapular nerve

50. B – Dorsal scapular nerve

> The **axillary nerve (A)** is one of the two terminal branches of the posterior cord and innervates the **teres minor** and deltoid muscles. The **dorsal scapular nerve (B)** arises from the anterior ramus of C5 and innervates the **levator scapulae** and **rhomboid muscles**. The **subscapular nerve (C)** has upper and lower components that come off the posterior cord to innervate the **teres major** and **subscapularis muscles**. The **suprascapular nerve (D)** arises from the superior trunk to innervate the **supraspinatus** and **infraspinatus muscles**.[3]

51. A – Decreased voltage and decreased duration

> The motor unit potential of myopathy tends to be of decreased voltage and decreased duration because in these conditions there is a reduced number of motor fibers per motor unit.[1]

52. C – The congenital form is inherited only from the maternal line.

> Frontal balding occurs in both men and women afflicted with myotonic dystrophy **(A is false)**. Lens opacities are found by slit lamp in 90% of patients **(B is false)**. The inheritance is autosomal dominant, and the defective gene segregates on chromosome 19 **(D is false)**. Myotonia may precede weakness by several years **(E is false)**. Answer C is correct: In the congenital (neonatal) form of myotonic dystrophy, the affected parent is always the mother.[1]

53. A – Cobalamin

> Subacute combined deficiency of the cord occurs from failure to transfer cobalamin (vitamin B_{12}) across the interstitial mucosa because of lack of intrinsic factor. Folic acid deficiency typically causes hematologic effects, and while folic acid is involved in B_{12} metabolism, it is rarely implicated in neurologic disease states **(B is incorrect)**. Nicotinic acid deficiency has been associated with encephalopathy **(C is incorrect)**. Pyridoxine (vitamin B_6) deficiency is associated with isoniazid therapy for tuberculosis and causes polyneuropathy **(D is incorrect)**. Thiamine deficiency is associated with the Wernicke-Korsakoff syndrome seen in chronic alcoholism **(E is incorrect)**.[1]

54. A – Chromosome 4

> The marker linked to the Huntington gene is localized to the short arm of chromosome 4 **(A)**. Neurofibromatosis type I is linked to chromosome 17 **(C is incorrect)**. Neurofibromatosis type II is linked to chromosome 22 **(D is incorrect)**.[1]

55. A – Left geniculocalcarine tract and corpus callosum

> The lesion described in **A** would render the patient blind in the right half of the visual field. Visual information reaches only the right occipital lobe but cannot be transferred to Wernicke's area across the callosum. Thus the ability to read aloud and to understand the written word is lost, but the ability to understand the spoken language, speak, write, dictate, and converse is retained.[1]

56. C – Contralateral paramedian branch of the basilar artery

Deviation of the eyes away from the lesion occurs in brainstem syndromes, for example, the medial midpontine syndrome **(occlusion of the paramedian branch of the midbasilar artery [C])**. Answers **B, D,** and **E** would cause deviation of the eyes to the left.[1]

57. E – Valproate

Of the antiepileptic drugs listed, **phenobarbital (C)** has the longest half-life of 96 ± 12 hours, followed by **ethosuximide (B)**, 40 ± 6 hours; **phenytoin (D)**, 24 ± 12 hours; **carbamazepine (A)**, 12 ± 4 hours; and **valproate (E)**, 8 ± 2 hours.[1]

58. C – Both
59. B – Syringomyelia
60. A – Amyotrophic lateral sclerosis

Despite the atrophy of the hands and forearms in amyotrophic lateral sclerosis (ALS), diffuse hyperreflexia is seen, with absence of sensory change.[1]

61. D – Decreased glycine levels (false)

Increased glycine levels have been found in neurons in seizure foci **(D is false)**.[1]

62. E – The finding of increased serum concentration of methylmalonic acid and homocysteine

Although **microbiologic assay (A)** is the most accurate way to measure serum cobalamin (B_{12}) levels, the serum level is not a measure of total body cobalamin (B_{12}). High **serum concentrations of cobalamin (B_{12}) metabolites (methylmalonic acid and homocysteine [E])** are the most reliable indicators of an intracellular cobalamin deficiency.[1]

63. D – Sensory changes usually develop after motor changes (false)

In radiation myelopathy, sensory changes usually precede the weakness **(D is false)**. The other responses are characteristics of radiation myelopathy (delayed progressive type).[1]

64. A – Motor nerve fiber irritability

Fasciculation potentials are a sign of **motor nerve fiber irritability (A)**. Fibrillation potentials are associated with **motor nerve fiber destruction (B)**. Insertional activity is typically seen with **denervating processes (C)**. **Muscle atrophy (D)** results in motor unit potentials of lower voltage and shorter duration. **Reinnervation of muscle units (E)** may result in "giant" motor unit potentials of unusually high amplitude.[1]

65. B – Fibrillation potential
66. A – Fasciculation potential
67. B – Fibrillation potential
68. C – Both
69. D – Neither

70. A – Fasciculation potential

Fibrillation potentials last from 1 to 5 milliseconds, may take the form of positive sharp waves, and are seen 10 to 25 days after the death of an axon. Fasciculation potentials have three to five phases. Both can be seen in poliomyelitis.[1]

71. B – Prolonged, low amplitude, and polyphasic

In early denervation, motor unit potentials may increase in size and amplitude and become longer in duration and polyphasic **(A)**. These so-called "giant" potentials are a result of motor units containing more than the usual number of motor fibers. In early reinnervation the motor units are low in amplitude, prolonged, and polyphasic **(B)**, representing a transitional configuration.[1]

72. A – Abnormal pupillary response to accommodation

Normal pupillary response to light and accommodation **(A is false, B is true)**, together with extraocular **(C)** and orbicularis oculi **(D)** muscle weakness, is highly suggestive of myasthenia gravis.[1]

73. E – All of the above

Acromegaly **(I)**, amyloidosis **(II)**, hypothyroidism **(III)**, and pregnancy **(IV)** are all risk factors for the carpal tunnel syndrome (median nerve entrapment neuropathy at the wrist).[1]

74. C – Polyopsia, polyuria, somnolence, and obesity are common features.

Neurologic involvement in sarcoidosis occurs in 5% of cases **(B is false)**. A granulomatous inflammatory response most prevalent at the base of the brain is seen **(D is false)**. Visual disturbances (due to lesions in and around the optic nerves and chiasm **[E is false]**) and polydipsia, polyuria, somnolence, or obesity (due to involvement of the pituitary and hypothalamus) are the usual features **(C is true)**. The facial nerve is the most common cranial nerve involved **(A is false)**.[1]

75. A – Increased total number of hours per day spent sleeping

The nocturnal sleep of a narcoleptic is often reduced, but frequent naps are taken during the day; hence, the total number of hours spent sleeping is similar to a normal individual **(A is false)**. The other responses are associated with narcolepsy.[1]

76. A – Bilateral internuclear ophthalmoplegia

The initial manifestation of MS in 25% of all patients is **optic neuritis (D)**, and ~50% of patients who present with optic neuritis will eventually develop MS. **Bilateral internuclear ophthalmoplegia occurring in a young person (A)**, however, is virtually diagnostic of MS.[1]

77. A – Inferior, superior, and medial recti

Upgaze or downgaze is usually more limited than lateral gaze. These deficits are caused by an inflammatory infiltration of the inferior and medial recti, leading to contractures of these muscles.[1]

78. A – Ephaptic transmission

The spasm is thought to be caused by nerve root compression and segmental demyelination, which leads to impulses conducted in one motor fiber being transmitted to neighboring fibers (ephaptic transmission **[A]**).[1]

79. A – Biopsy evidence of sarcoid granulomas in non-CNS tissue and neurologic findings

Although all of the options are seen in active neurosarcoidosis, the diagnosis is made on the basis of answer **A**.[1]

80. D – Opsoclonus-myoclonus
81. E – Sensory neuropathy
82. D – Opsoclonus-myoclonus
83. B – Eaton-Lambert syndrome
84. C – Moersch-Woltman (stiff-man) syndrome

The IgG antibody in patients with **Eaton-Lambert syndrome (B)** (associated with small-cell carcinoma of the lung) reacts with presynaptic voltage-gated calcium channels. The **Moersch-Woltman syndrome (C)** is characterized by involuntary muscle rigidity and spasms, and 60% of patients have autoantibodies to glutamic acid decarboxylase. Underlying tumors are often found. Most cases of **paraneoplastic sensory neuropathy (E)** are associated with small-cell carcinoma of the lung or lymphoma, and an antinuclear antibody (anti-Hu) is found in 70% of these patients. **Paraneoplastic opsoclonus (D)** in adults is associated with breast cancer and an antineuronal antibody (anti-Ri).[4]

85. D – Medial medullary occlusion
86. B – Lateral medullary syndrome (VA or PICA occlusion)
87. C – Lateral superior pontine syndrome (SCA occlusion)
88. A – Basilar syndrome

Medial medullary occlusion (D) is associated with contralateral hemiparesis sparing the face, contralateral loss of position and vibration sense, ipsilateral paralysis, and atrophy of the tongue. **Lateral medullary syndrome (VA or PICA occlusion [B])** is associated with contralateral pain and temperature loss in the body, ipsilateral Horner's syndrome, ipsilateral ataxia, ipsilateral paralysis of the palate and vocal cords, and ipsilateral pain and numbness in the face. **Lateral superior pontine syndrome (SCA occlusion [C])** is associated with ipsilateral cerebellar ataxia, contralateral loss of pain and temperature in the body, partial deafness, and nausea and vomiting. **Basilar syndrome (A)** is associated with bilateral motor weakness in all extremities, bilateral cerebellar ataxia, and diplopia.[1]

89. E – Subthalamic nucleus

> The lesion in hemiballismus is localized to the **contralateral subthalamic nucleus (E)**. Cerebellar incoordination and intention tremor are associated with damage to the **brachium conjunctivum (A)**. Huntington's chorea is associated with damage to the **caudate nucleus (B)**. Dysfunction of the **substantia nigra (D)** is involved in the pathogenesis of Parkinson's disease.[1]

90. D – Serratus anterior

> The long thoracic nerve arises from the posterior aspect of the anterior rami of C5, C6, and C7 and innervates the **serratus anterior muscle (D)**; lesions to the long thoracic nerve result in winging of the scapula. The **levator scapulae (B)** and **rhomboids (C)** are innervated by the dorsal scapular nerve, which is a branch off the posterior aspect of the anterior ramus of C5. **The latissimus dorsi (A)** is innervated by the thoracodorsal nerve, a side branch of the posterior cord. **The teres minor (E)** is innervated by the axillary nerve along with the deltoid muscle.[3]

91. D – Defect in release of acetylcholine quanta

> In Eaton-Lambert syndrome, the presynaptic vesicles are normal **(A is false)**, antibodies to the acetylcholine receptor are not present **(B is false)**, and the extent of receptor surface is actually increased **(C is false)**. There is, however, a defect in the release of acetylcholine quanta from the nerve terminals **(D)**.[1]

92. C – Iris hamartomas (false)

> Von Hippel-Lindau disease is associated with a **defect on chromosome 3 (A), dominant inheritance (B), pancreatic cysts (D)**, and **renal cell carcinomas (E)**. **Iris hamartomas (Lisch nodules [C])** are seen in neurofibromatosis type 1.[1]

93. B – Dominant parietal lobe

> Gerstmann's syndrome consists of finger agnosia, left–right confusion, acalculia, and agraphia. It is associated with lesions of the **dominant parietal lobe (B)**, usually in the inferior parietal lobule, angular gyrus, or subjacent white matter.[1]

94. E – The rate-limiting step in its synthesis is dopa decarboxylase (false)

> The rate-limiting step in dopamine synthesis is tyrosine hydroxylase (converts L-tyrosine to L-hydroxyphenylalanine [L-dopa]). The other responses regarding dopamine pharmacology are true.[1,5]

95. E – Sinemet (carbidopa-levodopa)
96. D – Eldepryl (selegiline)
97. C – Bromocriptine
98. B – Artane (trihexyphenidyl)
99. D – Eldepryl (selegiline)

Amantadine (A) is an antiviral agent that may release dopamine from striatal neurons. **Artane (trihexyphenidyl [B])** is an anticholinergic agent with side effects that include dry mouth and blurred vision. **Bromocriptine (C)** is an ergot derivative that agonizes D2 receptors. **Eldepryl (selegiline [D])** is a monoamine oxidase B inhibitor and slows progression of disability. **Sinemet (carbidopa-levodopa [E])** combines L-dopa with a dopa decarboxylase inhibitor.[1]

100. C – Area 22

Wernicke's area corresponds most closely to Brodmann's **area 22 (C)**. **Area 17 (A)** corresponds to primary visual cortex located on the banks of the calcarine fissure. **Area 19 (B)** represents tertiary visual function. **Areas 41 and 42 (D)** represent primary and secondary auditory cortex in Heschl's gyri and the superior temporal gyrus. **Area 44 (E)** corresponds to Broca's area located in the frontal operculum.[1,6]

101. A – I, II, III

The progressive **sensorimotor polyneuropathy (IV)** associated with diabetes mellitus is generally (but not universally) thought to be metabolic in origin. The pathophysiology of **ophthalmoplegia (I)**, **acute mononeuropathy (II)**, and **mononeuritis multiplex (III)** are generally thought to be vascular in origin.[1,4]

102. C – Increased strength after the Tensilon test

In a myasthenic patient presenting with acutely worsening weakness and respiratory failure, the differential includes myasthenic crisis and cholinergic crisis (due to anticholinesterase therapy). Muscarinic symptoms include **bradycardia (A)**, **diarrhea (B)**, **miosis (D)**, and **sweating (E)**. **Increased strength following the administration of Tensilon (edrophonium [C])** does not support the diagnosis of cholinergic crisis. Edrophonium is an anticholinesterase drug, which would increase the availability of acetycholine on administration. The weakness of a cholinergic crisis is unaffected by Tensilon (edrophonium).[1]

103. C – Maternal inheritance

The MELAS syndrome (mitochondrial myopathy, encephalopathy, lactic acidosis, and strokelike episodes) is a mitochondrial disease associated with a maternal inheritance.[1]

104. C – Central cord syndrome
105. A – Anterior cord syndrome
106. A – Anterior cord syndrome

107. B – Brown-Séquard syndrome

> The **anterior cord syndrome (A)** is associated with hypesthesia and hyp-algesia due to injury of the anterior and lateral spinothalamic tracts and is associated with hyperflexion injuries. Posterior column function is generally preserved. The **Brown-Séquard syndrome (B)** is associated with contralat-eral pain and temperature loss, ipsilateral dorsal column dysfunction, and ipsilateral hemiplegia. It is usually due to penetrating trauma and has the best prognosis of the incomplete syndromes. **Central cord syndrome (C)** is thought to be due to hyperextension in the setting of cervical stenosis. Cen-tral cord injuries cause decreased sensation over the upper limbs and shoul-ders and decreased motor function that is worse in the upper extremities.[2]

108. C – Both
109. B – Non-REM sleep
110. A – REM sleep
111. B – Non-REM sleep
112. B – Non-REM sleep
113. A – REM sleep

> Although most dreams occur in **rapid eye movement (REM) sleep (A)**, they can also occur in **non–REM (NREM) sleep (B)**. Adult somnambulism, K complexes, and sleep spindles all occur in **NREM sleep (B)** (the latter two in stage 2). Glucose metabolism in the brain is increased in **REM (A)** and de-creased in **NREM sleep (B)** in comparison to the waking state.[1]

114. B – Glycogen storage disease type V (McArdle's disease)
115. A – Glycogen storage disease type II (acid maltase deficiency)
116. A – Glycogen storage disease type II (acid maltase deficiency)
117. D – Neither

> **Glycogen storage disease type II (A)** results from acid maltase (α-1,4-glucosidase) deficiency and has three forms: infantile (classic Pompe's disease), juve-nile, and adult forms. Glycogen accumulates in lysosomes throughout the body. **Glycogen storage disease type V (McArdle's disease [B])** results from myo-phosphorylase deficiency. Glycogen cannot be converted to glucose-6-phosphate, and the blood lactate does not rise after ischemic exercise. Both types are autoso-mal recessive. Rarely, type V may be autosomal dominant.[1]

118. B – I, III (high urinary copper excretion and low ceruloplasmin levels)

> Wilson's disease is characterized by an **increased urinary copper excretion (I)**, low serum copper levels **(II is false)**, and **low ceruloplasmin levels (III)**. The computed tomography (CT) scan sometimes shows hypodense areas in the lenticular nuclei **(IV is false)**.[1]

119. A – A marked inflammatory response with destruction of nerve cells in the pons is seen (false)

Central pontine myelinolysis (CPM) occurs in the setting of **rapid correction of chronic hyponatremia (B)**, as is sometimes seen in **chronic alcoholism (C)**. **Quadriplegia, pseudobulbar palsy, and locked-in syndrome (D)** can occur with CPM. Microscopically, destruction of the medullated sheaths with relative sparing of the axis cylinders and preservation of nerve cells in the pons is seen. An inflammatory response is absent **(A is false)**.[1]

120. C – Both
121. A – Homocystinuria
122. A – Homocystinuria

Patients with **homocystinuria (A)** and those with **Marfan's syndrome (B)** have a tall, thin frame and arachnodactyly. Patients with homocystinuria (cystathione synthase deficiency) also show evidence of mental retardation and are prone to strokes.[1]

123. D – Nondominant parietal lobe

Dressing apraxia is a special type of anosognosia that is typically attributed to dysfunction of the **nondominant parietal lobe (D)**.[1]

124. E – Teres minor

The axillary nerve innervates the **teres minor (E)** and deltoid muscles. **Coracobrachialis (A)** is innervated by the musculocutaneous nerve. The **rhomboids (B)** are innervated by the dorsal scapular nerve. The suprascapular nerve innervates the **supraspinatus (C)** and infraspinatus muscles. The subscapular nerves innervate the **teres major (D)** and subscapularis muscles.[3]

125. A – Calcified cortical vessels (false)

Sturge-Weber syndrome is characterized by a **facial vascular nevus (B)** that is present at birth, with **seizures, hemisensory deficit (C)**, and hemiparesis **contralateral** to the side of the nevus. **Meningeal venous angiomas (D)** are also present ipsilateral to the skin lesion. Skull films may reveal **tramline calcification is present in the parieto-occipital cortical substance (E)**, not the vessels **(A is false)**.[1]

126. C – 50 m/s

The normal sensory conduction velocity in the median and ulnar nerves is approximately **50 m/s (C)**. The other answer choices are incorrect.[1]

127. E – The autonomic nervous system is usually involved (false)

> Charcot-Marie-Tooth disease, or peroneal muscular atrophy, is a slowly progressive, symmetric, inherited demyelinating condition of the peripheral nervous system. The usual pattern of inheritance is **autosomal dominant (A),** and the disease may cause weakness, atrophy, and ataxia of both the **upper and lower extremities (C)**, particularly of the **distal muscle groups (B)**—foot drop is common. No specific medical therapy is available at this time, and **steroids do not appear to have an effect on disease progression (D)**. The autonomic nervous system is usually not involved in Charcot-Marie-Tooth disease **(E is false)**.[1]

128. E – All of the above

> Clival chordomas may cause palsies of multiple cranial nerves. All of the cranial nerves listed could potentially be affected by a destructive lesion of the skull base (II, V, X, and XII).[1]

129. D – Protein of 35 mg/dL

> Lumbar puncture and CSF findings in tuberculous meningitis typically include **glucose less than 40 mg/dL (A)**, although glucose levels are typically not as low as those found in pyogenic meningitis. **CSF tends to be under increased pressure (C)**, and a **leukocytosis is usually present (E)** with a **predominance of lymphocytes after several days of the illness (B)**. The **protein level is elevated in tuberculous meningitis and is usually 100 to 200 mg/dL (D is false)**.[1]

130. A – Contralateral Horner's syndrome (false)

> PICA occlusion may result in Wallenberg's lateral medullary syndrome, which is characterized by **contralateral pain and temperature loss over the body (due to disruption of spinothalamic fibers [B])**, ipsilateral numbness over half of the face (due to descending tract and nucleus of the trigeminal nerve), **ipsilateral ataxia (etiology uncertain [C])**, **ipsilateral numbness of the limbs (due to injury to the cuneate and gracile nuclei [D])**, **ipsilateral paralysis of the palate (E)**, and **ipsilateral Horner's syndrome (due to injury of descending sympathetic fibers; A is incorrect)**.[1]

131. A – K complexes

> **K complexes (A)** are a characteristic of stage 2 sleep. **Delta waves (B)** are prevalent in stage 3 and 4 sleep. **Desynchronization of the EEG (C)** occurs in **REM sleep (A)**, and **somnambulism (E)** occurs almost exclusively in stage 4 sleep.[1]

132. B – Duchenne's muscular dystrophy
133. A – Becker's muscular dystrophy
134. E – Myotonic dystrophy
135. B – Duchenne's muscular dystrophy
136. C – Emery-Dreifuss muscular dystrophy
137. D – Landouzy-Dejerine (facioscapulohumeral) dystrophy
138. E – Myotonic dystrophy

139. D – Landouzy-Dejerine (facioscapulohumeral) dystrophy
140. E – Myotonic dystrophy
141. E – Myotonic dystrophy

> **Duchenne's (B) and Becker's (A)** muscular dystrophies are X-linked recessive disorders characterized by the absence of the gene product dystrophin in the former and the presence of a structurally abnormal form of the product in the latter. Weakness and pseudo-hypertrophy of certain muscles (notably the calf) occur. The onset is later and the course more benign in the **Becker's type (A)**. **Myotonic dystrophy (E)** is the most common adult form of muscular dystrophy and is characterized by an autosomal dominant inheritance, with the defective gene localized to chromosome 19q. Features include dystrophic changes in nonmuscular tissues (e.g., lens opacities) and a characteristic facies. **Landouzy-Dejerine dystrophy (D)** is usually transmitted by autosomal dominant inheritance, and the abnormal gene has been localized to chromosome 4. Congenital absence of a pectoral, brachioradialis, or biceps femoris muscle occasionally occurs. Characteristics of **Emery-Dreifuss dystrophy (C)**, a benign X-linked dystrophy, include contractures of the elbow flexors, neck extensors, and posterior calf muscles.[1]

142. B – Cortex

> Monoplegia without muscular atrophy is most often due to a lesion of the **cerebral cortex (B)**.[1]

143. C – II, IV (autoclaving at 132°C under pressure for 1 hour and immersion for 1 hour in bleach)

> Subacute spongiform encephalopathy, or Creutzfeldt-Jakob disease, is a progressive neurologic illness characterized by dementia and myoclonic jerks. The disease is thought to be due to a prion protein that is **resistant to formalin (I)**, **alcohol (III)**, boiling, and ultraviolet radiation. The protein can be **inactivated by autoclaving at 132°C under pressure for 1 hour (II)**, or by **immersion in bleach for 1 hour (IV)**.[1]

144. B – High-frequency loss

> Hearing loss caused by acoustic neuromas is most often **high-frequency (B)**, or high-tone, hearing loss.[6]

145. D – Middle trunk
146. B – Lower trunk
147. C – Medial cord
148. E – Upper trunk

149. A – Lateral cord

> Although **lower trunk lesions (B)** resemble **medial cord lesions (C)**, abnormalities of radially innervated C8 muscles are seen with the former, but not with the latter. Low-amplitude action potentials in the deltoid and biceps are seen in **upper trunk lesions (E)**. Median sensory responses from the index and middle finger are abnormal, and motor conduction velocities of the hand muscles are normal in **middle trunk lesions (D)**. **Lateral cord lesions (A)** cause weakness of the muscles supplied by the musculocutaneous nerve and the lateral root of the median nerve (innervates the forearm muscles). The intrinsic hand muscles innervated by the medial root of the median nerve are spared.[7]

150. A – Equal to that of the high-risk zone

> Several studies indicate that a person migrating from a high-risk to a low-risk zone of MS before age 15 will develop a risk that **is similar to the low-risk zone (B)**. If the migration takes place after age 15, the risk is **similar to that of natives of the high-risk zone (A)**.[1]

151. E – All of the above

> Botulism is a disease of the neuromuscular junction caused by a bacterial exotoxin. The botulinum toxin prevents the presynaptic release of acetylcholine from peripheral motor neurons. Early symptoms often include blurred vision and **diplopia (III)**. The presence of **ptosis (I)**, **strabismus (II)**, and palsies of extraocular muscles can sometimes confuse the diagnosis with myasthenias gravis. The pupils are often **unreactive (IV)** in botulism, which helps to clarify the diagnosis.[1]

152. D – Transcortical sensory aphasia

> **Transcortical motor and sensory aphasias (D)** are manifested by preserved repetition. **Broca's aphasia (A)** is characterized by a disruption of expressive speech with relative preservation of comprehension—repetition is impaired. **Wernicke's aphasia (E)** is characterized by fluent, articulate speech that lacks meaning with significant impairment of comprehension—repetition is impaired. **Conduction aphasia (B)** is characterized by fluent speech and a relative preservation of comprehension, but with significant impairment of repetition. **Global aphasia (C)** is characterized by impairment of speech, comprehension, and repetition.[1]

153. E – REM

> Narcoleptic sleep attacks tend to begin with **REM sleep (E)**, rather than with **non-REM (A–D)** sleep as in the general population. This finding suggests that narcolepsy is not a condition of excessive daytime drowsiness, but rather a "generalized disorder of sleep–wake function."[1]

154. A – Enterovirus

> The **enteroviruses (A)**, which include echovirus, Coxsackie, and polio, represent the most common cause of viral meningitis. **HIV (B)** may cause a mononucleosis-like syndrome, and **mumps (E)** can be associated with meningitis, although this is not as common as enterovirus meningitis. **Leptospirosis (C)** is a spirochete and therefore not a cause of viral meningitis.[1]

155. E – Tumors of the clivus

> Garcin's (hemibasal) syndrome has been reported with chondromas or chondrosarcomas of the clivus.[1]

156. C – High-tone loss occurs early in the disease (false)

> Ménière's disease is characterized by recurrent attacks of vertigo and **unilateral tinnitus and deafness (B)**. **Distention of the endolymphatic duct** is a characteristic pathologic change **(A)**. **Horizontal nystagmus may occur during an acute attack (D)**, and **low-pitched tinnitus is typical (E)**. Early in Ménière's disease, deafness affects mainly the low tones and fluctuates in severity. Later in the disease, high tones are affected **(C is false)**.[1]

157. E – Women are more frequently affected than men (false)

> The Eaton-Lambert syndrome is due to decreased calcium-dependent release of acetylcholine quanta at the neuromuscular junction. **A temporary increase in muscle power may be observed during the first few contractions (D)**, in contrast to myasthenia gravis. The disease process has been associated with **carcinoma of the stomach and colon (C); autonomic disturbances are often observed (A)**, but **fasciculations are not a presenting feature (B)**. Men are more often affected than women (5:1; **E is false**).[1]

158. A – Are more fatigable

> Type I (red) muscle fibers are richer in oxidative enzymes **(E)**, poorer in glycolytic enzymes, contain more mitochondria **(D)** and myoglobin, fire more tonically **(B)**, have slower rates of contraction and relaxation **(C)**, and are less fatigable **(A is false)** than type II (white) fibers.[1]

159. B – Anterior choroidal artery

> Infarction of the anterior choroidal artery may result in contralateral hemiplegia, hemihypesthesia, and homonymous hemianopia with sparing of cognitive and language functions. Historically, ligation of the **anterior choroidal artery (B)** was an early surgical treatment for patients with unilateral tremor and rigidity from Parkinson's disease.[1]

160. E – Symmetric neuropathy

> Mononeuropathy multiplex of diabetes is classically asymmetric **(E is false)**. In practice, however, a confluence of multiple mononeuropathies may lead to a symmetric picture. The other answer choices are characteristics of diabetic mononeuritis multiplex: **lower extremities are more commonly affected than upper extremities (A), neuropathy tends to be painful (B), proximal extremities are more commonly affected than distal extremities (C),** and **recovery is usual (D).**[1]

161. C – Lorazepam
162. B – Ethosuximide
163. F – Tegretol or valproic acid
164. A – ACTH
165. E – Valproic acid

> Benzodiazepines such as **lorazepam (C)** are the first-line agents for the treatment of status epilepticus. **Ethosuximide (B)** is typically used for the treatment of absence seizures. **ACTH (A)** is employed in the treatment of infantile spasms. **Tegretol (D)** and **valproic acid (E)** are acceptable alternatives for the treatment of complex partial seizures. **Valproic acid (E)** is sometimes used in the atypical petit mal syndrome of Lennox-Gastaut.[1]

166. C – It is usually painful (false)

> Pain with polymyositis occurs in only 15% of patients and often suggests an additional disorder, such as rheumatoid arthritis **(C is false)**. The other responses regarding polymyositis associated with carcinoma are true: **carcinoma affects 9% of patients with polymyositis (A),** it is **most commonly associated with lung and prostate cancer in men (B), muscle biopsies show no evidence of tumor cells (D),** and **proximal muscles are initially affected more than distal ones (E).**[1]

167. B – Bilateral location

> Cluster headaches typically are **recurrent for 6 to 12 weeks (C)** in a **unilateral (B is false) orbital (E)** location. The **male-to-female ratio is 4.5:1 to 6.7:1 (D)**. **Lacrimation, rhinorrhea (A),** flushing of the face, and other such parasympathetic-type responses often accompany the headache.[1]

168. B – Dry mouth

> The acute anticholinesterase effect of organophosphate poisoning results in **increased salivation (B is false)**, **bronchial spasms (A)**, **miosis (C)**, **sweating (D)**, abdominal cramps, and **vomiting (E)**. The mainstay of pharmacologic treatment consists of atropine and pralidoxime.[1]

169. B – Decreased GABA

> **Decreased glutamic acid decarboxylase (hence, decreased γ-aminobutyric acid [GABA] [B])** and **choline acetyltransferase (hence, decreased acetylcholine; E is false)** have been found in the striatum and lateral pallidum in Huntington's disease. Also reported has **been increased norepinephrine and somatostatin in the striatum (C and D are false). An excess of dopamine or an increased sensitivity of striatal dopamine receptors** has been postulated in the pathogenesis of Huntington's disease **(A is false)**.[1]

170. C – Bilateral medial temporo-occipital lobes

> Prosopagnosia refers to the inability to identify a familiar face while retaining the ability to identify its features and is associated with injury to the **bilateral medial temporo-occipital lobes (C)**.[1]

171. C – Poverty of spontaneous speech

> Injuries to the supplementary motor cortex are associated with **mutism**, contralateral motor neglect, and impairment of coordination **(C is correct)**.[1]

172. D – Tibialis anterior and extensor digitorum longus and brevis

> Lesions of the peroneal nerve produce weakness of the **tibialis anterior and extensor digitorum longus and brevis (D)**. The tibialis anterior is innervated by the deep peroneal nerve, while the flexor digitorum brevis is innervated by the medial plantar nerve, a branch of the tibial nerve **(E is incorrect)**. The abductor hallucis is innervated by the medial plantar nerve (a branch of the tibial nerve), and the gastrocnemius is innervated by the tibial nerve **(A is incorrect)**. The extensor digitorum longus and brevis are innervated by the deep peroneal nerve, whereas the abductor hallucis is innervated by a branch of the tibial nerve **(B is incorrect)**. **C is incorrect** because the gastrocnemius and flexor hallucis longus are innervated by the tibial nerve.[3]

173. D – Deficiency of sphingomyelinase

> Tay-Sachs disease is characterized by **macrocephaly (E)**, **abnormal startle response (A)**, and **cherry red spots in the retina (C)**. It is transmitted via **autosomal recessive inheritance (B)**. Deficiency of **hexoaminidase A characterizes Tay-Sachs disease (D is false)**, while sphingomyelinase deficiency is present in Niemann-Pick disease types A and B.[1]

174. A – Corticospinal tract dysfunction

> **Corticospinal and corticosensory functions**, visual acuity, and visual fields are relatively preserved throughout the course of Alzheimer's disease **(A is false)**.[1]

175. B – High-dose steroids form the mainstay of therapy

Neither conventional dose nor high-dose steroids have been shown to be helpful in the treatment of Guillain-Barré syndrome **(B is false)**. The other statements regarding the Guillain-Barré syndrome are true: **disturbances of autonomic function are common (A), hypo- or areflexia is characteristic (C), the mortality rate is 3% (D)**, and **the peak severity is 10 to 14 days after onset in 80% of cases.**[1]

176. D – Lateral horn cells at C8 to T3 to the superior cervical ganglion

The pathway from the **lateral horn cells at C8 to T3 to the superior cervical ganglion (D)** constitutes the second-order neuron (preganglionic) in the sympathetic pathway to the pupil. Neurons from the **hypothalamus to the lateral horn cells at C8 to T3 (C)** constitute the first-order neurons (central), and neurons projecting from the **superior cervical ganglion to the iris (E)** constitute the third-order neurons (postganglionic) in the sympathetic innervation of the pupil. Projections from the **Edinger-Westphal nucleus to the ciliary ganglion (B)** represent the parasympathetic system.[1]

177. C – Pyrimethamine and sulfadiazine

The treatment of choice for toxoplasmosis is oral **sulfadiazine and pyrimethamine (C)** for at least 4 weeks. Leucovorin is sometimes given as an adjuvant to counteract the antifolate effects of pyrimethamine. **Penicillin and nafcillin (A and D)** are β-lactam antibiotics and are not an appropriate treatment for toxoplasmosis. **Praziquantel (B)** is used for the treatment of cysticercosis; albendazole is another option for cysticercosis treatment. Thiabendazole **(E)** is most commonly employed in the treatment of trichinosis.[1]

178. D – The EEG shows characteristic periodic waves that occur every 2 to 3 seconds.

Subacute sclerosing panencephalitis (SSPE), characterized by a progressive mental decline with seizures, myoclonus, and ataxia, **mainly affects children and adolescents (B is false)**. SSPE is thought to be the result of chronic measles infection. The lesions are found in **both the cerebral cortex and white matter (C is false)**. Eosinophilic inclusions are found in both the **cytoplasm and nuclei of neurons and glial cells (A is false)**. Elevated gamma globulin in the CSF is typical—that is, **CSF protein tends to be increased (E is false)**. The EEG shows **characteristic 2 to 3 per second waves (D is true)**.[1]

179. B – Intravenous methylprednisolone followed by oral prednisone

Treatment with **oral prednisone (C) alone** actually increased the risk of new episodes of optic neuritis in a large randomized controlled study of optic neuritis treatment. **Intravenous methylprednisolone therapy followed by oral prednisone speeds recovery of visual loss (B is correct)**.[1]

180. C – Multiple sclerosis

> **Schilder's disease (C)** is a demyelinating illness of children and young adults that has several features in common with chronic relapsing MS.[1]

181. A – External branch of the superior laryngeal nerve

> The cricothyroid, supplied by the **external laryngeal nerve (A)**, is the only intrinsic laryngeal muscle not supplied by the **recurrent laryngeal nerve (D). Cranial nerves VII (E) and IX (C)** do not provide motor innervation to the larynx.[3]

182. A – Defect in learning and loss of past memories

> In Korsakoff's psychosis, retentive memory is impaired out of proportion to other cognitive functions in an otherwise alert patient.[1]

183. E – Mental retardation (false)

> Werdnig-Hoffmann disease is infantile spinal muscular atrophy, or SMA type I. SMA type I is characterized by neonatal **hypotonia (C)** and **areflexia (A)**. Inheritance is **autosomal recessive (B)** and has been linked to **chromosome 5q (D)**. **Mental retardation is not a feature of the spinal muscular atrophy of infancy and childhood (E)**, but may be associated with late-onset varieties of spinal muscular atrophy.[1]

184. B – I, III (block norepinephrine and serotonin reuptake)

> Tricyclic antidepressants such as imipramine and amitriptyline block the **reuptake of both norepinephrine and serotonin (I and III)**. Selective serotonin reuptake inhibitors such as citalopram or fluoxetine prevent the **reuptake of serotonin only (III)**. Monoamine oxidase inhibitors such as iproniazid and phenelzine prevent the **oxidative deamination of monoamines (II)**.[5]

185. C – Both
186. D – Neither
187. C – Both
188. A – Amyotrophic lateral sclerosis
189. C – Both

> Despite the muscle weakness and atrophy seen in ALS, hyperreflexia and mild lower extremity spasticity are characteristic. Lower extremity spasticity and hand atrophy can be seen in both conditions. Cervical spondylotic myelopathy tends not to present as a purely motor syndrome.[1]

190. F – Wegner's granulomatosis
191. C – Systemic lupus erythematosus
192. E – Temporal arteritis
193. D – Takayasu's syndrome
194. B – Polyarteritis nodosa

195. A – Cogan's syndrome

> **Cogan's syndrome (A)** represents a nonsyphilitic interstitial keratitis that eventually leads to deafness that may be accompanied by a systemic vasculitis resembling polyarteritis nodosa. **Polyarteritis nodosa (B)** is a systemic vasculitis that causes inflammatory necrosis of arteries and arterioles throughout the body, but spares the lungs (contrast with Churg-Strauss). Involvement of the vasa nervorum may lead to mononeuritis multiplex in **polyarteritis nodosa (B)**—kidney involvement and skin purpura are common. **Systemic lupus erythematosus (C)** may also cause a noninfectious vasculitis and is associated with positive antinuclear antibody titers and a malar rash. **Takayasu's syndrome (D)** is a vasculitis involving the aortic arch and its proximal branches—affected arteries become pulseless; blurring of vision is common. **Temporal arteritis (E)** typically presents with headache and may lead to blindness due to occlusion of ophthalmic artery branches. **Wegener's granulomatosis (E)** is a rare granulomatous vasculitis that is characterized by involvement of the respiratory tracts accompanied by a necrotizing glomerulonephritis. The presence of antineutrophil cytoplasmic antibodies (c-ANCA) is relatively sensitive and specific for **Wegner's granulomatosis (E)**.[1]

196. A – Defect in retentive memory out of proportion to other cognitive functions (false)

> Defects in learning and memory out of proportion to other cognitive functions **(A)** are features of Korsakoff's psychosis, not Wernicke's encephalopathy. The other responses are features of Wernicke's encephalopathy: **gait ataxia (B)**, **gaze palsy (C)**, **metal confusion (D)**, and **nystagmus (E)**.[1]

197. C – Loss of temperature sensation

> Parietal lobe lesions are characterized by **loss of position sense (B)**, impaired ability to **localize touch and pain stimuli (atopognosia [E])**, **astereognosis (A)**, and **impairment of two-point discrimination (D)**. **Perception of pain, touch, pressure, vibratory, and thermal stimuli is relatively intact (C)**.[1]

198. C – Right inferior occipitotemporal region

> A lesion in the right inferior occipitotemporal region sparing the optic radiation and striate cortex causes the purest form of achromatopsia.[1]

199. C – Third-order Horner's syndrome

> Horner's syndrome can be confirmed by the failure of the miotic pupil to dilate in response to 2 to 10% cocaine drops. If the later application of the adrenergic mydriatic hydroxyamphetamine has no effect, then the lesion localizes to the **third-order neuron (postganglionic part [C])**. A first- or second-order lesion **(A or B)** is indicated by a failure of the miotic pupil to dilate to cocaine drops, followed by dilation (after 24 hours) with 1% hydroxyamphetamine.[1]

200. C – Stage 4

Somnambulism, or sleep-walking, occurs almost exclusively in **stage 4 (non-REM) sleep (C)**.[1]

201. D - Imipramine

Nocturnal enuresis with daytime continence occurs frequently during childhood. The most effective medical therapy is **imipramine (D)**, a tricyclic antidepressant.[1]

202. B – Apraxia of the left hand to command

Sectioning of the corpus callosum causes a disconnection syndrome by isolating the language function of the left hemisphere from the right hemisphere. Therefore, when given a verbal command (processed by the left hemisphere), the patient will be able to execute the command with the right hand (controlled by left hemisphere), but will have difficulty executing the command with the left hand (controlled by right hemisphere). Therefore, the best answer is **B, apraxia of the left hand to command**.[1]

203. C – Good comprehension, nonfluent speech, poor repetition
204. A – Good comprehension, fluent speech, poor repetition
205. F – Poor comprehension, nonfluent speech, poor repetition
206. B – Good comprehension, nonfluent speech, good repetition
207. D – Poor comprehension, fluent speech, good repetition
208. E – Poor comprehension, fluent speech, poor repetition

Conduction aphasia is similar to **Wernicke's aphasia (E)** in that there is a fluent paraphasic speech with impaired repetition. In contrast to patients with Wernicke's aphasia, however, those with **conduction aphasia (A)** have little or no difficulty in comprehension. **Broca's aphasia (C)** is characterized by nonfluent agrammatical speech with relatively preserved comprehension; repetition is impaired. The **transcortical aphasias (B and D)** are characterized by good repetition. **Global aphasia (F)** is characterized by impaired speech, impaired comprehension, and impaired repetition.[1]

209. C – Both
210. D – Neither
211. B – Polymyositis
212. A – Dermatomyositis
213. B – Polymyositis
214. A – Dermatomyositis

215. D – Neither

Both idiopathic **polymyositis (PM [B])** and **dermatomyositis (DM [A])** are more common in women. About 9% of patients with PM and 15% of those with DM have an underlying carcinoma. Single-fiber necrosis is seen in **PM (B)**, whereas a perifascicular muscle fiber degeneration and atrophy are seen in **DM (A)**. IgG, IgM, complement, and membrane attack complexes are deposited in the small vessels in **DM (A)**, whereas in **PM (B)** the endomysial inflammatory exudate contains a large number of T cells and few B cells. Both disorders are readily responsive to corticosteroids and other immunosuppressants.[1]

216. A – Carbamazepine

Carbamazepine (A) is a sodium channel modulator that may lead to SIADH and hyponatremia. **Gabapentin (B)** causes somnolence as a major side effect. **Levetiracetam (C)** has a low risk of side effects, but may cause somnolence, particularly in the elderly. **Phenytoin (D)** has a myriad of side effects including allergy, ataxia, diplopia, stupor, hirsutism, gingival hyperplasia, cerebellar degeneration, peripheral neuropathy, and decreased vitamin K. **Topiramate (E)** has cognitive impairment, dizziness, and ataxia as its major side effects.

217. C – Ictal SPECT scans show decreased tracer signal in the seizure focus (false)

Single-photon emission computed tomography (SPECT) is used in seizure localization for patients with partial epilepsy. Both ictal and interictal SPECT studies can be acquired and compared for seizure localization **(A)**. Perfusion follows changes in metabolism during seizures **(D)**, and therefore there tends to be increased SPECT tracer signal in affected brain tissue on an ictal SPECT study **(C is false)**. PET scans tend to be interictal studies; ictal SPECT scans are generally easier to acquire than ictal PET scans **(B)**. The major limitation of ictal SPECT scanning is that tracer needs to be injected within 1–2 minutes of seizure onset **(E)**.[8]

218. C – Neurocysticercosis (false)

Mononeuritis multiplex is a condition that involves the acute or subacute involvement of multiple peripheral nerves. Common causes of mononeuritis multiplex include **polyarteritis nodosa (D)**, Wegner's granulomatosis, **diabetes (A)**, cryoglobulinemia, **sarcoidosis (E)**, Lyme disease, and **HIV (B)**. Rare causes include **sarcoidosis (E)**, paraneoplastic syndromes, amyloidosis, leprosy, lupus, rheumatoid arthritis, and Sjögren's syndrome.

219. B – 3, 4.5

The FDA initially approved intravenous rtPA for use in acute ischemic stroke within 3 hours of symptom onset following the NINDS trial in 1995. In 2009, the FDA approved the use of intravenous rtPA in patients up to 4.5 hours from symptom onset. Choice **B** is correct.[8]

220. C – 6 hours

> In the PROACT II study, patients with MCA occlusions within **6 hours (C)** of symptom onset treated with intra-arterial recombinant prourokinase had improvements in recanalization and functional independence in comparison to patients receiving placebo.[8]

221. D – 8 hours

> Benefit with mechanical thrombectomy has been demonstrated up to **8 hours (D)** from symptom onset. This offers an advantage over the **4.5-hour (B)** window of intravenous tPA and the **6-hour (C)** window of intra-arterial thrombolytic therapy.[8]

222. D – NIH stroke score of > 20

> Patients eligible for intravenous tPA should be treated before pursuing endovascular therapy. If the patient **fails to improve with intravenous tPA (C)**, presents **outside the therapeutic window for intravenous tPA (E)**, or has a **contraindication to intravenous tPA (A)**, endovascular therapy may be considered. A **diffusion-perfusion mismatch (B)** suggests that there is salvageable tissue present in the ischemic penumbra, which is desirable for endovascular therapy. An **NIH stroke score of > 20 (D)** suggests a severe stroke and may be a relative contraindication to endovascular therapy.[8]

References

1. Ropper AH, Brown RH. Principles of Neurology, 8th ed. New York: McGraw-Hill; 2005
2. Winn HR, ed-in-chief. Neurological Surgery, 5th ed. Philadelphia, PA: W.B. Saunders; 2003
3. Moore KL, Dalley AF. Clinically Oriented Anatomy, 5th ed. Baltimore, MD: Lippincott Williams and Williams; 2006
4. Rowland LP, ed. Merritt's Textbook of Neurology, 9th ed. Baltimore, MD: Williams & Wilkins; 1995
5. Brunton LL, Lazo JS, Parker KL, eds. Goodman & Gilman's the Pharmacological Basis of Therapeutics, 11th ed. New York: McGraw-Hill; 2006
6. Citow JS, Macdonald RL, Refai D, eds. Comprehensive Neurosurgery Board Review. New York: Thieme Medical Publishers; 2009
7. Youmans JR, ed-in-chief. Neurological Surgery, 4th ed. Philadelphia, PA: W.B. Saunders; 1992
8. Quinones-Hinojosa A, ed. Schmidek & Sweet Operative Neurosurgical Techniques, 6th ed. Philadelphia, PA: Elsevier; 2012

3A   Neuroanatomy—Questions

⇨ For questions **1** to **4**, match the following structures with the description. Each response may be used once, more than once, or not at all.

    A. Dorsal longitudinal fasciculus
    B. Lateral lemniscus
    C. Medial lemniscus
    D. Medial longitudinal fasciculus

1. Connection of posterior columns to thalamus

2. Carries fibers involved with eye movements and has vestibular input

3. A part of the auditory pathway

4. Connects the periventricular hypothalamus and mammillary bodies to the midbrain's central gray matter

5. Stimulation of caudal regions of the paramedian pontine reticular formation (PPRF) produces
    A. Conjugate horizontal deviation of the eyes to the opposite side
    B. Conjugate horizontal deviation of the eyes to the same side
    C. Deviation of only the contralateral eye to the same side
    D. Deviation of only the ipsilateral eye to the opposite side
    E. Deviation of only the ipsilateral eye to the same side

⇨ For questions **6** to **9**, match the description with the eye movements.
    A. Conjugate horizontal deviation to the opposite side
    B. Conjugate horizontal deviation to the same side
    C. Vertical eye movements
    D. None of the above

6. Stimulation of the caudal PPRF

7. Stimulation of the rostral PPRF

8. Stimulation of the superior colliculus

9. Stimulation of the middle frontal gyrus

10. Which of the following is *true* of the occipital eye field?
   A. It is localized to a relatively small area.
   B. It subserves pursuit eye movements that are largely voluntary.
   C. Lesions in this area are associated with transient deviation of the eyes away from the side of the lesion.
   D. The threshold for excitation in this area is lower than in the frontal eye fields.
   E. With lesions in this area, the patient can direct the eyes to a particular location on command.

11. The intracranial dura is innervated by
   I.   Cranial nerve V
   II. Upper cervical spinal nerves
   III. Cranial nerve X
   IV. Cranial nerve VII
   A. I, II, III
   B. I, III
   C. II, IV
   D. IV
   E. All of the above

12. Descending fibers of the medial longitudinal fasciculus (MLF) arise from all of the following structures *except* the
   A. Inferior colliculus
   B. Cajal's interstitial nucleus
   C. Medial vestibular nucleus
   D. Pontine reticular formation
   E. Superior colliculus

13. Which structure does *not* pass through the orbital tendinous ring (Zinn's anulus)?
   A. Frontal nerve
   B. Superior division of III
   C. Abducens nerve
   D. Nasociliary nerve
   E. Inferior division of III

14. All of the following can be seen in ulnar nerve entrapment at the wrist *except*
   A. Motor deficits in the adductor pollicis
   B. Motor deficits in the deep head of the flexor pollicis brevis
   C. Motor deficits in the third and fourth lumbricals
   D. Sensory deficits in the dorsum of the hand
   E. Sensory deficits in the palmar surface of the hypothenar eminence

15. The thalamus is fed by (the)
   I.   Medial posterior choroidal artery
   II. Anterior choroidal artery
   III. Basilar artery branches
   IV. Middle cerebral artery branches
   A. I, II, III
   B. I, III
   C. II, IV
   D. IV
   E. All of the above

16. The anterior choroidal artery supplies portions of each of the following structures *except* the
    A. Amygdala
    B. Globus pallidus
    C. Hippocampus
    D. Hypothalamus
    E. Internal capsule

⇨ For questions **17** to **21**, match the following structures with the description. Each response may be used once, more than once, or not at all.
    A. Central tegmental tract
    B. Lamina terminalis
    C. Medial forebrain bundle
    D. Stria medullaris
    E. Stria terminalis

17. Connects the amygdala to the hypothalamus

18. The closed rostral end of the neural tube

19. Connects the gustatory brainstem nucleus to the thalamus

20. Connects the septal area, hypothalamus, olfactory area, and anterior thalamus to the habenula

21. Connects the septal area, hypothalamus, olfactory area, and hippocampus to the midbrain, pons, and medulla

22. Efferent fibers from the dentate nuclei
    A. Are somatopically arranged in the thalamus with the head represented laterally and caudal body parts medially
    B. Influence activity of motor neurons in the contralateral cerebral cortex
    C. Leave the cerebellum via the middle cerebellar peduncle
    D. Mainly terminate in the red nucleus
    E. Project to the ipsilateral ventral lateral thalamic nuclei

23. The pulvinar has well-defined projections to the
    I. Occipital cortex
    II. Parietal cortex
    III. Temporal cortex
    IV. Frontal cortex
    A. I, II, III
    B. I, III
    C. II, IV
    D. IV
    E. All of the above

24. Each of the following is true of the fornix *except*
    A. It is the main efferent fiber system of the hippocampus.
    B. Postcommissural fibers of the fornix project to the mammillary bodies.
    C. The columns of the fornix lie anterior to the anterior commissure.
    D. The body of the fornix runs to the rostral margin of the thalamus.
    E. The fornical commissure (psalterium) is rostral to the anterior commissure.

25. The efferent projections of the arcuate nucleus are most closely associated with the
    A. Mammillary bodies
    B. Median eminence
    C. Nucleus of the diagonal band
    D. Posterior hypophysis
    E. Supraoptic nucleus

26. Regions of the striate cortex that do not contain ocular dominance columns are those representing the
    I. Fovea
    II. Blind spot of the retina
    III. Macula
    IV. Monocular temporal crescent of the visual field
    A. I, II, III
    B. I, III
    C. II, IV
    D. IV
    E. All of the above

27. Each of the following is true of the supplemental motor cortex (MII) *except*
    A. Some of the neurons project directly to the spinal cord.
    B. The body is somatopically represented.
    C. The neurons in this area exhibit movement-related activity only if the motor task is performed with the contralateral limbs.
    D. The threshold for stimulation is higher than for the primary motor cortex (MI).
    E. Unilateral ablations produce no permanent deficit in the maintenance of posture or capacity for movement.

28. Each of the following is true of dorsolateral fibers entering the dorsolateral spinal cord *except*
    A. Root fibers of spinal ganglia separate into a medial and lateral bundle.
    B. The central processes of each dorsal root ganglion divide into both ascending and descending branches.
    C. The lateral bundle conveys impulses from free nerve endings.
    D. The medial bundle consists of thinly myelinated or unmyelinated fibers, whereas the lateral bundle is thickly myelinated.
    E. The medial bundle conveys impulses from Golgi tendon organs.

29. Which of the following does the ulnar nerve innervate?
    I. Pronator quadratus
    II. Flexor pollicis longus
    III. Opponens pollicis
    IV. Adductor pollicis
    A. I, II, III
    B. I, III
    C. II, IV
    D. IV
    E. All of the above

⇨ For questions **30** to **40**, match the thalamic nucleus with the cortical area(s) to which it projects. Each response may be used once, more than once, or not at all.

    A. Areas 1, 2, 3
    B. Area 4
    C. Striatum
    D. Areas 5, 7
    E. Area 17
    F. Areas 18, 19
    G. Areas 41, 42
    H. Cingulate gyrus
    I. Prefrontal cortex

30. Anterior nuclear group

31. Lateral dorsal nucleus

32. Lateral geniculate nucleus

33. Lateral posterior nucleus

34. Medial geniculate nucleus

35. Mediodorsal nucleus

36. Pulvinar

37. Centromedian nucleus

38. Ventral lateral nucleus

39. Ventral posterolateral nucleus

40. Ventral posteromedial nucleus

⇨ For questions **41** to **43**, match the description with the structure.

    A. Supraopticohypophysial tract
    B. Tuberoinfundibular tract
    C. Both
    D. Neither

41. Efferent fibers project to the neurohypophysis.

42. Efferent fibers project to the anterior pituitary.

43. Efferent fibers project to the hypophyseal portal vessels.

⇨ For questions **44** to **49**, match the following structures with the description. Each response may be used once, more than once, or not at all.

    A. Ansa lenticularis
    B. Fasciculus retroflexus
    C. Lenticular fasciculus (FF H2)
    D. Postcommissural fornix
    E. Precommissural fornix
    F. Thalamic fasciculus (FF H1)

44. Connects the globus pallidus interna to the thalamus (travels around the internal capsule)

45. Connects the globus pallidus interna to the thalamus (travels through the internal capsule)

46. Combination of the ansa lenticularis, lenticular fasciculus, and cerebellothalamic tract

47. Connects the habenula to the midbrain and interpeduncular nuclei

48. Connects the hippocampus to the septal nuclei

49. Connects the hippocampus to the hypothalamus, mammillary bodies, anterior thalamus, septal nuclei, and cingulate gyrus

50. Which of the following structures is *not* present on a transverse section of the medulla taken at midolive?
A. Accessory cuneate nucleus
B. Dorsal nucleus of X
C. Nucleus ambiguus
D. Nucleus of the solitary tract
E. Superior vestibular nucleus

51. Which of the following fiber tracts is *not* a part of the limbic system?
A. Diagonal band of Broca
B. Fornix
C. Mammillothalamic tract
D. Medial forebrain bundle
E. Thalamic fasciculus

52. The secondary somatic sensory area (SII) is located on the
A. Medial surface of the superior frontal gyrus
B. Medial surface of the superior parietal lobule
C. Superior bank of the lateral sulcus
D. Ventral posterolateral nucleus of the thalamus
E. Same area as the primary somatic sensory area

53. Which of the following is *not* seen with a lesion of the facial nerve immediately distal to the geniculate ganglion?
A. Hyperacusis
B. Impairment of lacrimation
C. Impairment of salivary secretions
D. Loss of taste in the anterior two-thirds of the tongue
E. Paralysis of ipsilateral facial muscles

54. The external urethral sphincter is innervated by
A. Parasympathetic pelvic nerves
B. Somatic pudendal nerves
C. Sympathetic hypogastric nerves
D. **A** and **B**
E. **B** and **C**

55. Regions of the brain devoid of a blood–brain barrier (circumventricular organs) include each of the following *except*

A. Indusium griseum
B. Median eminence
C. Organum vasculosum of the lamina terminalis
D. Pineal gland
E. Subfornical organ

56. Uncrossed fibers of the optic tract terminate on which layers of the lateral geniculate?

A. 1, 3, and 5
B. 1, 4, and 6
C. 2, 3, and 5
D. 2, 4, and 6
E. 2, 5, and 6

57. Substances can cross the blood–brain barrier via

I. Active transport
II. Carrier-mediated transport
III. Diffusion
IV. Vesicular transport

A. I, II, III
B. I, III
C. II, IV
D. IV
E. All of the above

⇨ For questions **58** to **61**, match the following structures with the description. Each response may be used once, more than once, or not at all.

A. Arcuate fasciculus
B. Diagonal band of Broca
C. Tapetum
D. Uncinate fasciculus

58. Connects septal nuclei to the amygdala

59. Connects Wernicke's area to Broca's area

60. Connects temporal and occipital lobes

61. Connects the temporal lobe to the frontal lobe

⇨ For questions **62** to **67**, match the description with the structure.

A. Paraventricular nucleus
B. Supraoptic nucleus
C. Both
D. Neither

62. Located in the supraoptic region

63. Located in the tuberal region

64. Consists of several distinct cell groups

65. Composed mainly of uniformly large cells

66. Immunohistocytochemically large cells in this nucleus contain either vasopressin or oxytocin.

67. Regions of this nucleus give rise to descending axons projecting to the brainstem and all levels of the spinal cord.

68. Each of the following is true of corticobulbar fibers *except*
   A. Fibers projecting to the posterior column nuclei leave the pyramids and enter these nuclei via the medial lemniscus or reticular formation.
   B. Fibers projecting to trigeminal sensory nuclei and the nucleus solitarius are derived predominantly from frontoparietal cortical areas.
   C. Pseudobulbar palsy can result from unilateral lesions involving corticobulbar fibers.
   D. The supranuclear innervation of motor cranial nerve nuclei is largely bilateral.
   E. Unilateral lesions involving corticobulbar fibers produce paralysis of contralateral lower facial muscles only.

69. The palmar interosseus muscles
   A. Abduct the fingers
   B. Adduct the fingers
   C. Extend the metacarpophalangeal joints and flex the interphalangeal joints
   D. Flex the metacarpophalangeal joints and extend the interphalangeal joints
   E. Perform none of the above

70. The sciatic nerve supplies each of the following muscles in part or in whole *except* the
   A. Adductor magnus
   B. Biceps femoris (short head)
   C. Gluteus maximus
   D. Semimembranosus
   E. Semitendinosus

71. The syndrome of posteroinferior cerebellar artery (PICA) occlusion consists of each of the following *except*
   A. Contralateral loss of pain and temperature in the body
   B. Contralateral loss of pain and temperature in the face
   C. Ipsilateral paralysis of the pharynx and larynx
   D. Ipsilateral Horner's syndrome
   E. Persistent hiccup

⇨ For questions **72** to **77**, match the region of the internal capsule with the description. Each response may be used once, more than once, or not at all.
   A. Anterior limb of the internal capsule
   B. Genu of the internal capsule
   C. Posterior limb of the internal capsule
   D. None of the above

72. Location of the corticobulbar fibers

73. Location of corticospinal fibers

74. Location of anterior thalamic radiation

75. Location of superior thalamic radiation

76. Location of medial forebrain bundle fibers

77. Location of corticofugal fibers

⇨ For questions **78** to **85**, match the following ganglia with the description. Each choice may be used once, more than once, or not at all.

    A.   Ciliary ganglion
    B.   Gasserian ganglion
    C.   Geniculate ganglion
    D.   Otic ganglion
    E.   Scarpa's ganglion
    F.   Sphenopalatine ganglion
    G.   Spiral ganglion
    H.   Submandibular ganglion

78. Auditory system

79. Vestibular system

80. Parotid gland

81. Parasympathetic to eye

82. Majority of facial sensation

83. Taste

84. Lacrimation

85. Salivation (nonparotid)

86. Each of the following characterizes a pathway involved in the pupillary light reflex *except*

    A.   Crossed and uncrossed fibers of the optic tract terminate on the lateral geniculate body.
    B.   Efferent fibers from the pretectal olivary nucleus cross in the posterior commissure and end in visceral cell columns of the oculomotor nerve complex.
    C.   Efferent fibers from the pretectal olivary nucleus cross ventral to the cerebral aqueduct and end in the visceral cell columns of the oculomotor complex.
    D.   Postganglionic fibers from the ciliary ganglion project to the sphincter of the iris.
    E.   Preganglionic fibers from the nuclei of the oculomotor complex travel with fibers of the third nerve and synapse in the ciliary ganglion.

87. The choroid plexus of the fourth ventricle can be found
    I.   In the caudal aspect of the roof (inferior medullary velum)
    II.   In the cranial aspect of the roof (superior medullary velum)
    III. In the lateral recess (of Luschka)
    IV. On the floor
A. I, II, III
B. I, III
C. II, IV
D. IV
E. All of the above

88. The median nerve innervates each of the following muscles *except* the
A. Adductor pollicis
B. Flexor carpi radialis
C. Opponens pollicis
D. Palmaris longus
E. Pronator teres

89. Afferent sources of fiber pathways to the septal nuclei include the
    I.   Amygdala
    II.   Habenular nuclei
    III. Hippocampus
    IV. Basal ganglia
A. I, II, III
B. I, III
C. II, IV
D. IV
E. All of the above

90. The anterior choroidal artery supplies parts of the
    I.   Caudate nucleus
    II.   Optic tract
    III. Thalamus
    IV. Anterior limb of the internal capsule
A. I, II, III
B. I, III
C. II, IV
D. IV
E. All of the above

91. A lesion affecting the left optic tract will be manifested by a deficit in the
A. Nasal half of the visual field of both eyes
B. Nasal half of the right visual field and temporal half of the left visual field
C. No deficit unless the right optic tract was also affected
D. Temporal half of the visual field of both eyes
E. Temporal half of the right visual field and nasal half of the left visual field

92. Which of the following is *not* an afferent connection of the basal ganglia?
A. Cerebral cortex to globus pallidus
B. Cerebral cortex to putamen
C. Substantia nigra to caudate nucleus
D. Subthalamic nucleus to globus pallidus
E. Thalamus to caudate nucleus

93. Most of the fibers of the stria terminalis originate from the
    A. Amygdala
    B. Anterior hypothalamus
    C. Arcuate nucleus
    D. Habenula
    E. Septal nuclei

⟹ For questions **94** to **96**, match the following structures with the description. Each response may be used once, more than once, or not at all.
    A. Trapezoid body
    B. Probst's commissure
    C. Inferior collicular commissure

94. Connects inferior colliculi

95. Connects nuclei of lateral lemniscus

96. Connects ventral cochlear nucleus to superior olive

⟹ For questions **97** to **103**, match the region of the hypothalamus with the description. Each response may be used once, more than once, or not at all.
    A. Anterior hypothalamus
    B. Lateral hypothalamus
    C. Posterior hypothalamus
    D. Ventromedial hypothalamus

97. Bilateral lesions here produce hyperphagia.

98. Bilateral lesions here produce poikilothermia.

99. Tumors in this region can result in hyperthermia.

100. Together with the lateral region, this area controls sympathetic responses.

101. Lesions here produce emotional lethargy and sleepiness.

102. The feeding center

103. Together with the medial region, this area controls parasympathetic responses.

⟹ For questions **104** to **107**, match the following structures with the description. Each response may be used once, more than once, or not at all.
    A. Nodose ganglion
    B. Jugular ganglion
    C. Petrosal ganglion
    D. Superior ganglion of cranial nerve (CN) IX

104. Ear sensation to CN IX

105. Ear sensation to CN X

106. Carotid sinus and body input

107. Visceral input to CN X

108. The telencephalon gives rise to each of the following *except* the
   A. Amygdala
   B. Caudate
   C. Claustrum
   D. Globus pallidus
   E. Putamen

109. Weakness of the coracobrachialis muscle results from impairment of the
   A. Axillary nerve
   B. Dorsal scapular nerve
   C. Median nerve
   D. Musculocutaneous nerve
   E. Suprascapular nerve

110. Cells that give rise to commissural fibers that interconnect homologous cortical areas via the corpus callosum are found in layer
   A. I
   B. II
   C. III
   D. IV
   E. V

111. Neural crest derivatives include all of the following *except* the
   A. Adrenal medulla
   B. Dorsal root ganglion of cranial and spinal nerves
   C. Neurons of the cerebral cortex
   D. Pigmented layers of the retina
   E. Sympathetic ganglia of the autonomic nervous system

112. Which of the following progressions from primary vesicle to secondary vesicle to adult derivative is correct?
   A. Mesencephalon to rhombencephalon to medulla
   B. Prosencephalon to diencephalon to midbrain
   C. Prosencephalon to telencephalon to thalami
   D. Rhombencephalon to metencephalon to cerebellum
   E. Rhombencephalon to myelencephalon to pons

113. Major striatal efferent projections include
   A. Amygdala and globus pallidus
   B. Globus pallidus and substantia nigra
   C. Substantia nigra and amygdala
   D. Substantia nigra and thalamus
   E. Thalamus and globus pallidus

114. Fibers from the nucleus ambiguus make contribution to
       I.   Cranial nerve IX
       II.   Cranial nerve XI
       III. Cranial nerve X
       IV. Cranial nerve VII
   A. I, II, III
   B. I, III
   C. II, IV
   D. IV
   E. All of the above

115. Functional components of the facial and intermediate nerves include
     I.   General somatic afferent fibers
     II. General visceral afferent fibers
     III. Special visceral afferent fibers
     IV. Special visceral efferent fibers
     A.   I, II, III
     B.   I, III
     C.   II, IV
     D.   IV
     E.   All of the above

116. The infundibular recess of the third ventricle is located
     A.   Dorsal to the mammillary bodies
     B.   Dorsal to the habenula
     C.   Lateral to the infundibulum
     D.   Ventral to the infundibulum
     E.   Ventral to the mammillary bodies

117. Lesions of the lateral lemniscus produce
     A.   Bilateral complete deafness
     B.   Bilateral partial deafness, greater in the contralateral ear
     C.   Bilateral partial deafness, greater in the ipsilateral ear
     D.   Unilateral, contralateral deafness
     E.   Unilateral, ipsilateral deafness

118. The superior orbital fissure is traversed by which combination of cranial nerves?
     A.   III, IV, and VI only
     B.   III, IV, VI, and V1 only
     C.   III, IV, VI, V1, and V2 only
     D.   II, III, IV, VI, V1, and V2 only
     E.   II, III, IV, VI, and V1 only

⇨ For questions **119** to **123**, match the nerve with the foramen or fissure it traverses. Each response may be used once, more than once, or not at all.
     A.   Inferior orbital fissure
     B.   Foramen magnum
     C.   Foramen ovale
     D.   Superior orbital fissure
     E.   None of the above

119. Nasociliary nerve

120. Lacrimal nerve

121. Maxillary nerve

122. Mandibular nerve

123. Spinal accessory nerve

⇨ For questions **124** to **126**, match the following structures with the description. Each response may be used once, more than once, or not at all.
     A.   Pudendal nerve
     B.   Splanchnic nerve
     C.   Nervi erigentes

124. Parasympathetic

125. Sympathetic

126. Somatic

⇨ For questions **127** to **130**, match the structure involved in audition with the description. Each response may be used once, more than once, or not at all.

    A.   Cochlear nucleus
    B.   Inferior colliculus
    C.   Lateral lemniscus
    D.   Medial geniculate
    E.   Superior olivary nucleus

127. Fibers arising here are grouped into three acoustic striae.

128. The most proximal source of tertiary auditory fibers

129. Projects fibers into the lateral lemniscus

130. Fibers from this structure project bilaterally to stapedius motor neurons.

131. The fibers of the stria medullaris of the thalamus arise in the

    I.   Hypothalamus
    II.   Lateral preoptic region
    III.   Septal nuclei
    IV.   Amygdala

    A.   I, II, III
    B.   I, III
    C.   II, IV
    D.   IV
    E.   All of the above

132. Each of the following is true of striatal afferents *except*

    A.   Cells in the centromedian nucleus project to the caudate.
    B.   Corticostriate projections use glutamate as their transmitter.
    C.   Nigrostriatal fibers arise from cells in the pars compacta.
    D.   Serotonergic projections arise from the dorsal nucleus of the raphe.
    E.   Thalamostriate fibers arise largely from cells in the centromedian parafascicular nucleus

⇨ For questions **133** to **139**, match the trigeminal nucleus with the description. Each response may be used once, more than once, or not at all.

    A.   Mesencephalic nucleus
    B.   Motor nucleus
    C.   Principal sensory nucleus
    D.   Spinal trigeminal nucleus
    E.   Trigeminal ganglion

133. Consists of a pars oralis, pars interpolaris, and pars caudalis

134. Lesions in this structure can result in a loss of pain and temperature sense.

135. Afferent fibers of this nucleus convey proprioceptive information.

136. Second-order neurons of the ventral trigeminothalamic tract are found in the principal sensory nucleus and here.

137. Second-order neurons of the dorsal trigeminothalamic tract are found here.

138. This nucleus and the motor nucleus are involved in the jaw jerk.

139. Cells here have large receptive fields and respond to a wide range of pressure stimuli.

140. Which is *true* of dentate nucleus projections?
   A. They indirectly project to the ipsilateral cerebellar cortex.
   B. They indirectly project to the ipsilateral primary motor cortex.
   C. They leave the cerebellum via the middle cerebellar peduncle.
   D. They project somatotopically on the ventral anterior thalamic nucleus.
   E. They project to the ipsilateral red nucleus.

⇨ For questions **141** to **144**, match the following nerves with the description. Each response may be used once, more than once, or not at all.
   A. Superior gluteal nerve
   B. Inferior gluteal nerve
   C. Sciatic nerve
   D. Femoral nerve

141. Adductor magnus

142. Sartorius

143. Tensor fascia lata

144. Gluteus maximus

⇨ For questions **145** to **149**, match the component of the brachial plexus with the description. Each response may be used once, more than once, or not at all.
   A. Lateral cord
   B. Medial cord
   C. Posterior cord
   D. Radial nerve
   E. Ulnar nerve

145. The nerve that supplies the teres major originates here.

146. The medial cutaneous nerve of the forearm originates here.

147. The axillary nerve is a branch of this structure.

148. The musculocutaneous nerve is a branch of this structure.

149. The middle and lower trunks both contribute to this structure.

150. Each of the following is true of fiber tracts leaving the cerebellum and terminating in the thalamus *except*

A. Fibers terminate on the ventral lateral and ventral posterolateral thalamic nuclei.

B. In the thalamus, the extremities are represented dorsally and the back ventrally.

C. In the thalamus, the head is represented medially and the caudal thorax laterally.

D. Some fibers project to the rostral interlaminar nuclei.

E. These fibers originate from both the dentate and the interposed nuclei.

151. All of the following subcortical nuclei are considered part of the limbic system *except* the

A. Amygdala

B. Centromedian nucleus of the thalamus

C. Epithalamus

D. Hypothalamus

E. Septal nuclei

152. Central nervous system melanocytes are concentrated in the

A. Choroid plexus

B. Red nuclei

C. Region of the amygdala

D. Septum pellucidum

E. Ventral medulla

153. A lesion in the medial lemniscus produces

A. Contralateral loss of pain and temperature

B. Contralateral loss of position and vibration

C. Ipsilateral loss of pain and temperature

D. Ipsilateral loss of position and vibration

E. Loss of pain and temperature bilaterally

154. Each of the following is considered a part of the diencephalon *except* the

A. Fornix

B. Hypothalamus

C. Mammillary bodies

D. Pineal gland

E. Stria medullaris thalami

For questions **155** to **162**, match the following structures with the description. Each response may be used once, more than once, or not at all.

A. Maxillary branch of CN V

B. Nasopalatine nerve

C. Mandibular branch of CN V

D. Abducens nerve

E. Mental nerve

F. Middle meningeal artery

155. Inferior orbital fissure

156. Superior orbital fissure

157. Foramen spinosum

158. Foramen rotundum

159. Foramen ovale

160. Dorello's canal

161. Incisive foramen

162. Mental foramen

⇨ For questions **163** to **170**, match the vestibular nucleus with the description. Each response may be used once, more than once, or not at all.
  A. Inferior vestibular nucleus
  B. Interstitial nucleus of the vestibular nerve
  C. Lateral vestibular nucleus
  D. Medial vestibular nucleus
  E. Superior vestibular nucleus

163. The largest of the vestibular nuclei

164. Cells of the superior vestibular ganglion, which innervate the utricular macule, project to this nucleus.

165. Cells of the inferior vestibular ganglion, which innervate the posterior part of the saccular macule, project to this nucleus.

166. Gives rise to the vestibulospinal tract

167. Ascending fibers from this nucleus are predominantly crossed and project bilaterally to the extraocular nerve nuclei.

168. Gives rise to the uncrossed ascending fibers in the medial longitudinal fasciculus projecting to the oculomotor and trochlear nuclei

169. Cells of this nucleus lie among fibers of the vestibular root.

170. Secondary vestibulocerebellar projections arise from the caudal aspect of the inferior vestibular nucleus and this nucleus.

⇨ For questions **171** to **175**, match the trigeminal nucleus with the description. Each response may be used once, more than once, or not at all.
  A. Mesencephalic nucleus
  B. Motor nucleus
  C. Principal sensory nucleus
  D. Spinal trigeminal nucleus
  E. Trigeminal ganglion

171. The most rostral of the nuclei

172. Extends the most caudally

173. Afferent fibers of this nucleus convey pressure and kinesthetic sense from the teeth.

174. Central processes from the trigeminal ganglion cells ascend to this nucleus.

175. Central processes from the trigeminal ganglion cells descend to this nucleus.

176. The solitary tract is formed from fibers of cranial nerve(s)

    I.   IX
    II.   X
    III. VII
    IV. XII
A. I, II, III
B. I, III
C. II, IV
D. IV
E. All of the above

177. A femoral nerve injury results in weakness of
A. Hip extension
B. Hip flexion
C. Knee flexion
D. Thigh abduction
E. Thigh adduction

178. The pars tuberalis is a part of the
A. Anterior lobe of the pituitary
B. Diaphragma sellae
C. Intermediate lobe of the pituitary
D. Pituitary stalk
E. Posterior lobe of the pituitary

179. The dentate nuclei project to each of the following, directly or indirectly, *except* the
A. Cerebellar cortex
B. Inferior olive
C. Red nucleus
D. Reticulotegmental nucleus
E. Subthalamic nucleus

180. Fibers in the superior cerebellar peduncle synapse in which of the following thalamic nuclei?

    I.   Ventral anterior
    II.   Ventral lateral
    III. Rostral interlaminar nuclei
    IV. Ventral lateral posterior (VLp)
A. I, II, III
B. I, III
C. II, IV
D. IV
E. All of the above

181. The limbic lobe is composed of all the following *except* the
A. Amygdala
B. Cingulate gyrus
C. Dentate gyrus
D. Parahippocampal gyrus
E. Subcallosal gyrus

182. The most significant contribution to the nasal septum is made by the
- **A.** Ethmoid and frontal bones
- **B.** Ethmoid and sphenoid bones
- **C.** Ethmoid and vomer bones
- **D.** Frontal and vomer bones
- **E.** Sphenoid and vomer bones

183. The posterior interosseus nerve innervates the
- **A.** Abductor pollicis brevis
- **B.** Abductor pollicis longus
- **C.** Adductor pollicis
- **D.** Flexor pollicis longus
- **E.** Opponens pollicis

184. The internal cerebral vein receives each of the following veins *except* the
- **A.** Choroidal vein
- **B.** Epithalamic vein
- **C.** Great cerebral vein of Galen
- **D.** Septal vein
- **E.** Thalamostriate vein

185. The striate cortex corresponds to area
- **A.** 17 ′
- **B.** 18
- **C.** 19
- **D.** 41
- **E.** 42

186. The internal capsule is supplied by branches of the
-     I.   Middle cerebral artery
-     II.   Anterior cerebral artery
-     III.   Internal carotid artery
-     IV.   Posterior cerebral artery
- **A.** I, II, III
- **B.** I, III
- **C.** II, IV
- **D.** IV
- **E.** All of the above

⇨ For questions **187** to **191**, match the association or commissural fiber bundle with the description. Each response may be used once, more than once, or not at all.
- **A.** Anterior commissure
- **B.** Arcuate fasciculus
- **C.** Cingulate fasciculus
- **D.** Corpus callosum
- **E.** Uncinate fasciculus

187. Connects the orbital frontal gyri with anterior parts of the temporal lobe

188. Connects the medial frontal and parietal lobes with the parahippocampal region

189. Connects the superior and middle frontal gyri to the temporal lobe

190. The tapetum is derived from these fibers.

191. Interconnects regions of the middle and inferior temporal gyri between hemispheres

⇨ For questions **192** to **194**, match the following structures with the description. Each response may be used once, more than once, or not at all.

    A. Restiform body
    B. Juxtarestiform body
    C. Brachium conjunctivum
    D. Brachium pontis

192. Superior cerebellar peduncle

193. Middle cerebellar peduncle

194. Portion of the inferior cerebellar peduncle containing only afferent fibers from the inferior olive and pons

195. A discrete unilateral lesion of the abducens nucleus produces paralysis of movement of
    A. Both eyes away from the lesion
    B. Both eyes toward the lesion
    C. The contralateral eye toward the lesion
    D. The ipsilateral eye away from the lesion
    E. The ipsilateral eye toward the lesion

196. Postganglionic parasympathetic fibers destined for the lacrimal gland are derived from the
    A. Geniculate ganglion
    B. Otic ganglion
    C. Pterygopalatine ganglion
    D. Sublingual ganglion
    E. Submandibular ganglion

197. Fibers originating in the substantia nigra synapse on each of the following structures *except* the
    A. Caudate
    B. Globus pallidus
    C. Putamen
    D. Superior colliculus
    E. Thalamus

198. The blood–brain barrier is formed by (the)
    A. Astrocytic foot processes
    B. Basement membrane
    C. Ependymal lining cells
    D. Microglia
    E. Tight junctions of the capillary endothelium

199. Which of the following ligaments is a continuation of the posterior longitudinal ligament?
  A. Anterior atlanto-occipital membrane
  B. Apical ligament
  C. Cruciate ligament
  D. Tectorial ligament
  E. Transverse ligament

⇨ For questions **200** to **204**, match the percentage of corticospinal fibers with the description. Each response may be used once, more than once, or not at all.
  A. 3%
  B. 30%
  C. 40%
  D. 60%
  E. 90%

200. Betz cells account for this proportion of the corticospinal fibers.

201. The approximate percentage of corticospinal fibers arising from area 4

202. The approximate percentage of corticospinal fibers arising from area 6

203. The approximate percentage of corticospinal fibers arising from the parietal lobe

204. The approximate percentage of corticospinal fibers that are poorly myelinated

205. The facial nerve innervates all of the following muscles *except* the
  A. Anterior belly of the digastric
  B. Buccinator
  C. Platysma
  D. Stapedius
  E. Stylohyoid

206. The nucleus pulposus of the intervertebral disk is formed from the
  A. Chondrification of the centrum of the vertebral body
  B. Myotome
  C. Notochord
  D. Primitive streak
  E. Sclerotome

207. The primary olfactory cortex is located in the
  A. Anterior perforated substance
  B. Entorhinal cortex
  C. Mediodorsal nucleus of the thalamus
  D. Orbitofrontal cortex
  E. Pyriform cortex

208. Each of the following cell groups is derived from the alar plate *except* the
  A. Nucleus ambiguus
  B. Principal sensory nucleus of CN V
  C. Solitary nucleus
  D. Spinal trigeminal nucleus
  E. Vestibular nucleus

209. A unilateral lesion of the trochlear nerve produces maximal diplopia on
   A. Downgaze to the opposite side
   B. Downgaze to the same side
   C. Upgaze to the opposite side
   D. Upgaze to the same side
   E. Lateral gaze to the opposite side

⇨ For questions **210** and **211**, match the following structures with the description. Each response may be used once, more than once, or not at all.
   A. Superior olive
   B. Inferior olivary complex
   C. Both
   D. Neither

210. Part of the auditory system

211. Part of the cerebellar system

⇨ For questions **212** to **216**, match the following structures with the description.
   A. Superior salivatory nucleus
   B. Inferior salivatory nucleus
   C. Both
   D. Neither

212. General visceral efferent fibers arise here.

213. Preganglionic parasympathetic fibers from this nucleus travel with the intermediate nerve.

214. Preganglionic parasympathetic fibers from this nucleus travel with the lesser petrosal nerve.

215. Located in the reticular formation

216. Fibers originating here eventually divide into two groups that pass to the pterygopalatine and submandibular ganglia, respectively.

⇨ For questions **217** and **218**, match the following structures with the description. Each response may be used once, more than once, or not at all.
   A. Parasympathetic
   B. Sympathetic
   C. Both

217. Short ciliary nerves

218. Long ciliary nerves

⇨ For questions **219** to **225**, match the ascending spinal tract with the description. Each response may be used once, more than once, or not at all.
   A. Anterior spinothalamic tract
   B. Cuneocerebellar tract
   C. Dorsal spinocerebellar tract
   D. Lateral spinothalamic tract
   E. Ventral spinocerebellar tract

219. Arises from the dorsal nucleus of Clarke

220. The upper limb equivalent of the dorsal spinocerebellar tract

221. Transmits light touch

222. Crossed; cells of origin receive input from group Ib afferents

223. Crossed within one or two spinal segments; cells in laminae I, IV, and V give rise to most of the axons in this tract

224. Enters the cerebellum via the superior cerebellar peduncle

225. First-order neurons are found from L1 to S2.

⇨ For questions **226** to **230**, match the descending spinal tract with the description. Each response may be used once, more than once, or not at all.
    A. Corticospinal tract
    B. Reticulospinal tract
    C. Rubrospinal tract
    D. Tectospinal tract
    E. Vestibulospinal tract

226. The majority of fibers descend only to cervical levels.

227. Cells of origin reside in the pontine tegmentum and medulla.

228. Divides into three tracts at the spinomedullary junction

229. Associated with the control of tone in flexor muscle groups

230. Associated with the control of tone in extensor muscle groups

⇨ For questions **231** to **240**, match the peripheral nerve with the muscle it innervates. Each response may be used once, more than once, or not at all.
    A. Deep peroneal   **E.** Sciatic
    B. Femoral   **F.** Superficial peroneal
    C. Inferior gluteal   **G.** Superior gluteal
    D. Obturator   **H.** Tibial

231. Adductor brevis

232. Biceps femoris

233. Extensor hallucis longus

234. Gluteus medius

235. Gluteus maximus

236. Gastrocnemius

237. Iliopsoas

238. Flexor digitorum longus

239. Peroneus longus and brevis

240. Quadriceps

241. Movement of molecules across the blood–brain barrier involves
   A. Active transport requiring energy
   B. Carrier-mediated transport
   C. Both
   D. Neither

242. Which of the following most closely characterizes the tuberohypophysial tract?
   A. Arcuate nucleus to median eminence
   B. Arcuate nucleus to posterior hypophysis
   C. Dorsomedial nucleus to posterior hypophysis
   D. Supraoptic nucleus to median eminence
   E. Supraoptic nucleus to posterior hypophysis

⇨ For questions **243** to **250**, match the following structures with the description. Each response may be used once, more than once, or not at all.
   A. Apical ligament
   B. Alar ligaments
   C. Dentate ligaments
   D. Tectorial membrane
   E. Superior cruciate ligaments
   F. Inferior cruciate ligaments
   G. Anterior atlanto-occipital membrane
   H. Transverse ligament

243. Dens to basion

244. Dens to lateral foramen magnum

245. Pia to dura

246. Continuous with posterior longitudinal ligament

247. Continuous with anterior longitudinal ligament

248. Between C1 lateral masses

249. Transverse ligament to basion

250. Transverse ligament to axis

251. Which hypothalamic nucleus is the principle source of hypothalamic descending fibers responsible for autonomic control?
   A. Mammillary nucleus
   B. Medial preoptic nucleus
   C. Paraventricular nucleus
   D. Periventricular nucleus
   E. Supraoptic nucleus

252. All of the following targets of descending hypothalamic autonomic fibers participate in parasympathetic control *except*
   A. Dorsal motor nucleus of the vagus
   B. Edinger-Westphal nucleus
   C. S2-S4 nucleus
   D. Superior and inferior salivatory nuclei
   E. T1-L2 of the spinal cord

⇨ For questions **253** to **259**, match the following structures to the appropriate answer choice.

    A. Sympathetic system
    B. Parasympathetic system
    C. Both
    D. Neither

253. Anterior and medial hypothalamus

254. Dorsal motor nucleus of the vagus

255. Edinger-Westphal nucleus

256. Posterior and lateral hypothalamus

257. Preganglionic neurons from T1-L2 of the spinal cord

258. S2-S4 parasympathetic nucleus

259. Superior and inferior salivatory nuclei

260. Which of the following answer choices best describes the decussation of the dorsal column–medial lemniscal system?
    A. Second-order neurons as the anterior white commissure
    B. Second-order neurons as the internal arcuate fibers
    C. Second-order neurons as the lateral lemniscus
    D. Second-order neurons as the medial lemniscus
    E. Second-order neurons as the pyramidal decussation

261. Melanocytes are most often found in which of the following anatomical locations?
    A. Basal forebrain
    B. Leptomeninges of the cerebral convexities
    C. Leptomeninges of the ventral medulla
    D. Substantia nigra
    E. None of the above

262. All of the following features are associated with injury to the nondominant hemisphere *except*
    A. Anosognosia
    B. Contralateral hemineglect
    C. Disorientation to time and direction
    D. Global aphasia
    E. Visuospatial deficits

263. Which of the following statements is *true* regarding the anterolateral system?
    A. First-order fibers decussate in the anterior white commissure of the spinal cord.
    B. Projections of first-order neurons form Lissauer's tract (dorsolateral fasciculus).
    C. Second-order interneurons project to Clarke's column conveying pain and temperature sensation.
    D. Thinly myelinated C fibers are fast conducting fibers.
    E. Unmyelinated A-delta fibers are slow conducting fibers.

264. Proprioception from the lower extremities is mediated by
    A. Dorsal column–medial lemniscal system
    B. Clarke's column and dorsal spinocerebellar tract
    C. Nucleus cuneatus and cuneocerebellar tract
    D. Nucleus gracilis and dorsal spinocerebellar tract
    E. Nucleus of Clarke homologue and rostral spinocerebellar tract

265. All of the following statements regarding the mammillothalamic tract are true *except* that it
    A. Is also known as the tract of Vicq d'Azyr
    B. Is a part of the proposed Papez circuit
    C. Is a thin bundle of unmyelinated fibers
    D. Projects from the mammillary body to the anterior nuclear group of the thalamus
    E. Serves as a landmark for deep brain stimulation implantation

266. The membrane of Liliequist separates which of the following subarachnoid cisterns?
    A. Ambient cistern and crural cistern
    B. Ambient cistern and quadrigeminal cistern
    C. Interpeduncular and chiasmatic cistern
    D. Interpeduncular and prepontine cistern
    E. Lamina terminalis cistern and interpeduncular cistern

⇨ For questions **267** to **271**, match the pair of structures with the structure that separates them.
    A. Choroid fissure
    B. Foramen of Luschka
    C. Foramen of Magendie
    D. Lamina terminalis
    E. Velum interpositum

267. Lamina terminalis cistern and third ventricle

268. Crural cistern and temporal horn of lateral ventricle

269. Velum interpositum cistern and third ventricle

270. Lateral recess of fourth ventricle and lateral cerebellomedullary cistern

271. Fourth ventricle and cisterna magna

3B Neuroanatomy— Answer Key

1. C
2. D
3. B
4. A
5. B
6. B
7. C
8. A
9. A
10. E
11. A
12. A
13. A
14. D
15. A
16. D
17. E
18. B
19. A
20. D
21. C
22. B
23. A
24. C
25. B
26. C

27. C
28. D
29. D
30. H
31. H
32. E
33. D
34. G
35. I
36. F
37. C
38. B
39. A
40. A
41. A
42. D
43. B
44. A
45. C
46. F
47. B
48. E
49. D
50. E
51. E
52. C

53.	B	92.	A
54.	B	93.	A
55.	A	94.	C
56.	C	95.	B
57.	A	96.	A
58.	B	97.	D
59.	A	98.	C
60.	C	99.	A
61.	D	100.	C
62.	C	101.	C
63.	D	102.	B
64.	A	103.	A
65.	B	104.	D
66.	C	105.	B
67.	A	106.	C
68.	C	107.	A
69.	B	108.	D
70.	C	109.	D
71.	B	110.	C
72.	B	111.	C
73.	C	112.	D
74.	A	113.	B
75.	C	114.	A
76.	D	115.	E
77.	C	116.	E
78.	G	117.	B
79.	E	118.	B
80.	D	119.	D
81.	A	120.	D
82.	B	121.	A
83.	C	122.	C
84.	F	123.	B
85.	H	124.	C
86.	A	125.	B
87.	B	126.	A
88.	A	127.	A
89.	A	128.	E
90.	A	129.	E
91.	E	130.	E

131. A	170. D
132. A	171. A
133. D	172. D
134. D	173. A
135. A	174. C
136. D	175. D
137. C	176. A
138. A	177. B
139. C	178. A
140. A	179. E
141. C	180. C
142. D	181. A
143. A	182. C
144. B	183. B
145. C	184. C
146. B	185. A
147. C	186. A
148. A	187. E
149. C	188. C
150. B	189. B
151. B	190. D
152. E	191. A
153. B	192. C
154. A	193. D
155. A	194. A
156. D	195. B
157. F	196. C
158. A	197. B
159. C	198. E
160. D	199. D
161. B	200. A
162. E	201. B
163. D	202. B
164. C	203. C
165. A	204. C
166. C	205. A
167. D	206. C
168. E	207. E
169. B	208. A

209.	A	241.	C
210.	A	242.	A
211.	B	243.	A
212.	C	244.	B
213.	A	245.	C
214.	B	246.	D
215.	C	247.	G
216.	A	248.	H
217.	C	249.	E
218.	B	250.	F
219.	C	251.	C
220.	B	252.	E
221.	A	253.	B
222.	E	254.	B
223.	D	255.	B
224.	E	256.	A
225.	E	257.	A
226.	D	258.	B
227.	B	259.	B
228.	A	260.	B
229.	C	261.	C
230.	E	262.	D
231.	D	263.	B
232.	E	264.	B
233.	A	265.	C
234.	G	266.	C
235.	C	267.	D
236.	H	268.	A
237.	B	269.	E
238.	H	270.	B
239.	F	271.	C
240.	B		

Neuroanatomy—Answers and Explanations

1. **C** – Medial lemniscus
2. **D** – Medial longitudinal fasciculus
3. **B** – Lateral lemniscus
4. **A** – Dorsal longitudinal fasciculus

The **dorsal longitudinal fasciculus (A)**, or dorsolateral fasciculus, carries fibers from the hypothalamus to the autonomic nuclei and reticular formation of the brainstem's central gray matter to influence activities such as chewing, swallowing, and shivering. The **lateral lemniscus (B)** is part of the auditory pathway, carrying second-order fibers arising from the cochlear nucleus that ascend to the inferior colliculus. The **medial lemniscus (C)** connects the second-order neurons of nucleus gracilis and cuneatus (dorsal columns) to the ventral posterior lateral nucleus of the thalamus. The **medial longitudinal fasciculus (D)** carries projections from the superior colliculus to the oculomotor, trochlear, and abducens nuclei and contributes to reflex movements of the eyes in response to visual, auditory, and somatic stimuli.[1]

5. **B** – Conjugate horizontal deviation to the same side

The paramedian pontine reticular formation (PPRF) mediates horizontal eye movements in response to head movement. Stimulation of the caudal PPRF causes **conjugate horizontal deviation of the eyes to the same side (B)**.[1,2]

6. **B** – Conjugate horizontal deviation to the same side
7. **C** – Vertical eye movements
8. **A** – Conjugate horizontal deviation to the opposite side

9. A –   Conjugate horizontal deviation to the opposite side

The center for horizontal gaze (the abducens nucleus) and the center for vertical gaze (the rostral interstitial nucleus of the medial longitudinal fasciculus [RiMLF]) are joined physiologically by the paramedian pontine reticular formation (PPRF), which lies rostral to the abducens nucleus. Stimulation of the caudal and rostral PPRF produces **conjugate horizontal eye deviation (B)** and **vertical eye movements (C)**, respectively. Fibers from the caudal PPRF project to the ipsilateral abducens nucleus, and fibers from the rostral PPRF project uncrossed fibers to the RiMLF, which in turn projects to the ipsilateral oculomotor nuclear complex. Lesions of the caudal PPRF may cause paralysis of horizontal eye movements, whereas lesions of the rostral PPRF can cause paralysis of vertical eye movements. Extensive lesions may affect both types of eye movements. Stimulation of the frontal eye field, located in the caudal part of the middle frontal gyrus, usually results in **conjugate deviation of the eyes to the opposite side (A)**. Stimulation of the superior colliculus results in **contralateral conjugate deviation of the eyes (A)**.[1,2]

10. E –   With lesions of this area, the patient can direct the eyes to a particular location on command.

The occipital eye fields are not as well defined as the frontal eye fields and contribute to smooth pursuit movements when tracking objects. With lesions of the occipital eye fields, which are located near the junction of the occipital lobes with the posterior temporal and parietal lobes, the patient **can direct the eyes to a particular location on command (E)**.[2]

11. A –   I, II, III (cranial nerve V, upper cervical spinal nerves, and cranial nerve X)

The supratentorial dura is innervated by **CN V**. V1 supplies the anterior cranial fossa, V2 supplies the middle fossa, and V3 supplies the supratentorial posterior fossa. The infratentorial dura is innervated by the **upper cervical roots (C2, C3)** and **CN X**.[3]

12. A –   Inferior colliculus (false)

The MLF carries fibers arising from **Cajal's interstitial nucleus (B)**, the **medial vestibular nucleus (C)**, the **paramedian pontine reticular formation (D)**, as well as the **superior colliculus (E)**. Projections from the **inferior colliculus (A)** do not contribute the MLF.[1,2]

13. A –   Frontal nerve

The annular tendon of Zinn divides the superior orbital fissure (SOF) into lateral, central, and inferior segments. The lateral sector contains the trochlear, **frontal (A)**, and lacrimal nerves, which all pass outside the annular tendon of Zinn. The superior ophthalmic vein also passes inferior to the nerves in this portion of the fissure to reach the cavernous sinus. The central portion of the SOF (oculomotor foramen) contains the **oculomotor nerve (B and E)**, **nasociliary nerve (D)**, **abducens nerve (C)**, and roots of the ciliary ganglion—all of which pass through the annulus of Zinn. The optic nerve and ophthalmic artery course medially to the oculomotor foramen through part of the annular tendon that is attached to the optic foramen.[4]

14. D – Sensory deficits in the dorsum of the hand

> The sensory branch to the dorsum of the hand leaves the ulnar nerve in the forearm and is never involved in ulnar nerve entrapment at the wrist. The superficial head of the abductor pollicis brevis is innervated by the median nerve.[5]

15. A – I, II, III (medial posterior choroidal artery, anterior choroidal artery, and basilar artery branches)

> The thalamus is also fed by thalamoperforators arising from the posterior communication (PComm) arteries. There is generally no contribution to thalamic blood supply by the middle cerebral artery or its branches.[3]

16. D – Hypothalamus (false)

> The anterior choroidal artery is a branch of the internal carotid artery that arises 2–4 mm distal to the PComm artery. It courses posteromedially to supply several structures including the **amygdala (A)**, **hippocampus (C)**, **internal capsule (E)**, and **globus pallidus (B)**. The anterior choroidal artery does not provide blood supply to the **hypothalamus (D)**, which is supplied by perforators arising from the anterior cerebral artery and anterior communicating (AComm) arteries.[3]

17. E – Stria terminalis
18. B – Lamina terminalis
19. A – Central tegmental tract
20. D – Stria medullaris
21. C – Medial forebrain bundle

> The **central tegmental tract (A)** connects the gustatory brainstem nucleus (rostral nucleus solitarius) to the thalamus. The **medial forebrain bundle (C)** is a bidirectional pathway between the hypothalamus/septal area and the midbrain, pons, and medulla that is thought to be involved in motivation and sense of smell. The **stria medullaris thalami (D)** connects the hypothalamus, septal area, and olfactory area to the habenula. The fibers of the **stria terminalis (E)** project from the amygdala to the hypothalamus. The **lamina terminalis (B)** represents the rostral boundary of the neural tube.[1,3]

22. B – Influence activity of motor neurons in the contralateral cerebral cortex

> The bulk of the fibers from the dentate nucleus pass around the red nucleus and project to the contralateral thalamus via the superior cerebellar peduncle, whereas the bulk of fibers from the interposed nuclei project to the caudal two thirds of the red nucleus. In the thalamic nuclei, the head is represented medially and the caudal parts of the body laterally.[1]

23. A – I, II, III (occipital, parietal, and temporal cortex)

> The pulvinar of the thalamus is involved in the integration of visual, auditory, and somatosensory information. For this reason, it necessarily shares projections with the association areas of the occipital, parietal, and temporal lobes. They include projections to the occipital cortex (areas 17, 18, and 19), the inferior parietal lobule (areas 39 and 40), and the superior temporal gyrus.[1,2]

24. C – The columns of the fornix lie anterior to the anterior commissure (false)

> The fornix is the **main efferent pathway from the hippocampal formation (A)**. At the level of the anterior commissure, the fornix is divided into a precommissural and postcommissural part, which lie anterior and posterior to the anterior commissure, respectively **(C is false)**. The precommissural fibers arise primarily from the pyramidal cells of the hippocampus and project to the septal area and basal forebrain while the **postcommissural fibers arise from the subiculum and project primarily to the mammillary bodies (B)**. The **body of the fornix runs to the rostral margin of the thalamus (D)**; the crura of the fornix meet in the midline at the **forniceal commissure (psalterium), which is rostral to the anterior commissure (E)**.[1,2]

25. B – Median eminence

> The efferent projections of the arcuate nucleus have been traced to the external layer of the median eminence. Chemical substances from the arcuate nucleus (including dopamine) play a major role in the regulation of hormonal output from the anterior pituitary.[2]

26. C – II, IV (blind spot of the retina and monocular temporal crescent)

> The blind spot of the retina and the monocular temporal crescent, both receiving only monocular visual input, do not contain ocular dominance columns.[2]

27. C – The neurons in this area exhibit movement-related activity only if the motor task is performed with the contralateral limbs (false)

> Motor tasks performed with either the ipsilateral or the contralateral limbs can elicit movement-related activity in the supplementary area **(C is false)**. The other responses are correct: **some neurons of the SMA project directly to the spinal cord (A), the body is somatopically represented (B), the threshold for stimulation is higher than for primary motor cortex (D)**, and **unilateral ablations produce no permanent deficit in the maintenance of posture or capacity for movement (E)**.[2]

28. D – The medial bundle consists of thinly myelinated fibers or unmyelinated fibers, whereas the lateral bundle is thickly myelinated (false)

> The **dorsal roots separate into a lateral and medial bundle (A)**. The medial bundle of dorsal root afferents entering the dorsolateral spinal cord consists of large myelinated fibers while the **lateral bundle consists of thin, unmyelinated fibers (D is false)**. The **lateral bundle conveys information from free nerve endings (C)** while the **medial bundle transmits impulses from encapsulated receptors, such as Golgi tendon organs (E)**, to the posterior columns.[2,3]

29. D – IV (adductor pollicis)

> The pronator quadratus and flexor pollicis longus are innervated by the anterior interosseous nerve (a purely motor branch of the median nerve). The opponens pollicis (a thenar muscle) is innervated by the median nerve. The adductor pollicis is innervated by the ulnar nerve.[6]

30. H – Cingulate gyrus
31. H – Cingulate gyrus
32. E – Area 17
33. D – Areas 5, 7
34. G – Areas 41, 42
35. I – Prefrontal cortex
36. F – Areas 18, 19
37. C – Striatum
38. B – Area 4
39. A – Areas 1, 2, 3
40. A – Areas 1, 2, 3

The ventral posteromedial (VPM) and ventral posterolateral (VPL) nuclei of the thalamus are part of the lateral tier of the lateral thalamic nuclei and are part of the sensory thalamus. They receive input from the trigeminothalamic (VPM) and lateral spinothalamic tracts (VPL) and relay this information to the primary sensory cortex in the postcentral gyrus of the parietal lobe, **Brodmann's areas 1, 2, and 3 (A)**. The ventral lateral nucleus of the thalamus (VL) is also part of the ventral tier of the lateral nuclear group and receives afferents from the basal ganglia and cerebellum. The VL nucleus influences somatic motor activity via projections to the supplementary motor area (Brodmann's area 6) as well as the **primary motor cortex, Brodmann's area 4 (B)**. The centromedian nucleus is classified with the intralaminar nuclei of the thalamus, which represent the rostral continuation of the brainstem reticular activating system into the thalamus. The centromedian nucleus is primarily concerned with sensorimotor integration receiving afferents from the globus pallidus, premotor, and primary motor area and sending the majority of its projections to the **striatum (C)**. The lateral posterior nucleus (LP) of the thalamus is part of the dorsal tier of the lateral nuclear group, is closely related to the pulvinar, and is involved with sensory integration. The LP sends projections primarily to the **superior parietal lobule, Brodmann's areas 5 and 7 (D)**. The lateral geniculate nucleus (LGN) receives fibers of the optic tract and projects to **primary visual cortex, Brodmann's area 17 (E)**. The pulvinar of the thalamus is a member of the dorsal tier of the lateral nuclear group and integrates visual, auditory, and somatosensory information, projecting to **association areas of the occipital, temporal, and parietal lobes—Brodmann's areas 18 and 19 (F)**. The medial geniculate nucleus (MGN) receives auditory pathway input and projects to **primary auditory cortex, Brodmann's areas 41 and 42 (G)**. The anterior nuclear group of the thalamus is closely associated with the limbic system, and as such sends its projections to the **cingulate gyrus (H)**. The lateral dorsal (LD) nucleus of the thalamus is part of the dorsal tier of the lateral nuclear group, but represents the caudal continuation of the anterior nuclear group, and may be involved in the expression of emotions, projecting to the **cingulate gyrus (H)** of the limbic system. The medial dorsal (MD) or dorsomedial (DM) nucleus of the thalamus is a member of the medial nuclear group and functions in the processing of emotion. The MD nucleus sends its projections primarily to the **prefrontal cortex (I)**.[1]

41. A – Supraopticohypophyseal tract

42. D –   Neither
43. B –   Tuberoinfundibular tract

> Axons of the **tuberoinfundibular tract (B)** project to the median eminence near the sinusoids of the hypophyseal portal system; their products are carried to the anterior pituitary and influence hormone production at the adenohypophysis (anterior pituitary gland). The **supraopticohypophyseal (A)** tract consists of neurosecretory projections from the supraoptic and paraventricular nuclei that produce antidiuretic hormone and oxytocin, which are released directly into the bloodstream, constituting the neurohypophysis or posterior pituitary gland.[1]

44. A –   Ansa lenticularis
45. C –   Lenticular fasciculus (FF H2)
46. F –   Thalamic fasciculus (FF H1)
47. B –   Fasciculus retroflexus
48. E –   Precommissural fornix
49. D –   Postcommissural fornix

> The **ansa lenticularis (A)** represents a bundle of pallidothalamic fibers that courses posteriorly, looping around the posterior limb of the internal capsule from the globus pallidus to the thalamus. Another group of pallidothalamic fibers, the **lenticular fasciculus (C)**, projects from the globus pallidus and traverses the posterior limb of the internal capsule to reach the thalamus. The **thalamic fasciculus (F)** represents the confluence of the **ansa lenticularis (A)** and the **lenticular fasciculus (C)** as they reach the thalamus. The **fasciculus retroflexus (B)** connects the habenula to the midbrain and interpeduncular nuclei.

> The fornix is the main efferent pathway from the hippocampal formation. At the level of the anterior commissure, the fornix is divided into a precommissural and postcommissural part, which lie anterior and posterior to the anterior commissure, respectively. The **precommissural fibers (E)** arise primarily from the pyramidal cells of the hippocampus and project to the septal area and basal forebrain while the **postcommissural fibers (D)** arise from the subiculum of the hippocampus and project primarily to the mammillary bodies and hypothalamus.[1,3]

50. E –   Superior vestibular nucleus

> The superior vestibular nucleus is found at the level of the pons.[2]

51. E –   Thalamic fasciculus

> The thalamic fasciculus contains pallidothalamic fibers and ascending fibers from the contralateral deep cerebellar nuclei. It is not a component of the limbic system.[1,2]

52. C –   Superior bank of the lateral sulcus

> The secondary somatosensory cortex (SII, Brodmann's area 43) is located on the superior bank of the lateral fissure at the inferior extent of the primary motor and sensory areas.[1]

53. B – Impairment of lacrimation

Fibers innervating the lacrimal gland arise from postganglionic fibers from the pterygopalatine ganglion, which is linked to the geniculate ganglion via the greater superficial petrosal nerve. A lesion distal to the geniculate ganglion would not **impair lacrimation (B is false)**. A lesion to the facial nerve just distal to the geniculate ganglion would cause **paralysis of ipsilateral facial muscles** due to disruption of somatic motor neurons **(E)**, **hyperacusis** due to disruption of the facial nerve proximal to the take-off of the nerve to the stapedius muscle **(A)**, and **impairment of salivary secretions** and **loss of taste in the anterior two-thirds of the tongue** due to disruption of the facial nerve proximal to the take-off of the chorda tympani nerve **(C and D)**.[1]

54. B – Somatic pudendal nerves

The external urethral sphincter is innervated by somatic motor fibers supplied by the pudendal nerve (S2–S4). The internal urinary sphincter is innervated by sympathetic fibers supplied by the vesical (pelvic) nerve plexus.[6]

55. A – Indusium griseum (false)

Regions of the brain devoid of a blood–brain barrier include the **median eminence (B)**, **the organum vasculosum of the lamina terminalis (C)**, **the pineal gland (D)**, **the subfornical organ (E)**, the area postrema, and the neurohypophysis. The indusium griseum (or supracallosal gyrus) is a vestigial convolution of the dentate gyrus.[1,2,3]

56. C – 2, 3, and 5

Uncrossed fibers of the optic tract terminate in **layers 2, 3, and 5 (C)** of the lateral geniculate nucleus while crossed fibers terminate in **layers 1, 4, and 6 (B)**.[2,3]

57. A – I, II, III (active transport, carrier-mediated transport, and diffusion)

Substances can cross the blood–brain barrier (formed by capillary endothelial tight junctions) via active transport, carrier-mediated transport, or diffusion. Substances do not cross the blood–brain barrier via vesicular transport mechanisms.[2,3]

58. B – Diagonal band of Broca
59. A – Arcuate fasciculus
60. C – Tapetum
61. D – Uncinate fasciculus

The **arcuate fasciculus (A)** connects Wernicke's to Broca's area. The **diagonal band of Broca (B)** connects the septal (paraolfactory) area to the amygdala. The **tapetum (C)** is a posterior section of the corpus callosum connecting the temporal and occipital lobes. The **uncinate fasciculus (D)** connects the anterior temporal lobe to the orbitofrontal gyrus.[3]

62. C – Both
63. D – Neither

64. A – Paraventricular nucleus
65. B – Supraoptic nucleus
66. C – Both
67. A – Paraventricular nucleus

> The **supraoptic (B)** and **paraventricular (A)** nuclei of the hypothalamus are both located in the supraoptic region and synthesize vasopressin (antidiuretic hormone [ADH], arginine vasopressin [AVP]) and oxytocin. The supraoptic nucleus is comprised of uniformly large cells (magnocellular). The paraventricular nucleus contains a diverse group or neurons, some of which project to the brainstem and spinal cord. Neither of these structures is located in the tuberal region, which contains the arcuate nucleus, the dorsomedial nucleus, the ventromedial nucleus, and the lateral hypothalamic nucleus.[1]

68. C – Pseudobulbar palsy can result from unilateral lesions involving corticobulbar fibers (false)

> Pseudobulbar palsy (characterized by weakness of the muscles involved in chewing, swallowing, breathing, and speaking, with loss of emotional control) results from bilateral lesions of the corticobulbar fibers.[1]

69. B – Adduct the fingers

> **Adduction of the fingers (B)** is performed by the palmar interosseus muscles, innervated by the deep branch of the ulnar nerve. **Finger abduction (A)** is performed by the dorsal interossei, also innervated by the ulnar nerve. The lumbricals (median nerve) **flex the metacarpophalangeal joints while extending the interphalangeal joints (D)** of the 2nd–5th digits.[6]

70. C – Gluteus maximus

> The **gluteus maximus (C)** is innervated by the inferior gluteal nerve. A portion of the **adductor magnus (A)** is also innervated by the obturator nerve. The sciatic nerve innervates all muscles of the posterior compartment of the thigh including **biceps femoris (B)**, **semimembranosus (D)**, and **semitendinosus (E)**.[6]

71. B – Contralateral loss of pain and temperature in the face[2]

> The syndrome of PICA occlusion, or Wallenberg lateral medullary syndrome, is characterized by **contralateral pain and temperature loss over the body (A)**, **ipsilateral Horner's syndrome (D)**, **ipsilateral paralysis of the pharynx and larynx (C)**, and **hiccup (E)**. Ipsilateral, not contralateral, loss of pain and temperature in the face occurs in the syndrome of posteroinferior cerebellar artery (PICA) occlusion **(B is false)**.[7]

72. B – Genu of the internal capsule
73. C – Posterior limb of the internal capsule
74. A – Anterior limb of the internal capsule
75. C – Posterior limb of the internal capsule
76. D – None of the above

77. C – Posterior limb of the internal capsule

> The **anterior limb of the internal capsule (A)** contains the anterior thalamic radiation and the prefrontal corticopontine tract. The **genu of the internal capsule (B)** contains corticobulbar and corticoreticular fibers. The **posterior limb of the internal capsule (C)** contains the superior thalamic radiation, the frontopontine tract, corticospinal fibers, as well as corticorubral and corticotectal projections. The medial forebrain bundle is not part of the internal capsule.[3]

78. G – Spiral ganglion
79. E – Scarpa's ganglion
80. D – Otic ganglion
81. A – Ciliary ganglion
82. B – Gasserian ganglion
83. C – Geniculate ganglion
84. F – Sphenopalatine ganglion
85. H – Submandibular ganglion

> The **ciliary ganglion (A)** receives parasympathetic fibers of CN III and projects to the pupillary constrictor and ciliary muscle mediating the efferent limb of the pupillary light and accommodation reflexes. The **gasserian ganglion (B)** is also known as the semilunar or trigeminal ganglion and is associated with CN V, which provides sensory innervation to the face. The **geniculate ganglion (C)** is associated with the facial nerve, and transmits information regarding taste (chorda tympani) and visceral sensation from the middle ear, nasal cavity, and soft palate, as well as a small area of skin over the external auditory meatus. The **otic ganglion (D)** conveys parasympathetic messages transmitted by CN IX to the parotid gland. **Scarpa's ganglion (E)** includes the superior and inferior vestibular ganglia and is involved in equilibrium. The **sphenopalatine ganglion (F)** is also known as the pterygopalatine ganglion and transmits parasympathetics from the facial nerve (via the greater superficial petrosal nerve and vidian nerve) to the lacrimal gland and glands of the nasal cavity and palate. The **spiral ganglion (G)** is associated with the organ of Corti and transmits information regarding sound to the dorsal and ventral cochlear nuclei via CN XIII. The **submandibular ganglion (H)** transmits parasympathetic signals from the facial nerve (chorda tympani) to the submandibular and sublingual glands.[1]

86. A – Crossed and uncrossed fibers of the optic tract terminate on the lateral geniculate body (false)

> The lateral geniculate body is not involved in the pupillary light reflex.[1]

87. B – I, III (in the caudal aspect of the roof and in the lateral recess)

> Choroid plexus is located in the caudal aspect of the roof of the fourth ventricle near the midline, and laterally extends through the lateral recesses of Luschka.[4]

88. A – Adductor pollicis (false)

> The **adductor pollicis (A)** is innervated by the ulnar nerve. The other structures listed are innervated by the median nerve: **flexor carpi radialis (B)**, **opponens pollicis (C)**, **palmaris longus (D)**, and **pronator teres (E)**.[6]

89. A – I, II, III (amygdala, habenular nuclei, and hippocampus)

The **amygdala** participates in limbic modulation of the hypothalamus by two major pathways that project to the septal nuclei: the stria terminalis and the ventral amygdalofugal pathway. The **habenular nuclei** send projections to the septal nuclei via the stria medullaris thalami. The **hippocampus** projects to the septal area via the fornix.[1]

90. A – I, II, III (caudate nucleus, optic tract, and thalamus)[2]

The anterior choroidal artery supplies ventrolateral parts of the posterior limb of the internal capsule and the retrolenticular internal capsule, not the **anterior limb**. The anterior limb of the internal capsule is supplied by the lateral striate branches of the middle cerebral artery and the medial striate artery. The anterior choroidal artery may supply a portion of the tail of the **caudate** and a portion of the **thalamus** as well as the **optic tract**. The syndrome of anterior choroidal artery infarction consists of contralateral hemiplegia, hemihypesthesia, and homonymous hemianopia.[3,7]

91. E – Temporal half of the right visual field and nasal half of the left visual field

A lesion to the optic tract results in a contralateral homonymous hemianopsia **(E)**, which would affect the temporal half of the contralateral visual field and the nasal half of the ipsilateral visual field. **B** describes a left-sided homonymous hemianopsia, which would occur with a lesion to the right optic tract. **D** describes a bitemporal hemianopsia as typically occurs with chiasmal lesions with compression of crossing fibers from the nasal retina (temporal field). A lesion of the occipital cortex typically results in a homonymous hemianopsia with macular sparing.[1]

92. A – Cerebral cortex to globus pallidus

The striatum (caudate and putamen) represent the major input centers for the basal ganglia. There are no direct cortical projections from the cerebral cortex to the **globus pallidus (A is false). Cortical inputs to the basal ganglia (corticostriate fibers) terminate in the caudate and putamen (B)** and represent the principle input to the basal ganglia. Thalamostriate fibers are the second major input to the basal **ganglia arising in the intralaminar nucleus of the thalamus and projecting to the striatum (E)**. Subcortical structures such as the **subthalamic nucleus project to the globus pallidus (D)**. Dopaminergic nigrostriatal fibers project from the **substantia nigra to the caudate nucleus (C)** and have been implicated in the pathophysiology of Parkinson's disease.[1]

93. A – Amygdala

The **amygdala (A)** projects to the hypothalamus via two pathways, the stria terminalis and the ventral amygdalohypothalamic tract. This is not to be confused with the stria medullaris which projects from the **habenula (D)** to the septal nuclei and anterior hypothalamus.[1]

94. C – Inferior collicular commissure
95. B – Probst's commissure

96. A – Trapezoid body

> The **trapezoid body (A)** connects the ventral cochlear nuclei to the contralateral superior olive. **Probst's commissure (B)** connects the nuclei of the lateral lemniscus. The **inferior collicular commissure (C)** connects the inferior colliculi.[3]

97. D – Ventromedial hypothalamus
98. C – Posterior hypothalamus
99. A – Anterior hypothalamus
100. C – Posterior hypothalamus
101. C – Posterior hypothalamus
102. B – Lateral hypothalamus
103. A – Anterior hypothalamus

> The preoptic and anterior hypothalamus is involved in regulation of body temperature. Lesions to the **anterior hypothalamus (A)** can result in hyperthermia. Lesions to the **anterior hypothalamus (A)** can also result in decreased parasympathetic tone. The **lateral hypothalamus (B)**, or "feeding center," causes an increase in appetite when stimulated. The **posterior hypothalamus (C)** is responsible for sympathetic tone; lesions to this area can result in inability to regulate temperature (poikilothermia), decreased sympathetic tone, lethargy, and sleepiness. The **ventromedial nucleus (D)** of the hypothalamus is responsible for satiety—lesions here may produce hyperphagia and weight gain.[1]

104. D – Superior ganglion of CN IX
105. B – Jugular ganglion
106. C – Petrosal ganglion
107. A – Nodose ganglion

> The inferior ganglion of CN IX is called the **petrosal ganglion (B)** and receives input from the carotid sinus and body as well as from taste receptors in the posterior one-third of the tongue. The **superior ganglion of CN IX (D)** contains the cell bodies of neurons that provide general somatic sensory innervation to the pinna of the ear and a portion of the external acoustic meatus. The inferior ganglion of cranial nerve CN X is called the **nodose ganglion (A)** and receives taste and other visceral information. The superior ganglion of CN X is called the **jugular ganglion (B)** and houses the cell bodies of general somatic afferent neurons innervating a portion of the external acoustic meatus and tympanic membrane via the vagus nerve. Both superior ganglia are involved with somatic sensation.[1,3]

108. D – Globus pallidus (false)

> The telencephalon is the anterior-most portion of the prosencephalon and gives rise to the cerebral hemispheres. The hippocampal formation, cerebral hemispheres and cortex, as well as the **amygdala (A)**, **caudate (B)**, **putamen (E)**, and **claustrum (C)** are telencephalic structures. The caudal portion of the prosencephalon, the diencephalon, gives rise to the thalamus, **globus pallidus (D)**, posterior hypophysis, infundibulum, optic nerve, retina, posterior commissure, and habenular commissure.[1,3]

109. D – Musculocutaneous nerve

The **musculocutaneous nerve (D)** innervates the muscles of the anterior compartment of the arm including the coracobrachialis, biceps brachii, and brachialis muscles. The **axillary nerve (A)** innervates the teres minor and deltoid muscles. The **dorsal scapular nerve (B)** innervates the rhomboids. The **median nerve (C)** innervates the muscles of the anterior compartment of the forearm except the flexor carpi ulnaris and the ulnar half of the flexor digitorum profundus, as well as five hand intrinsics on the thenar aspect of the hand. The **suprascapular nerve (E)** innervates the supraspinatus and infraspinatus muscles.[6]

110. C – III

Cells that give rise to commissural fibers that interconnect homologous cortical areas via the corpus callosum are found in **layer III (C)** of the cerebral cortex (the external pyramidal layer). **Layer I (A)** is the plexiform molecular layer and consists mainly of nerve cell processes. **Layer II (B)** is the external granular layer comprised mostly of small granule cells. **Layer IV (D)**, the internal granular layer, is important for afferent signaling and is thicker in the primary sensory area. **Layer V (E)**, the internal pyramidal layer, is the source of the majority of output fibers for the cerebral cortex. Layer VI is the fusiform layer and lies adjacent to underlying white matter and consists primarily of association neurons.[1]

111. C – Neurons of the cerebral cortex

The neural crest is a narrow strip of cells at the edge of the developing neural plate that gives rise to several structures including, neurons of the **dorsal root ganglia of cranial and spinal nerves (B)**, **adrenal medulla (A)**, **melanocytes of the retina (D)**, Schwann cells, meninges, as well as the **sympathetic and parasympathetic ganglia (E)**. **Cortical neurons (C)** are derived from neuroectoderm that forms from the neural tube.[1]

112. D – Rhombencephalon to metencephalon to cerebellum

The primary brain divisions include the rhombencephalon (hindbrain), mesencephalon (midbrain), and prosencephalon (forebrain). The rhombencephalon gives rise to the myelencephalon and metencephalon. The prosencephalon gives rise to the diencephalon and telencephalon. The myelencephalon gives rise to the medulla and inferior cerebral peduncles. The metencephalon gives rise to the pons, cerebellum, and middle and superior cerebellar peduncles. The mesencephalon gives rise to the cerebral peduncles, midbrain tectum, and tegmentum. The diencephalon gives rise to the epithalamus, thalamus, and hypothalamus. The telencephalon gives rise to the cerebral hemispheres including the corpus striatum and rostral aspect of the hypothalamus. **D** is the only correct response.[1]

113. B – Globus pallidus and substantia nigra

Efferent transmission from the striatum is limited to only two targets: **the globus pallidus and substantia nigra (B)** via the striatopallidal fibers and striatonigral fibers. The striatum does not have any direct projections to the **amygdala (A, C) or thalamus (D, E)**.[1]

114. A – I, II, III (cranial nerves IX, X, and XI)

The nucleus ambiguous contributes fibers to cranial nerves IX, X, and XI, but not VII. The contribution of the nucleus ambiguous to the **glossopharyngeal nerve (IX)** is special visceral efferent fibers to the stylopharyngeus and pharyngeal constrictor muscles as well as receiving general visceral afferent input from the middle ear, pharynx, tongue, and carotid sinus. The nucleus ambiguous provides special visceral efferent fibers to the **vagus nerve (X)** for muscles of the larynx and pharynx. The nucleus ambiguous provides special visceral efferent fibers to the **spinal accessory nerve (XI)** for the control of laryngeal muscles. The **facial nerve (VII)** is not associated with the nucleus ambiguous.[1]

115. E – All of the above

Functional components of the facial nerve and nervus intermedius include **special visceral efferent fibers** to the muscles of facial expression and stapedius muscles, general visceral efferent (parasympathetic) fibers to the lacrimal and sublingual glands, **special visceral afferent** input from the anterior two-thirds of the tongue, **general visceral afferent** inputs from the middle ear, nasal cavity, and soft palate, as well as **general somatic afferents** from the external auditory meatus and posterior auricular area.[1]

116. E – Ventral to the mamillary bodies

The infundibular recess of the third ventricle is located in the floor of the third ventricle **ventral to the mamillary bodies (E)**.[3]

117. B – Bilateral partial deafness, greater in the contralateral ear

The majority of second-order neurons from the cochlear nuclei decussate in the trapezoid body to the contralateral superior olivary nucleus, while a smaller number of fibers ascend to the ipsilateral superior olivary nucleus. This bilateral input to the superior olivary nuclei contributes to sound localization and determination of directional intensity. The lateral lemniscus is the main ascending pathway of the auditory system in the brainstem. Due to the presence of both crossed and uncrossed fibers, a lesion to the lateral lemniscus causes **bilateral partial deafness, worse in the contralateral ear (B)**.[1]

118. B – III, IV, VI, and V1 only

The lateral sector of the superior orbital fissure (SOF) contains the **trochlear (IV), frontal (branch of V1)**, and **lacrimal nerves (branch of V1)**, which all pass outside the annular tendon of Zinn. The superior ophthalmic vein also passes inferior to the nerves in this portion of the fissure to reach the cavernous sinus. The central portion of the SOF (oculomotor foramen) contains the **oculomotor nerve (III), nasociliary nerve (branch of V1), abducens nerve (VI)**, and roots of the ciliary ganglion—all of which pass through the annulus of Zinn. The optic nerve and ophthalmic artery course medially to the oculomotor foramen passing through the optic foramen. The maxillary nerve (V2) exits the cranial vault via foramen rotundum before entering the orbit via the inferior orbital fissure, not the superior orbital fissure.[4]

119. D – Superior orbital fissure
120. D – Superior orbital fissure
121. A – Inferior orbital fissure
122. C – Foramen ovale
123. B – Foramen magnum

> The **superior orbital fissure (D)** transmits cranial nerves (CN) III, IV, V1, and VI. The **inferior orbital fissure (A)** transmits CN V2 (maxillary nerve) into the orbit after it has exited the skull via the foramen rotundum. The **foramen ovale (C)** transmits CN V3 (mandibular nerve), and the **foramen magnum (B)** transmits CN XI as it ascends to join the vagus nerve prior to exiting the skull through the jugular foramen.[1]

124. C – Nervi erigentes
125. B – Splanchnic nerve
126. A – Pudendal nerve

> The **pudendal nerve (A)** arises from S2, 3, and 4 and provides somatic innervation to the skin of the perineum and of the muscles of the perineum and pelvic floor including the external urethral and anal sphincters. The sacral **splanchnic nerves (B)** provide sympathetic innervation to the pelvis. The **nervi erigentes (C)**, or pelvic splanchnic nerves, provide parasympathetic innervation to the structures of the pelvis.[6]

127. A – Cochlear nucleus
128. E – Superior olivary nucleus
129. E – Superior olivary nucleus
130. E – Superior olivary nucleus

> First-order neurons of the auditory pathway project from the spiral ganglion and terminate in the ipsilateral **cochlear nucleus (A)**. Second-order fibers from the cochlear nucleus may either ascend to the ipsilateral superior olivary nucleus or decussate in the trapezoid body to form three acoustic striae: the dorsal, intermediate, and ventral acoustic striae. The **superior olivary nucleus (E)** projects third-order neurons into both the ipsilateral and bilateral **lateral lemniscus (C)**. The **inferior colliculus (B)** receives input from the lateral lemniscus and is involved in sound localization. The inferior colliculus then projects to the ipsilateral **medial geniculate nucleus (D)** via the brachium of the inferior colliculus. The medial geniculate nucleus gives off the auditory radiations, which project to the auditory cortex.[1]

131. A – I, II, III (hypothalamus, lateral preoptic region, septal nuclei)

> The stria medullaris thalami is a bidirectional pathway that connects the hypothalamus, preoptic region, and septal nuclei with the habenula. The stria medullaris does not contain fibers from the amygdala.[1]

132. A – Cells in the centromedian nucleus project to the caudate (false)

> Cells in the centromedian nucleus project to the putamen (**A is false**), and cells in the parafascicular nucleus project to the caudate. The other responses are true. Corticostriate projections use glutamate as their transmitter, nigrostriatal fibers arise from cells in the pars compacta, serotonergic projections arise from the dorsal nucleus of the raphe, and thalamostriate fibers arise largely from cells in the centromedian parafascicular nucleus.[1,2]

133. D – Spinal trigeminal nucleus
134. D – Spinal trigeminal nucleus
135. A – Mesencephalic nucleus
136. D – Spinal trigeminal nucleus
137. C – Principal sensory nucleus
138. A – Mesencephalic nucleus
139. C – Principle sensory nucleus

> The **mesencephalic nucleus (A)** is unique because it is a sensory ganglion containing the cell bodies of pseudounipolar neurons that are responsible for conveying proprioceptive information from the muscles of the face. The **motor nucleus of the trigeminal nerve (B)** contains the cell bodies of the neurons that innervate the muscles of mastication. **The principle sensory nucleus (C)** is homologous to the nucleus gracilis and nucleus cuneatus and sends the dorsal trigeminothalamic tract to the ipsilateral VPM of the thalamus, conveying tactile and pressure sense. The **spinal trigeminal nucleus (D)** is the largest of the trigeminal sensory nuclei, and consists of a pars oralis, pars interpolaris, and pars caudalis. The ventral trigeminothalamic tract carries projections from the main sensory nucleus to the thalamus regarding tactile and pressure sense, and carries projections from the **spinal trigeminal nucleus (D)** regarding pain and temperature sense. The **trigeminal ganglion (E)** houses cell bodies of pseudounipolar sensory neurons; it lies in Meckel's cave in the petrous temporal bone.[1]

140. A – They indirectly project to the ipsilateral cerebellar cortex.

> Efferent fibers from the dentate nucleus leave via the superior cerebellar peduncle (**C is false**), decussate in the caudal mesencephalon, and project to the contralateral red nucleus (**B and E are false**) and ventral lateral and ventral posterolateral thalamic nuclei (**D is false**). These thalamic nuclei then project to the primary motor cortex. Fibers forming the descending part of the superior cerebellar peduncle project to reticular nuclei and the inferior olivary nucleus, which in turn projects back to the ipsilateral cerebellar cortex (**A is true**).[1]

141. C – Sciatic nerve
142. D – Femoral nerve
143. A – Superior gluteal nerve

144. B – Inferior gluteal nerve

> The **superior gluteal nerve (A)** innervates gluteus medius, gluteus minimus, and the tensor of the fascia lata, which adduct and medially rotate the thigh. The **inferior gluteal nerve (B)** innervates gluteus maximus, which extends the thigh at the hip. The **sciatic nerve (C)** innervates no gluteal muscles, all muscles of posterior thigh, and all the muscles of the leg and foot. The adductor magnus is in the medial compartment of the thigh and is considered to be one of the five adductors of the thigh. The medial compartment of the thigh is innervated primarily by the obturator nerve. The adductor part of adductor magnus is innervated by the obturator nerve, but the hamstrings part of adductor magnus is innervated by the **sciatic nerve (C)**. The **femoral nerve (D)** innervates the muscles of the anterior thigh, which consist primarily of hip flexors and knee extensors such as pectineus, iliacus, sartorius, and quadriceps femoris (rectus femoris, vastus lateralis, vastus medialis, and vastus intermedius).[6]

145. C – Posterior cord
146. B – Medial cord
147. C – Posterior cord
148. A – Lateral cord
149. C – Posterior cord

> The **lateral cord (A)** is formed by the anterior divisions of the superior and middle trunks and gives rise to the lateral pectoral nerve, the musculocutaneous nerve, and the lateral root of the median nerve. The **medial cord (B)** consists of the anterior division of the inferior trunk and gives rise to the medial pectoral nerve, the medial cutaneous nerve of the arm, and the medial cutaneous nerve of the forearm; the **medial cord (B)** ultimately terminates into the ulnar nerve and the medial root of the median nerve. The **posterior cord (C)** receives contributions from the posterior divisions of the superior, middle, and inferior trunks, and ultimately branches into the axillary and radial nerves. The **posterior cord (C)** gives off the upper and lower subscapular nerves (teres major muscle) and the thoracodorsal nerve (latissimus dorsi muscle). The **radial nerve (D)** is the larger terminal branch of the posterior cord and innervates the extensor compartments of the arm and forearm. The **ulnar nerve (E)** is the larger terminal branch of the medial cord and innervates flexor carpi ulnaris, the ulnar half of flexor digitorum profundus, and most of the intrinsic muscles of the hand.[6]

150. B – In the thalamus, the extremities are represented dorsally and the back ventrally (false)

> The extremities are represented ventrally and the back dorsally in the thalamus **(B is false)**. The other statements regarding cerebellar projections to the thalamus are true. Fibers terminate on the ventral lateral and ventral posterolateral thalamic nuclei **(A)**, in the thalamus the head is represented medially and the caudal thorax represented laterally **(C)**, some fibers project to the rostral interlaminar nuclei **(D)**, and these fibers originate from the dentate and interposed nuclei **(E)**. Fibers from the fastigial nucleus project to either the lateral or inferior vestibular nuclei or the brainstem reticular formation.[1]

151. B – Centromedian nucleus of the thalamus[2]

> The **centromedian nucleus of the thalamus (B)** is most closely related to motor functions in that it receives input from the motor and premotor cortex and from the globus pallidus and projects mainly to the striatum. The other responses are considered part of the limbic system including the **amygdala (A)**, **epithalamus (C)**, **hypothalamus (D)**, and **septal nuclei (E)**.[1]

152. E – Ventral medulla

> Melanocytes are located in the pia mater and are concentrated in the region of the ventral medulla and upper spinal cord. These may represent the cells of origin for melanomas seen in patients with no history of primary skin melanoma.[8]

153. B – Contralateral loss of position and vibration

> Information regarding position and vibration is carried in the dorsal columns via first-order sensory neurons that then synapse in the nucleus gracilis or nucleus cuneatus. These second-order neurons decussate in the caudal medulla as the internal arcuate fibers before ascending in the medial lemniscus before synapsing in the ventral posterior lateral nucleus of the thalamus. A lesion to the medial lemniscus would cause **contralateral loss of position and vibration sense (B)**. A lesion to the dorsal columns at the level of the spinal cord would cause an **ipsilateral loss of position and vibration sense (D)**. The decussation for the spinothalamic tract (pain and temperature) occurs in the anterior commissure of the spinal cord, so a unilateral lesion to the spinal cord or brainstem would cause **contralateral loss of pain and temperature sensation (A)**.[9]

154. A – Fornix (false)

> The diencephalon is the caudal portion of the prosencephalon (forebrain) and gives rise to the epithalamus (**habenula [D]**, **stria medullaris [E]**, and **pineal gland [D]**), thalamus, and **hypothalamus (B)**. The telencephalon is the rostral portion of the prosencephalon and gives rise to the cerebral hemispheres including the hippocampal formation and **fornix (A)**.[1]

155. A – Maxillary branch of CN V
156. D – Abducens nerve
157. F – Middle meningeal artery
158. A – Maxillary branch of CN V
159. C – Mandibular branch of CN V
160. D – Abducens nerve
161. B – Nasopalatine nerve
162. E – Mental nerve

> The superior orbital fissure transmits cranial nerves (CN) III, IV, V1, and **VI (D)**. The inferior orbital fissure transmits **CN V2 (maxillary nerve [A])** into the orbit after it has exited the skull via foramen rotundum. The foramen ovale transmits **CN V3 (mandibular nerve [C])**. The **nasopalatine nerve (B)** traverses the incisive foramen and the **mental nerve (E)** traverses the mental foramen. The **middle meningeal artery (F)** enters the skull via foramen spinosum. The **abducens (D)** nerve traverses Dorello's canal as part of its long intracranial course.[1]

163. D – Medial vestibular nucleus
164. C – Lateral vestibular nucleus
165. A – Inferior vestibular nucleus
166. C – Lateral vestibular nucleus
167. D – Medial vestibular nucleus
168. E – Superior vestibular nucleus
169. B – Interstitial nucleus of the vestibular nerve
170. D – Medial vestibular nucleus

> The **inferior vestibular nucleus (A)** receives fibers from the inferior vestibular ganglion and sends projections to the reticular formation and cerebellum. **The interstitial nucleus of the vestibular nerve (B)** consists of cell bodies that lie among fibers of the vestibular root. The **lateral vestibular nucleus (C)**, Deiter's nucleus, receives input from the superior vestibular ganglion and forms the lateral vestibulospinal tract, which projects to all spinal levels and is responsible for extensor tone. The **medial vestibular nucleus (D)**, Schwalbe's nucleus, is the largest of the vestibular nuclei and sends projections to contralateral extraocular nuclei via the MLF. The **superior vestibular nucleus (E)**, Bechterew's nucleus, gives rise to uncrossed ascending fibers to the oculomotor and trochlear nuclei traveling in the MLF. Second-order vestibulocerebellar projections arise from the caudal aspect of the inferior cerebellar nucleus and the **medial vestibular nucleus (D)**.[1,2]

171. A – Mesencephalic nucleus
172. D – Spinal trigeminal nucleus
173. A – Mesencephalic nucleus
174. C – Principal sensory nucleus
175. D – Spinal trigeminal nucleus

> The **mesencephalic nucleus (A)** is unique because it is a sensory ganglion containing the cell bodies of pseudounipolar neurons that are responsible for conveying proprioceptive information from the muscles of the face; it is the most rostral of the nuclei listed. The **motor nucleus of the trigeminal nerve (B)** contains the cell bodies of the neurons that innervate the muscles of mastication. **The principal sensory nucleus (C)** is homologous to the nucleus gracilis and nucleus cuneatus and sends the dorsal trigeminothalamic tract to the ipsilateral VPM of the thalamus, conveying tactile and pressure sense; it receives ascending processes from trigeminal ganglion cells. The **spinal trigeminal nucleus (D)** is the largest of the trigeminal sensory nuclei and consists of a pars oralis, pars interpolaris, and pars caudalis. The pars caudalis of the **spinal trigeminal nucleus (D)** is the most caudal of the nuclei listed and receives descending fibers from the trigeminal ganglion cells. The ventral trigeminothalamic tract carries projections from the main sensory nucleus to the thalamus regarding tactile and pressure sense, and carries projections from the **spinal trigeminal nucleus (D)** regarding pain and temperature sense. The **trigeminal ganglion (E)** houses cell bodies of pseudounipolar sensory neurons. It lies in Meckel's cave in the petrous temporal bone.[1]

176. A – I, II, III (IX, X, and VII)

> The solitary tract is formed by visceral afferent fibers from the vagus, glosso-pharyngeal, and facial (intermediate) nerves. The hypoglossal nerve (CN XII) is associated with the hypoglossal nucleus, not the nucleus of the solitary tract.[1]

177. B – Hip flexion

> The femoral nerve innervates the muscles of the anterior thigh, which consist primarily of **hip flexors (B)** and knee extensors such as pectineus, iliacus, sartorius, and quadriceps femoris (rectus femoris, vastus lateralis, vastus medialis, and vastus intermedius).[6]

178. A – Anterior lobe of the pituitary

> The pars tuberalis, a part of the anterior pituitary (adenohypophysis), surrounds the lower portion of the pituitary stalk and is derived from Rathke's pouch, along with pars distalis and pars intermedia. The neurohypophysis (median eminence, pituitary stalk, and pars nervosa) arises from the infundibulum.[1]

179. E – Subthalamic nucleus

> The major output from the dentate nucleus is via the brachium conjuncti-vum to the contralateral VL nucleus of the thalamus. The VL sends projections to the motor and premotor areas of the cerebral cortex, which then project back to the **cerebellar cortex (A)**. A portion of the fibers leave the dentate nucleus via the brachium conjunctivum, decussate and synapse on the **red nucleus (C)**. The red nucleus then sends projections to the ipsilateral **inferior olivary nucleus (B)**. Indirect projections also arrive in the **reticulo-tegmental nucleus (D)**, so the dentate may participate in regulation of sac-cadic eye movements. The dentate nucleus does not send projections to the **subthalamic nucleus (E)**.[1,2]

180. C – II, IV (ventral lateral and ventral lateral posterior)

> The superior cerebellar peduncle contains mostly efferent fibers from the cer-ebellum including the dentorubrothalamic, interpositorubrothalamic (both in the brachium conjunctivum), fastigiothalamic, and fastigiovestibular tracts. The **ventral lateral (VL)** and **ventral anterior (VA)** nuclei serve as motor relay stations. The VL nucleus is divided into an anterior and posterior portion: ventral lateral anterior (VLa) and **ventral lateral posterior (VLp)**. The VLp receives projections from the contralateral dentate nucleus via the brachium conjunctivum. The VLp should not be confused with the ventral posterior lateral nucleus (VPL), which is a sensory relay station that receives spinotha-lamic inputs. The ventral anterior nucleus of the thalamus (VA) receives input from the substantia nigra and the globus pallidus, not the cerebellum. **The rostral intralaminar nuclei** receive their input from the ascending sensory systems and basal ganglia primarily, not the cerebellum.[1]

181. A – Amygdala

The **amygdala (A)** is part of the limbic system but not the limbic lobe. The limbic system consists of the limbic lobe plus all subcortical nuclei and pathways. The limbic lobe consists of the **cingulate gyrus (B)**, **subcallosal gyrus (E)**, **parahippocampal gyrus (D)**, and hippocampal formation. The hippocampal formation includes the **dentate gyrus (C)**, the hippocampus proper, and the subiculum.[1]

182. C – Ethmoid and vomer bones

The nasal septum is comprised of a bony part and a cartilaginous part. The bony nasal septum is comprised primarily of perpendicular plate of the ethmoid bone and the vomer bone.[6]

183. B – Abductor pollicis longus

The posterior interosseous nerve (PIN) is the motor branch of the radial nerve in the forearm providing innervation to all muscles located in the posterior compartment of the forearm including the **abductor pollicis longus (B)**. **The abductor pollicis brevis (A)** and **opponens pollicis (E)** are thenar muscles innervated by the recurrent branch of the median nerve. The **adductor pollicis (C)** is a thenar muscle innervated by the deep branch of the ulnar nerve. The anterior interosseous nerve, a branch of the median nerve, innervates the **flexor pollicis longus (D)**, the radial half of the flexor digitorum profundus, and the pronator quadratus.[6]

184. C – Great cerebral vein of Galen

The paired internal cerebral veins are formed by the union of the **thalamostriate (E)**, **choroidal (A)**, **septal (D)**, **epithalamic (B)**, and lateral ventricular veins. They run in the tela choroidea in the roof of the third ventricle before coursing over the thalamus into the quadrigeminal cistern where they join to contribute to the **vein of Galen (C)**.[3]

185. A – 17

The striate cortex refers to the primary visual cortex, **Brodmann's area 17 (A)**. **Areas 18 (B) and 19 (C)** are visual association cortex. **Areas 41 (D) and 42 (E)** are primary auditory cortex.[1]

186. A – I, II, III (anterior cerebral artery, middle cerebral artery, internal carotid artery)

The internal capsule receives blood supply from the **anterior cerebral artery** via the recurrent artery of Huebner, the **middle cerebral artery** via lenticulostriate perforators, and the **internal carotid artery** via the anterior choroidal artery. The **posterior cerebral artery** does not contribute to the internal capsule.[3]

187. E – Uncinate fasciculus
188. C – Cingulate fasciculus
189. B – Arcuate fasciculus
190. D – Corpus callosum

191. A – Anterior commissure

> The **anterior commissure (A)** connects the temporal lobes of the two hemi-spheres. The **arcuate fasciculus (B)** links Broca's area to Wernicke's area. The **cingulate fasciculus (C)** connects the anterior perforated substance to the parahippocampal gyrus. The **corpus callosum (D)** connects the bilateral cerebral hemispheres; the tapetum is a subset of fibers connecting the temporal and occipital lobes. The **uncinate fasciculus (E)** connects the anterior temporal lobe to the orbitofrontal gyrus.[1,3]

192. C – Brachium conjunctivum
193. D – Brachium pontis
194. A – Restiform body

> The **restiform (A)** and **juxtarestiform (B)** body make up the inferior cerebellar peduncle. The **restiform body (A)** contains afferent fibers from the spinal cord and brainstem. The **juxtarestiform body (B)** contains mostly afferent fibers but also some efferent fibers from the cerebellum. The **brachium conjunctivum (C)** travels in the superior cerebellar peduncle and represents the principle efferent pathway from the cerebellum (dentorubrothalamic and interpositorubrothalamic pathways). The **brachium pontis (D)** is the middle cerebellar peduncle and consists of afferent fibers from the pons—pontocerebellar fibers.[1,3]

195. B – Both eyes toward the lesion

> The abducens nucleus contains two subsets of neurons. One set is made up of motor neurons and projects to the ipsilateral lateral rectus muscle, and the other population is made up of interneurons that project to the contralateral oculomotor nucleus via the MLF. Therefore, damage to the abducens nucleus causes **lateral gaze paralysis ipsilateral to the side of the lesion (B)**. A lesion to the abducens nerve causes an **ipsilateral lateral rectus palsy (E)**. It is the only cranial nerve in which lesions of the root fibers and nucleus do not produce the same effects.[1]

196. C – Pterygopalatine ganglion

> Postganglionic parasympathetic fibers destined for the lacrimal gland are de-rived from the **pterygopalatine ganglion (C)**. Preganglionic parasympathetic fibers from the superior salivatory nucleus run in the nervus intermedius (along with pseudounipolar SVA taste fibers from the tongue and GSA fibers from the ear). The parasympathetics for the lacrimal gland run with the great-er superficial petrosal nerve, which branches in the facial canal proximal to the geniculate ganglion. The fibers of the GSPN join the fibers of the nerve of the pterygoid canal (vidian nerve) and synapse in the **pterygopalatine gan-glion (C)**. These fibers reach the lacrimal gland via the lacrimal nerve. The **geniculate ganglion (A)** is associated with general and special visceral affer-ent and general somatic afferent fibers traveling with the facial nerve and me-diates taste and nasopharyngeal sensation. The **otic ganglion (B)** transmits parasympathetic signals from the glossopharyngeal nerve (IX) to the parotid gland. The **submandibular (D)** and **sublingual (E)** ganglia convey parasym-pathetics transmitted from CN VII via the chorda tympani nerve.[1]

197. B – Globus pallidus (false)

> The substantia nigra sends projections to the **thalamus (E)**, the striatum (**caudate [A] and putamen [C]**), the **superior colliculus (D)**, and tegmental area. The substantia nigra does not send direct projections to the **globus pallidus (B)**.[1]

198. E – Tight junctions of capillary endothelium

> The blood–brain barrier is formed by tight junctions of capillary endothelium.[1]

199. D – Tectorial ligament

> The **tectorial ligament (D)** is the rostral extension of the posterior longitudinal ligament. The **anterior atlanto-occipital membrane (A)** is the rostral extension of the anterior longitudinal ligament. The **apical ligament (B)** extends from the tip of the dens to the basion. The **transverse ligament (E)** extends between the tubercles of the lateral masses of C1 and holds the dens against the anterior arch of C1. The **cruciate ligaments (C)** emerge from the transverse ligament, connecting the transverse ligament to the posterior basion and posterior body of C2.[3]

200. A – 3%
201. B – 30%
202. B – 30%
203. C – 40%
204. C – 40%

> Giant pyramidal cells, or Betz cells, make up approximately **3%** of corticospinal fibers and are located exclusively in primary motor cortex. Approximately **30%** arise from area 4, **30%** from area 6, and the remainder **(40%)** arise from the parietal lobe. Approximately **40%** of corticospinal tract axons are poorly myelinated.[1]

205. A – Anterior belly of the digastric muscle (false)

> The facial nerve innervates all of the muscles of facial expression including the **buccinator (B)** and **platysma (C)**. The facial nerve also innervates the posterior belly of the digastric, the **stylohyoid (E)**, and mylohyoid muscles. The nerve to the **stapedius (D)** leaves CN VII in the facial canal to innervate the stapedius muscle. CN V innervates the **anterior belly of the digastric (A)** and the muscles of mastication.[3]

206. C – Notochord

> The nucleus pulposus of the intervertebral disks are formed by **notochord remnants (C)**. Notochord remnants are also thought to be the cells of origin for chordomas.[3]

207. E – Pyriform cortex

> The **pyriform cortex (E)** (lateral olfactory gyrus) and periamygdaloid area constitute the primary olfactory cortex, and the **entorhinal cortex (B)** constitutes the secondary olfactory cortical area.[1]

208. A – Nucleus ambiguus[2,6]

> The ventral basal plate and dorsal alar plate are divided by the sulcus limitans. The basal plate tends to differentiate toward motor functions and the alar plate tends to differentiate toward sensory functions (**A**lar = **A**fferent). The **nucleus ambiguus (A)** contains special visceral efferent motor fibers involved in the swallowing reflex and is a basal plate derivative. The basal plate of the metencephalon gives rise to the nucleus of the abducens nerve, parasympathetics of the facial nerve, and motor nuclei of trigeminal and facial nerves. The alar plate of the metencephalon gives rise to the neurons of the **trigeminal (B, D)** and **vestibulocochlear (E)** nerves. Basal plate of the mesencephalon gives rise to the red nucleus, substantia nigra, oculomotor, and trochlear nuclei. The **nucleus of the tractus solitarius (C)** receives afferent fibers and is a product of the alar plate.[1]

209. A – Downgaze to the opposite side

> The trochlear nerve is unique because it is the only cranial nerve to originate totally from the contralateral nucleus and the only cranial nerve to emerge from the dorsal aspect of the brainstem. A lesion to the trochlear nerve causes an ipsilateral superior oblique palsy, while a lesion to the trochlear nucleus causes a contralateral superior oblique palsy. Normal contraction of the superior oblique muscle results in intorsion with simultaneous depression and lateral movement of the eye (down and out). This diplopia is exacerbated by downward, medial (contralateral) gaze, particularly when descending stairs or reading.[1]

210. A – Superior olive

211. B – Inferior olivary complex

> The **superior olivary nuclear complex (A)** is involved in the processing of auditory information and helps determine the direction that a sound is coming from and the sound's intensity. The **inferior olivary nucleus** (B) is a relay nucleus of the cortico-olivocerebellar pathway, functions as a cerebellar relay nucleus, and is important for learning new motor tasks.[1]

212. C – Both

213. A – Superior salivatory nucleus

214. B – Inferior salivatory nucleus

215. C – Both

216. A – Superior salivatory nucleus

> The **superior (A)** and **inferior (B) salivatory nuclei** both transmit general visceral efferent parasympathetic fibers and are located in the brainstem reticular formation. The **superior salivatory nucleus (A)** sends its fibers via the nervus intermedius of the facial nerve; a portion of its fibers travel to the pterygopalatine ganglion via the GSPN and vidian nerve, and another portion travels to the submandibular ganglion via the chorda tympani nerve. The **inferior salivatory nucleus (B)** sends its fibers with the lesser petrosal nerve of the glossopharyngeal nerve (IX) to ultimately reach the otic ganglion and parotid gland.[1]

217. C – Both
218. B – Sympathetic

The short ciliary nerves are mainly composed of parasympathetic fibers from the ciliary ganglion to the eye, but some sympathetic fibers are also present. The long ciliary nerves carry sympathetic fibers that mediate pupillary dilatation.[1]

219. C – Dorsal spinocerebellar tract
220. B – Cuneocerebellar tract
221. A – Anterior spinothalamic tract
222. E – Ventral spinocerebellar tract
223. D – Lateral spinothalamic tract
224. E – Ventral spinocerebellar tract
225. E – Ventral spinocerebellar tract

The **lateral spinothalamic tract (D)** arises from cells in laminae I, IV, and V, and transmits pain and temperature sensation. Fibers in this tract cross in the anterior white commissure, usually within one spinal segment. The **anterior spinothalamic tract (A)** also arises from cells in laminae I, IV, and V, and crosses in a decussation that involves several segments. It transmits light touch. The **dorsal spinocerebellar tract (C)** is uncrossed and arises from cells of the dorsal nucleus of Clarke (from C8 to L2). The ventral **spinocerebellar tract (E)** is crossed, whereas the **cuneocerebellar (B)** tract is uncrossed. The latter three tracts transmit unconscious exteroceptive impulses concerned with movement and posture. The **cuneocerebellar tract (B)** transmits impulses from the upper extremity, whereas the **dorsal spinocerebellar tract (C)** transmits impulses from the lower extremity.[2]

226. D – Tectospinal tract
227. B – Reticulospinal tract
228. A – Corticospinal tract
229. C – Rubrospinal tract
230. E – Vestibulospinal tract

The **corticospinal tract (A)** divides into a large crossed lateral corticospinal tract, small uncrossed anterior corticospinal tract, and a minute (~2% of fibers) uncrossed anterolateral corticospinal tract at the junction of the medulla and spinal cord. The **tectospinal tract (D)** arises from cells in the superior colliculus, terminates in the upper four cervical levels, and mediates reflex postural movements in response to visual stimuli. The **rubrospinal tract (C)** arises from the magnocellular region of the red nucleus, and its most important function is in the control of flexor muscle tone. The **vestibulospinal tract (E)** arises mainly from the lateral vestibular nucleus. This tract facilitates spinal reflex activity and spinal mechanisms that control extensor tone. The tectospinal and rubrospinal tracts are both crossed, whereas the vestibulospinal tract is uncrossed. The **reticulospinal tracts (B)** arise from the pontine tegmentum (pontine reticulospinal tract) and the medulla (medullary reticulospinal tract). The former is uncrossed, whereas the latter consists of crossed and uncrossed components. Stimulation of the brainstem reticular formation can facilitate and inhibit voluntary movement, cortically induced movement, and reflex activity, among other effects.[2]

231. D – Obturator nerve
232. E – Sciatic nerve
233. A – Deep peroneal nerve
234. G – Superior gluteal nerve
235. C – Inferior gluteal nerve
236. H – Tibial nerve
237. B – Femoral nerve
238. H – Tibial nerve
239. F – Superficial peroneal nerve
240. B – Femoral nerve

The **superior gluteal nerve (G)** innervates gluteus medius, gluteus minimus, and the tensor of the fascia lata, which adduct and medially rotate the thigh. The **inferior gluteal nerve (C)** innervates gluteus maximus, which extends the thigh at the hip. The **sciatic nerve (E)** innervates no gluteal muscles, all muscles of posterior thigh, and all the muscles of the leg and foot (via its branches). The adductor magnus is in the medial compartment of the thigh and is considered to be one of the five adductors of the thigh. The medial compartment of the thigh is innervated primarily by the **obturator nerve (D)**. The adductor part of adductor magnus is innervated by the obturator nerve, but the hamstrings part of adductor magnus is innervated by the **sciatic nerve (E)**. The **femoral nerve (B)** innervates the muscles of the anterior thigh, which consist primarily of hip flexors and knee extensors such as iliopsoas, pectineus, iliacus, sartorius, and quadriceps femoris (rectus femoris, vastus lateralis, vastus medialis, and vastus intermedius). A portion of the adductor magnus is also innervated by the obturator nerve. The sciatic nerve branches into the **tibial nerve (H)**, which supplies the muscles of the posterior compartment of the leg such as gastrocnemius and flexor digitorum longus, and the **peroneal nerve**. The peroneal nerve has a superficial and a deep branch. The **superficial peroneal nerve (F)** supplies the muscles of the lateral compartment of the leg such as peroneus longus and brevis. The **deep peroneal nerve (A)** supplies the muscles of the anterior compartment of the leg including the extensor hallucis longus.[6]

241. C – Both

Molecules also move across the blood–brain barrier by diffusion. Substances that cross the blood–brain barrier by diffusion include water and alcohol. D-glucose and large neutral amino acids are transported into the brain by carrier-mediated transport. Active transport is used to move weak organic acids, halides, and extracellular K^+ from the brain and cerebrospinal fluid into plasma.[2]

242. A – Arcuate nucleus to median eminence

The tuberohypophysial or tuberoinfundibular tract arises from the tuberal region (mainly the arcuate nucleus) and can be traced to the **median eminence (A)** and infundibular stem where hormones are released into the hypophyseal portal system. The supraopticohypophyseal tract carries oxytocin or vasopressin from the **supraoptic and periventricular nuclei to the posterior hypophysis (E)**.[1]

243. A – Apical ligament
244. B – Alar ligaments
245. C – Dentate ligaments
246. D – Tectorial membrane
247. G – Anterior atlanto-occipital membrane
248. H – Transverse ligament
249. E – Superior cruciate ligaments
250. F – Inferior cruciate ligaments

The **tectorial membrane (D)** is the rostral extension of the posterior longitudinal ligament. The **anterior atlanto-occipital membrane (G)** is the rostral extension of the anterior longitudinal ligament. The **apical ligament (A)** extends from the tip of the dens to the basion. The **alar ligament (B)** extends from the dens to the lateral foramen magnum. The **transverse ligament (H)** extends between the tubercles of the lateral masses of C1 and holds the dens against the anterior arch of C1. The **cruciate ligaments** emerge from the transverse ligament, connecting the transverse ligament to the posterior basion (**superior cruciate ligaments [E]**) and posterior body of C2 (**inferior cruciate ligaments [F]**). The **dentate ligaments (C)** are bilateral extensions of pia connecting the lateral spinal cord to the dura.[3]

251. C – Paraventricular nucleus

Descending hypothalamic autonomic fibers arise from multiple hypothalamic nuclei, but the principle source of these descending autonomic fibers is the parvocellular part of the **paraventricular nucleus (C)**. Some of the paraventricular neurons project to both sympathetic and parasympathetic targets. The **mammillary nucleus (A)** is associated with the processing of information related to emotional expression. The **medial preoptic nucleus (B)** regulates the release of reproductive hormones from the adenohypophysis. The **periventricular nucleus (D)** produces hypothalamic releasing and inhibiting hormones. The **supraoptic nucleus (E)** contributes to the production of ADH and oxytocin.[1]

252. E – T1-L2 of the spinal cord (false)

The hypothalamus sends descending autonomic projections to a variety of structures. Fibers from the posterior and lateral hypothalamus project to the preganglionic sympathetic neurons from T1-L2 of the spinal cord to provide sympathetic control (**E is false**). Fibers from the anterior and medial hypothalamus project to the **Edinger-Westphal nucleus (B)**, the **superior and inferior salivatory nuclei (D)**, the **dorsal motor nucleus of vagus (A)**, and the **S2-S4 parasympathetic nucleus (C)** to drive parasympathetic control.[1]

253. B – Parasympathetic system
254. B – Parasympathetic system
255. B – Parasympathetic system
256. A – Sympathetic system
257. A – Sympathetic system
258. B – Parasympathetic system

259. B – Parasympathetic system

> The hypothalamus sends descending autonomic projections to a variety of structures. Fibers from the posterior and lateral hypothalamus project to the preganglionic sympathetic neurons from T1-L2 of the spinal cord to provide **sympathetic control (A)**. Fibers from the anterior and medial hypothalamus project to the Edinger-Westphal nucleus, the superior and inferior salivatory nuclei, the dorsal motor nucleus of vagus, and the S2-S4 parasympathetic nucleus to drive **parasympathetic control (B)**.[1]

260. B – Second-order neurons as the internal arcuate fibers

> In the dorsal column–medial lemniscal system, first-order neurons terminate in the nucleus gracilis and cuneatus, where the cell bodies of second-order neurons are located. These second-order neurons form the **internal arcuate fibers (B)** that curve ventromedially and decussate through the reticular formation. These same second-order neurons then ascend in the caudal medulla as the **medial lemniscus (D)**, ultimately synapsing with third-order neurons in the ventral posterior lateral nucleus of the thalamus. Fibers of the spinothalamic tract decussate as second-order neurons in the **anterior white commissure (A)** of the spinal cord. The **lateral lemniscus (C)** contains both second- and third-order neurons, and is the major ascending auditory pathway in the brainstem. The **pyramidal decussation (E)** is associated with the descending motor system.[1]

261. C – Leptomeninges of ventral medulla

> Melanocytes are most often found in the **leptomeninges of the ventral medulla (C)** and cervical cord. These are the presumed cells of origin for focal or disseminated CNS melanoma when there is no history of a primary skin lesion. The pigmentation in the **substantia nigra (D)** is due to accumulation of neuromelanin, a catecholamine waste product, in dopaminergic neurons. The other responses are incorrect.

262. D – Global aphasia (false)

> The deficits seen in injuries to the nondominant hemisphere may be due, in part, to deficits of perception and attention. These patients may be unaware of their deficit **(anosognosia [A])**. They may also neglect objects and persons on the contralateral side of their body or contralateral visual field **(contralateral hemi-neglect [B])**. **Disorientation to time and direction (C)** is characteristic, and may even occur when the patient is oriented to person and place. **Visuospatial problems (E)** are common including difficulty remembering shapes and even faces (prosopagnosia). True aphasias are associated with injury to the dominant hemisphere **(D is false)**.[7]

263. B – Projections of first-order neurons form Lissauer's tract (dorsolateral fasciculus)

The anterolateral system transmits information about pain, temperature, and crude touch to the brain. The first-order fibers consist mainly of **thinly myelinated, fast conducting A-delta fibers (E is false)** and **unmyelinated, slow conducting C fibers (D is false)**. These first-order pseudounipolar neurons enter the dorsal horn and **form the tract of Lissauer or dorsolateral fasciculus (B)**, which ascend or descend one to three spinal levels. The **second-order neurons then decussate in the anterior white commissure (A is false)** before ascending to their targets. The **anterolateral system does not interact with Clarke's column (nucleus dorsalis)**, which is located in lamina VII of spinal cord levels C8-L2,3 and is involved in proprioception **(C is false).**[1]

264. B – Clarke's column and dorsal spinocerebellar tract

Proprioceptive information from the trunk and lower limb is carried by first-order pseudounipolar neurons to the **nucleus dorsalis (Clarke's column)**, which is located in lamina VII of spinal cord levels C8-L2,3. Clarke's column contains second-order neurons that project rostrally to form the **dorsal spinocerebellar tract (B)**. Lower limb proprioception is carried in the lateral Clarke's column neurons, not in the **posterior columns (A)**. The **nucleus cuneatus and cuneocerebellar tract (C)** carry proprioceptive information from the neck and upper limbs to the cerebellum. The **nucleus of Clarke homologue in the cervical region and the rostral spinocerebellar tract (E)** carry proprioceptive information from the head and upper limb to the cerebellum. **Choice B** is a better answer than **choice D.**[1,3]

265. C – Is a thin bundle of unmyelinated fibers (false)

The mammillothalamic tract, also known as the **tract of Vicq d'Azyr (A)**, is a **heavily myelinated (C is false)** bundle of fibers that projects from the medial and lateral mammillary nucleus of the **mammillary body to the anterior nuclear group of the thalamus (D)**. The **Papez circuit (B)** consists of the hippocampus, fornix, mammillary body, mammillothalamic tract, anterior nucleus of the thalamus, and cingulated gyrus. The mammillothalamic tract can be a **useful landmark during planning for subthalamic nucleus targeting (E)**, as it is usually situated at the level of the anterior border of the STN.[1,5]

266. C – Interpeduncular and chiasmatic cistern

On pneumoencephalogram, air is prevented from ascending in the subarachnoid space around the optic chiasm by a thick layer of arachnoid, Liliequist's membrane. The two cisterns separated by the membrane of Liliequist are the **chiasmatic cistern and the interpeduncular cistern (C).**[10]

267. D – Lamina terminalis
268. A – Choroid fissure
269. E – Velum interpositum
270. B – Foramen of Luschka

271. C – Foramen of Magendie

> This is a list of structures that separate portions of the ventricular system from the subarachnoid cisterns. The crural cistern and temporal horn of the lateral ventricle meet at the choroid fissure **(A)**, where they are separated by the arachnoid and a single pial layer—the anterior and lateral posterior choroidal arteries traverse the choroid fissure to supply the choroid plexus. The lateral recess of the fourth ventricle opens into the lateral cerebellomedullary cistern through the **foramen of Luschka (B)**; a fine incomplete arachnoid membrane is present here. The fourth ventricle opens in the midline into the cisterna magna via the **foramen of Magendie (C)**. A thin membrane containing neural elements, the **lamina terminalis (D)**, separates the lamina terminalis cistern from the anterior part of the third ventricle. The cistern of the velum interpositum and third ventricle are separated by arachnoid and ependyma **(the velum interpositum [E])**. The velum interpositum cistern contains the medial posterior choroidal arteries and internal cerebral veins.[10]

References

1. Patestas MA, Gartner LP. A Textbook of Neuroanatomy. Malden, MA: Blackwell Publishing; 2006
2. Carpenter MB. Core Text of Neuroanatomy, 4th ed. Baltimore, MD: Williams & Wilkins; 1991
3. Citow JS, Macdonald RL, Refai D, eds. Comprehensive Neurosurgery Board Review. New York: Thieme Medical Publishers; 2009
4. Rhoton AL. Cranial Anatomy and Surgical Approaches. Philadelphia: Lippincott, Williams, and Wilkins; 2013
5. Quinones-Hinojosa A, ed. Schmidek & Sweet Operative Neurosurgical Techniques, 6th ed. Philadelphia, PA: Elsevier; 2012
6. Moore KL, Dalley AF. Clinically Oriented Anatomy, 5th ed. Baltimore, MD: Lippincott Williams and Williams; 2006
7. Ropper AH, Brown RH. Principles of Neurology, 8th ed. New York: McGraw-Hill; 2005
8. Miller DC. Modern Surgical Neuropathology. New York: Cambridge University Press; 2009
9. Blumenfeld H. Neuroanatomy through Clinical Cases, 2nd ed. Sunderland, MA: Sinauer Associates; 2011
10. Yasargil MG. Microneurosurgery, Volume I. New York: Thieme; 1984

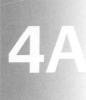 **Neurobiology—Questions**

For questions **1** to **5**, match the substances with the description.
- **A.** Bone growth factors
- **B.** Recombinant human bone morphogenic proteins
- **C.** Both
- **D.** Neither

1. A strong mitogen

2. A potent inducer of bone cell differentiation

3. Act on differentiated mesenchymal cells of the chondro-osseous lineage

4. Act on undifferentiated mesenchymal cells

5. Polypeptides

6. Which of the following is the correct representation of the subunits of the acetyl-choline (ACh) receptor at the neuromuscular junction?
   - **A.** $\alpha\beta\gamma\delta$
   - **B.** $\alpha 2\beta\gamma\delta$
   - **C.** $\alpha\beta 2\gamma\delta$
   - **D.** $\alpha\beta\gamma 2\delta$
   - **E.** $\alpha\beta\gamma\delta 2$

7. Which of the following is true of the α subunit of the nicotinic acetylcholine receptor?
   - **A.** It contains four hydrophobic transmembrane portions.
   - **B.** The binding site is not located on the α subunit.
   - **C.** The cytoplasmic loop is the most highly conserved portion of the subunit.
   - **D.** The N terminal is extracellular, and the C terminal is intracellular.
   - **E.** The transmembrane portion is the least conserved segment.

8. The number of binding sites on the nicotinic acetylcholine receptor is
   A. 1
   B. 2
   C. 3
   D. 4
   E. 5

⇨ For questions **9** and **10**, match the description with the receptor.
   A. α subunit of GABA$_A$ receptor
   B. β subunit of GABA$_A$ receptor
   C. Both
   D. Neither

9. Binds γ-aminobutyric acid (GABA)

10. Binds benzodiazepines

⇨ For questions **11** to **16**, match the receptor with the description. Each response may be used once, more than once, or not at all.
   A. GABA receptor
   B. Glutamate receptor
   C. Glycine receptor
   D. Nicotinic ACh receptor
   E. Serotonin (5-HT) receptor

11. Most closely linked with synaptic plasticity and cell death

12. GABA and this receptor are permeable to chloride ions

13. Binds strychnine

14. Binds benzodiazepine

15. One type of this receptor is both ligand and voltage regulated

16. One type of this receptor is blocked by magnesium ions

⇨ For questions **17** to **21**, match the description with the receptor.
   A. Kainate receptor only
   B. N-methyl-ᴅ-aspartate (NMDA) receptor only
   C. Quisqualate/α-amino-3-hydroxy-5-methyl-4-isoxazoleproprionic acid (AMPA) receptor only
   D. **A** and **B**
   E. **A**, **B**, and **C**

17. Significantly permeable to calcium ions

18. Permeable to monovalent cations

19. Ligand-gated

20. Voltage-gated

21. Blocked by magnesium ions

22. Which of the following is true of acetylcholine (ACh) release from the neuromuscular junction?
A. One molecule of ACh equals 10,000 quanta
B. One quanta contains 10,000 molecules of ACh
C. One quanta equals 1 molecule of ACh
D. One vesicle contains 10,000 quanta
E. One vesicle contains 10 molecules

23. Pro-opiomelanocortin is a precursor of
   I. Adrenocorticotropic hormone (ACTH)
   II. α-melanocyte-stimulating hormone (MSH)
   III. β-endorphin
   IV. β-lipotropin
A. I, II, III
B. I, III
C. II, IV
D. IV
E. All of the above

24. Removal of calcium ions from the cytosol in a presynaptic nerve terminal following an action potential is thought to occur by
   I. Active transport
   II. Binding to cytosolic proteins
   III. Transport into intracellular calcium storage vesicles
   IV. Reversal of flow through voltage-gated calcium channels
A. I, II, III
B. I, III
C. II, IV
D. IV
E. All of the above

25. Each of the following occurs in phototransduction *except*
A. Activated rhodopsin activates a G protein.
B. Activation of cyclic guanosine monophosphate (cGMP) phosphodiesterase increases hydrolysis of cGMP to 5′-GMP.
C. Current through a cGMP-activated sodium channel decreases.
D. Rhodopsin is activated when light converts bound 11-*cis*-retinal to all-*trans*-retinal.
E. The decreased concentration of cGMP results in depolarization of the plasma membrane.

26. Each of the following is true of G proteins *except*
A. Each G protein is regulated by only one type of receptor.
B. Each G protein may regulate multiple effectors.
C. The α subunit binds guanosine triphosphate (GTP).
D. The β and γ subunits help anchor the α subunit to the plasma membrane.
E. The β and γ subunits modulate guanosine diphosphate (GDP)/GTP exchange.

⇨ For questions **27** to **33**, match the second messenger with the description. Each response may be used once, more than once, or not at all.

- **A.** Calcium
- **B.** 1,2-Diacylglycerol (DAG)
- **C.** Cyclic adenosine monophosphate (cAMP)
- **D.** Cyclic guanine monophosphate (cGMP)
- **E.** Inositol-1,4,5-trisphosphate (IP3)
- **F.** B and E

27. D1 receptors act by this second messenger

28. Increased by nitric oxide

29. Generated by the action of phospholipase C

30. Synergistically activates protein kinase C with calcium

31. Binds to calmodulin

32. Photoreception utilizes this second messenger

33. Opens a calcium channel in the endoplasmic reticulum, releasing free calcium into the cytosol

34. Each of the following is true of the Na$^+$/K$^+$ pump *except* that it

- **A.** Contributes to the resting potential of the cell
- **B.** Hyperpolarizes the membrane
- **C.** Is electrogenic
- **D.** Transports three Na$^+$ ions out for two K$^+$ ions in
- **E.** Utilizes two molecules of adenosine triphosphate (ATP) for every three Na$^+$ ions transported

35. Each of the following is true of events occurring during the action potential *except*

- **A.** A sudden increase in conductance of Na results in depolarization.
- **B.** Chloride permeability increases during depolarization.
- **C.** During hyperpolarization, the conductance of Na is lower than normal, and the conductance of K is higher than normal.
- **D.** The decrease in Na permeability, occurring as the action potential reaches a peak, results from inactivation of Na channels.
- **E.** The presence of voltage-dependent K channels is to allow faster repolarization.

36. The velocity of an action potential increases with a

- **A.** High transmembrane resistance, low internal resistance, and high membrane capacitance
- **B.** High transmembrane resistance, low internal resistance, and low membrane capacitance
- **C.** Low transmembrane resistance, high internal resistance, and high membrane capacitance
- **D.** Low transmembrane resistance, low internal resistance, and high membrane capacitance
- **E.** Low transmembrane resistance, low internal resistance, and low membrane capacitance

37. Which of the following is true of myelination?
A. It has no effect on transmembrane resistance but increases membrane capacitance.
B. It decreases both transmembrane resistance and membrane capacitance.
C. It decreases transmembrane resistance and increases membrane capacitance.
D. It increases transmembrane resistance and decreases membrane capacitance.
E. It increases both transmembrane resistance and membrane capacitance.

For questions **38** to **40**, match the description with the potential.
A. End-plate potential
B. Miniature end-plate potential
C. Both
D. Neither

38. Usually depolarizes muscle cells past threshold

39. Occurs in unstimulated cells

40. Produces a miniature action potential

41. Inhibitory postsynaptic potentials are produced when a transmitter opens channels permeable to
A. Cl^- only
B. Cl^- or K^+
C. Na^+ only
D. Na^+ or Cl^-
E. Na^+ or K^+

42. Which of the following is true of axonal transport?
A. Dynamin does not use ATP.
B. Dynein is the motor for anterograde fast axonal transport.
C. Fast axonal transport occurs primarily along neurofilaments.
D. Kinesin is the motor for retrograde fast axonal transport.
E. Slow axonal transport occurs at 200 to 400 mm/day.

For questions **43** to **52**, match the description with the structure.
A. Golgi tendon organ
B. Muscle spindle
C. Both
D. Neither

43. Discharge increases with passive stretch

44. Discharge increases with active contraction

45. In series with extrafusal fibers

46. In parallel with extrafusal fibers

47. Sensitive to muscle tension

48. Sensitive to muscle length and velocity of length change

49. Innervated by group I (large myelinated) fibers

50. Innervated by group II (small myelinated) fibers

51. Conduction velocity of afferent fibers is > 120 m/s.

52. Contains dynamic nuclear bag, static nuclear bag, and nuclear chain fibers

53. Each of the following is true of decerebrate rigidity *except*
  - **A.** It results from tonic activity in the vestibulospinal and pontine reticulospinal neurons.
  - **B.** It is reduced by cutting dorsal roots.
  - **C.** It is reduced by destruction of the anterior lobe of the cerebellum.
  - **D.** It occurs with transection between the colliculi.
  - **E.** There is increased gamma motor neuron activity.

⇨ For questions **54** to **59**, match the reflex or response with the description. Each answer may be used once, more than once, or not at all.
  - **A.** Clasp-knife response
  - **B.** Flexion reflex
  - **C.** F response
  - **D.** H response
  - **E.** M response
  - **F.** Stretch reflex

54. An antidromic wave in motor fibers traveling to anterior horn cells

55. Has phasic and tonic components

56. A protective reflex involving polysynaptic reflex pathways

57. The electrical equivalent of the tendon reflex

58. The direct motor response obtained by stimulating a mixed motor sensory nerve

59. A length-dependent change in muscle force when the limb is passively moved

60. Contraction of the detrusor muscle of the bladder is achieved through activation of
  - **A.** Parasympathetic fibers from T9 to L1
  - **B.** Parasympathetic fibers from S2 to S4
  - **C.** Sympathetic fibers from T9 to L1
  - **D.** Sympathetic fibers from S2 to S4
  - **E.** Pudendal nerves

61. Which is true of events occurring after a typical axon is severed?
  - **A.** Chromatolysis is always associated with decreased protein synthesis.
  - **B.** Retraction bulbs form only at the proximal end of the cut nerve.
  - **C.** Terminal degeneration leads to the loss of presynaptic terminals.
  - **D.** Wallerian degeneration occurs before terminal degeneration.
  - **E.** Wallerian degeneration leads to loss of the proximal axon segment.

62. Agents that increase the formation of cerebrospinal fluid (CSF) include
  I.   Carbon dioxide
  II. Norepinephrine
  III. Volatile anesthetic agents
  IV. Carbonic anhydrase inhibitors
  A. I, II, III
  B. I, III
  C. II, IV
  D. IV
  E. All of the above

63. The main neurotransmitter of the Renshaw cell is thought to be
  A. Acetylcholine
  B. GABA
  C. Glutamate
  D. Glycine
  E. Histamine

⇨ For questions **64** to **68**, match the wave in the brainstem auditory evoked response with the structure with which it is most closely associated. Each response may be used once, more than once, or not at all.
  A. Wave I
  B. Wave II
  C. Wave III
  D. Wave IV
  E. Wave V

64. Auditory nerve

65. Cochlear nuclei

66. Inferior colliculus

67. Lateral lemniscus

68. Superior olivary nucleus

⇨ For questions **69** to **72**, match the wave in the somatosensory evoked potential with the description. Each response may be used once, more than once, or not at all.
  A. Erb's point
  B. N11
  C. N13/P13
  D. N19
  E. P22

69. Absence or delay implies cervical cord disease

70. Absence or delay implies peripheral nerve disease

71. Absence or delay implies a lesion in the lower medulla

72. Is found at the shoulder

➡ For questions **73** to **75**, match the rate of cerebral blood flow with the description. Each response may be used once, more than once, or not at all.

    A.   75 mL/100 g/min
    B.   55 mL/100 g/min
    C.   23 mL/100 g/min
    D.   17 mL/100 g/min
    E.   8 mL/100 g/min

73. Critical threshold below which functional impairment occurs

74. Irreversible infarction occurs below this flow rate

75. Normal cerebral blood flow

➡ For questions **76** to **83**, match the cerebellar cortical cell with the description. Each response may be used once, more than once, or not at all.

    A.   Basket cells
    B.   Golgi cells
    C.   Granule cells
    D.   Purkinje cells
    E.   Stellate cells

76. Axons of these cells mainly compose the molecular layer

77. Reside in the granular layer together with granule cells

78. Excitatory

79. Mossy fibers synapse here

80. Climbing fibers synapse here

81. The only cerebellar cortical output

82. Directly inhibit Purkinje cells together with stellate cells

83. Utilize glutamate

84. Which is true of the macule of the utricle and saccule when the head is held erect?

    A.   The utricular macule is oriented horizontally, and the saccular macule is oriented vertically.
    B.   The utricular macule is oriented vertically, and the saccular macule is oriented horizontally.
    C.   They are both oriented horizontally.
    D.   They are both oriented vertically.
    E.   None of the above is true.

85. The sensation of sharp, pricking pain is mediated by

    A.   Aα fibers
    B.   Aβ fibers
    C.   Aγ fibers
    D.   Aδ fibers
    E.   C fibers

86. Which is true of synaptic transmission in automatic ganglia?
   A. Neuronal ACh receptors contain four types of subunits.
   B. The slow excitatory postsynaptic potential (EPSP) is produced by muscarinic receptors closing Na^+ and Ca^{2+} channels while opening K^+ channels.
   C. The slow inhibitory postsynaptic potential (IPSP) is mediated by activation of muscarinic receptors that close K^+ channels.
   D. The fast EPSP is mediated by nicotinic ACh receptors.
   E. Peptides are never co-released with ACh.

87. Each of the following is true of the neural innervation of the bladder *except*
   A. Increased postganglionic sympathetic activity results in bladder wall contraction.
   B. Increased postganglionic sympathetic activity results in α-adrenergic inhibition of parasympathetics in the pelvic ganglion.
   C. Motor neurons in the ventral horn of the sacral spinal cord innervate the external sphincter.
   D. Parasympathetic activity promotes bladder emptying.
   E. The internal sphincter is innervated by sympathetic fibers.

88. Fibers from the superior salivatory nucleus synapse in the
   I.   Pterygopalatine ganglion
   II.   Geniculate ganglion
   III.   Submandibular ganglion
   IV.   Trigeminal ganglion
   A. I, II, III
   B. I, III
   C. II, IV
   D. IV
   E. All of the above

89. Ipsilateral cortico-cortical association fibers arise from cells in cortical layers
   A. I and II
   B. II and III
   C. III and IV
   D. IV and V
   E. V and VI

90. As the membrane of a motor neuron becomes increasingly depolarized,
   A. Both EPSP and IPSP decrease
   B. Both EPSP and IPSP increase
   C. EPSP decreases and IPSP increases
   D. EPSP increases and IPSP decreases
   E. There is no change in IPSP, but EPSP increases

91. Each of the following is true of Renshaw cells *except* that
   A. They are part of a negative feedback loop to the motor neurons.
   B. They facilitate Ia inhibitory interneurons that act on antagonist motor neurons.
   C. They inhibit motor neurons that innervate synergist muscles.
   D. They make divergent connections to motor neurons.
   E. They receive input from descending pathways.

⇨ For questions **92** to **96**, match the nucleus with the description. Each response may be used once, more than once, or not at all.

   A. Inferior vestibular nucleus
   B. Lateral vestibular nucleus
   C. Medial vestibular nucleus
   D. Superior vestibular nucleus
   E. None of the above

92. Involved in the control of posture

93. This nucleus and the medial vestibular nucleus are involved in mediating vestibulo-ocular reflexes

94. Also known as Deiters' nucleus

95. Integrates input from the vestibular labyrinth and the cerebellum

96. Decerebrate rigidity is due to the unopposed excitatory effect of the reticulospinal tract and the tract originating from this nucleus

97. Which of the following modifications of proteins does not occur in the Golgi complex?
   A. Attachment of fatty acids
   B. Formation of O-linked sugars
   C. Initiation of N-linked glycosylation
   D. Sugar phosphorylation
   E. Sulfation of tyrosine residues

⇨ For questions **98** to **104**, match the toxin with the description. Each response may be used once, more than once, or not at all.

   A. Binds to the ACh receptor
   B. Blocks reuptake of dopamine
   C. Blocks voltage-gated K^+ channels
   D. Blocks voltage-gated Na^+ channels
   E. Depletes norepinephrine (NE) from vesicles
   F. Inhibits GTP hydrolysis
   G. Prevents presynaptic release of quanta of ACh

98. α-bungarotoxin

99. Botulinum

100. Cholera

101. Cocaine

102. Reserpine

103. Tetraethylammonium (TEA)

104. Tetrodotoxin

105. At the equilibrium potential of potassium,
   A. The electrical force equals the chemical force
   B. The net electrical force is zero
   C. The net chemical force is zero
   D. There is no movement of K^+ ions across the membrane
   E. None of the above

106. Each of the following is true of G protein activation and deactivation *except*
    A. Activation of any G protein will inhibit the activation of other G proteins in the membrane
    B. Hydrolysis of bound GTP to GDP inactivates a G protein
    C. The βγ subunit stabilizes the binding of GDP
    D. The βγ subunit stabilizes the binding of GTP
    E. When activated, the α subunit's affinity for the βγ subunit decreases

107. The effect of succinylcholine at the neuromuscular junction is
    A. Amplified by increased muscle temperature
    B. Hyperpolarization
    C. Not reversed by anticholinesterase agents
    D. Not similar to that of decamethonium
    E. Similar to that of D-tubocurarine

➪ For questions **108** to **111**, match the area in the somatic sensory cortex with the receptors. Each response may be used once, more than once, or not at all.
    A. Area 1
    B. Area 2
    C. Area 3a
    D. Area 3b

108. Muscle stretch receptors in deep tissue

109. Pressure and joint position in deep tissue

110. Slowly and rapidly adapting receptors in the skin

111. Rapidly adapting receptors in the skin

112. Each of the following is true of the dorsal column medial lemniscal system *except*
    A. Proprioception from the leg is relayed in the dorsal columns
    B. Second-order neurons cross the midline in the medial lemniscus
    C. Thalamic neurons project to the primary somatic sensory cortex (SI)
    D. Thalamic neurons project to the secondary somatic sensory cortex (SII)
    E. Touch and vibration sense from the arm is relayed in the dorsal columns

➪ For questions **113** to **121**, match the region of the cerebellum with the clinical sign or symptom. Each response may be used once, more than once, or not at all.
    A. Cerebellar hemisphere, intermediate part (interposed nuclei)
    B. Cerebellar hemisphere, lateral part (dentate nuclei)
    C. Flocculonodular (lateral vestibular nucleus)
    D. Vermis (fastigial nucleus)
    E. None of the above

113. Truncal ataxia

114. Appendicular ataxia

115. Terminal tremor

116. Nystagmus

117. Scanning speech

118. Hypertonia

119. Hypotonia is seen in lesions of the interposed nuclei or of this portion

120. Decomposition of multijoint movements

121. Delay in initiating movements

122. In the formation of nitric oxide, nitric oxide synthetase acts on the substrate
    A. Arginine
    B. Citrulline
    C. Lysine
    D. Ornithine
    E. Tyrosine

123. The pineal gland synthesizes melatonin from
    A. Acetylcholine
    B. Dopamine
    C. Histidine
    D. Norepinephrine
    E. Serotonin

⇨ For questions **124** to **128**, match the receptor with the description. Each response may be used once, more than once, or not at all.
    A. Muscarinic receptor
    B. Nicotinic receptor
    C. Both
    D. Neither

124. Binds ACh

125. Found in skeletal muscle

126. Found in sympathetic neurons

127. Blocked by hexamethonium

128. Activates a second messenger system via G proteins

129. The EPSP in spinal motor neurons results from the opening of
    A. Cl^- channels only
    B. Cl^- and Na^+ channels
    C. K^+ channels only
    D. Na^+ and K^+ channels
    E. Na^+ and Cl^- channels

130. The response of the carotid sinus to an increase in blood pressure is a
    I. Decrease in peripheral resistance
    II. Decrease in heart rate
    III. Decrease in force of contraction
    IV. Decrease in blood pressure
    A. I, II, III
    B. I, III
    C. II, IV
    D. IV
    E. All of the above

➱ For questions **131** to **137**, match the description with the structure.
  A. Thick filaments
  B. Thin filaments
  C. Both
  D. Neither

131. Contains actin

132. Contains myosin

133. Contains tropomyosin

134. Contains troponin

135. Binds ADP during rest

136. Sarcomeres contain them

137. Attached to the Z disks

138. Which of the following is true of skeletal muscle contraction?
  A. Calcium binds to tropomyosin.
  B. Rotation of myosin heads pulls thin filaments toward the center of the sarcomere.
  C. The detachment of cross bridges does not require ATP.
  D. The dissociation of actin from myosin uses energy from the hydrolysis of GTP.
  E. When muscle relaxes, calcium diffuses into the sarcoplasmic reticulum from the intracellular space.

139. The resting potential of a neuron is approximately
  A. -90 mV
  B. -65 mV
  C. -50 mV
  D. $+50$ mV
  E. $+65$ mV

140. Each of the following agents or states promotes antidiuretic hormone (ADH) release *except*
  A. Alcohol
  B. Angiotensin II
  C. Decreased blood volume
  D. Vomiting
  E. Increased plasma osmolality

141. Each of the following is a criterion that a chemical messenger should fulfill to be considered a transmitter *except*
  A. A specific mechanism exists for removing it from its site of action
  B. It is present in the presynaptic terminal and is released in amounts sufficient to exert its action on the postsynaptic neuron or effector organ
  C. It is synthesized in the neuron
  D. The enzymes that catalyze the steps in its synthesis are cytoplasmic
  E. The exogenously applied substance should mimic the action of the endogenously released transmitter

142. Each of the following is considered a neurotransmitter *except*
- **A.** Epinephrine
- **B.** Glycine
- **C.** Histamine
- **D.** Serotonin
- **E.** Vasoactive intestinal polypeptide (VIP)

143. Each of the following organs is innervated by both the sympathetic and parasympathetic systems *except* the
- **A.** Gastrointestinal tract
- **B.** Heart
- **C.** Lungs and bronchi
- **D.** Salivary glands
- **E.** Sweat glands

144. Each of the following is true of gamma motor neurons *except*
- **A.** Their activation during active muscle contraction allows muscle spindles to sense changes in length
- **B.** Their activity is increased after lesions of the spinocerebellum
- **C.** They innervate intrafusal fibers
- **D.** Dynamic gamma motor neurons innervate dynamic nuclear bag fibers only
- **E.** Static gamma motor neurons innervate nuclear chain fibers and static nuclear bag fibers

145. Neurotransmitters that are found in major descending pain pathways from the pons and medulla are
- I. Dopamine
- II. Norepinephrine
- III. Acetylcholine
- IV. Serotonin
- **A.** I, II, III
- **B.** I, III
- **C.** II, IV
- **D.** IV
- **E.** All of the above

146. Cell groups that have concentric receptive fields include
- I. Retinal ganglion cells
- II. Simple cells of the primary visual cortex
- III. Lateral geniculate cells
- IV. Complex cells of the primary visual cortex
- **A.** I, II, III
- **B.** I, III
- **C.** II, IV
- **D.** IV
- **E.** All of the above

⇨ For questions **147** to **151**, match the sensory receptor with the description. Each response may be used once, more than once, or not at all.

    A. Free nerve endings
    B. Meissner's corpuscles
    C. Merkel's receptors
    D. Pacinian corpuscles
    E. Ruffini's corpuscles

147. A subcutaneous, slowly adapting receptor

148. A rapidly adapting receptor found in the dermal papillae

149. A receptor subserving pressure and with a small receptive field

150. A rapidly adapting receptor more sensitive to high-frequency stimulation than low-frequency stimulation

151. A nociceptor

152. A man in his early 40s presents with the insidious onset of persistent spasms of the proximal lower limbs and lumbar spinal muscles that initially caused difficulty walking, but now have left him bed bound with the legs locked in an extended position. His spasticity abates during sleep and during general anesthesia. His EMG is normal. He has no history, signs, or symptoms of cancer. What is the most likely autoantibody responsible?

    A. Anti-amphiphysin
    B. Anti-gephyrin
    C. Anti-glutamic acid decarboxylase
    D. Anti-Yo
    E. Anti-Ri

153. A 3-year-old child presents with abnormal eye movements and is diagnosed with an optic tract glioma. What other finding might you expect in this patient?

    A. Bilateral vestibular schwannomas
    B. Gain of function mutation in a tumor promoter
    C. Mutation associated with chromosome 22
    D. Mutation affecting the RAS signal-transduction pathway
    E. Mutation of the hamartin gene locus on chromosome 9

154. Which of the following cell cycle transitions represents the "point of no return" in the cell cycle?

    A. G_0/G_1
    B. G_1/S
    C. G_1/G_0
    D. G_2/M
    E. S/G_2

155. The main advantage of K_i-67 or MIB1 labeling over traditional hematoxylin and eosin (H&E) staining is

    A. MIB1 labeling index allows for the more accurate diagnosis of glioblastoma
    B. MIB1 labeling index does not provide any advantage over H&E staining
    C. MIB1 labels cells proliferating in multiple stages of the cell cycle
    D. Mitoses are more obvious with MIB1 staining
    E. World Health Organization (WHO) grading of fibrillary astrocytomas depends on MIB1 labeling index

⇨ For questions **156** to **163**, match each solute with the appropriate response. Each answer may be used once, more than once, or not at all.

    A. Value is higher in CSF than plasma.
    B. Value is higher in plasma than CSF.
    C. Value is equal in plasma and CSF.

156. Beta-2 transferrin

157. Calcium

158. Chloride

159. Glucose

160. Osmolality

161. Potassium

162. Sodium

163. Uric acid

164. Huntington's disease is associated with all of the following *except*
    A. Caudate atrophy
    B. Genetic abnormality localizes to chromosome 4
    C. Increased acetylcholine transferase activity
    D. Progressive choreoathetosis
    E. Trinucleotide CAG repeat

165. What is the equilibrium potential for sodium?
    A. -94 mV
    B. -90 mV
    C. -86 mV
    D. $+61$ mV
    E. $+267$ mV

166. All of the following statements regarding the O^6-methylguanine-DNA methyl-transferase (*MGMT*) gene in glioblastoma are true *except*
    A. Methylation of the *MGMT* gene's promoter region upregulates *MGMT* gene expression
    B. *MGMT* methylation predicts improved survival
    C. *MGMT* methylation predicts improved benefit from temozolomide
    D. The *MGMT* gene encodes a DNA repair protein
    E. The *MGMT* gene promotes chemotherapy resistance

⇨ For questions **167** to **171**, match the rate of cerebral blood flow to the approximate time to cell death. Each answer may be used once, more than once, or not at all.

    A. < 4 minutes
    B. 15 minutes
    C. 40 minutes
    D. 80 minutes
    E. Infinite

167. 0 mL/100 g/min

168. 10 mL/100 g/min

169. 15 mL/100 g/min

170. 18 mL/100 g/min

171. 55 mL/100 g/min

⇨ For questions **172** to **176**, match the description or signs and symptoms to the appropriate autoantibody.

    A.   Anti-glutamic acid decarboxylase
    B.   Anti-Hu
    C.   Anti-Ma
    D.   Anti-Ri
    E.   Anti-Yo

172. Associated with limbic encephalitis

173. Cerebellar degeneration, associated with ovarian and breast cancer

174. Sensory neuropathy, encephalitis, and cerebellar degeneration, associated with pulmonary carcinoma and lymphoma

175. Opsoclonus, associated with breast cancer

176. Stiff-man syndrome

4B Neurobiology— Answer Key

1.	A	27.	C
2.	B	28.	D
3.	A	29.	F
4.	B	30.	B
5.	C	31.	A
6.	B	32.	D
7.	A	33.	E
8.	B	34.	E
9.	C	35.	B
10.	A	36.	B
11.	B	37.	D
12.	C	38.	A
13.	C	39.	B
14.	A	40.	D
15.	B	41.	B
16.	B	42.	A
17.	B	43.	C
18.	E	44.	A
19.	E	45.	A
20.	B	46.	B
21.	B	47.	B
22.	B	48.	B
23.	E	49.	C
24.	A	50.	B
25.	E	51.	D
26.	A	52.	B

53.	C		92.	B
54.	C		93.	D
55.	F		94.	B
56.	B		95.	A
57.	D		96.	B
58.	E		97.	C
59.	A		98.	A
60.	B		99.	G
61.	C		100.	F
62.	B		101.	B
63.	D		102.	E
64.	A		103.	C
65.	B		104.	D
66.	E		105.	A
67.	D		106.	D
68.	C		107.	C
69.	B		108.	C
70.	A		109.	B
71.	C		110.	D
72.	A		111.	A
73.	C		112.	A
74.	E		113.	D
75.	B		114.	A
76.	C		115.	B
77.	B		116.	C
78.	C		117.	D
79.	C		118.	E
80.	D		119.	D
81.	D		120.	B
82.	A		121.	B
83.	C		122.	A
84.	A		123.	E
85.	D		124.	C
86.	D		125.	B
87.	A		126.	C
88.	B		127.	B
89.	B		128.	A
90.	C		129.	D
91.	B		130.	E

131.	B	154.	B
132.	A	155.	C
133.	B	156.	A
134.	B	157.	B
135.	A	158.	A
136.	C	159.	B
137.	B	160.	C
138.	B	161.	B
139.	B	162.	C
140.	A	163.	B
141.	D	164.	C
142.	E	165.	D
143.	E	166.	A
144.	B	167.	A
145.	C	168.	C
146.	B	169.	D
147.	E	170.	E
148.	B	171.	E
149.	C	172.	C
150.	D	173.	E
151.	A	174.	B
152.	C	175.	D
153.	D	176.	A

4C Neurobiology–Answers and Explanations

1. A – Bone growth factors
2. B – Recombinant human bone morphogenic proteins
3. A – Bone growth factors
4. B – Recombinant human bone morphogenic proteins
5. C – Both

> **Bone growth factors (A)** are strong mitogens and act on differentiated mesenchymal cells of the chondro-osseous lineage. **Recombinant human bone morphogenic proteins (B)** are potent inducers of bone cell differentiation and may act on undifferentiated mesenchymal cells. Both **bone growth factors (A)** and **bone morphogenic proteins (B)** are polypeptides.[1]

6. B – α2βγδ

> Acetylcholine receptors can be divided into muscarinic and nicotinic types. The muscarinic acetylcholine receptors are present in all postganglionic parasympathetic terminals and in the postganglionic sympathetic terminals innervating sweat glands. The muscarinic acetylcholine receptor is a G-protein-coupled receptor and therefore transmits its signals via a second messenger system. Nicotinic acetylcholine receptors function as cation-selective ion channels. Nicotinic acetylcholine receptors are present at the neuromuscular junction and at the preganglionic terminals of sympathetic and parasympathetic fibers. Autonomic nicotinic acetylcholine receptors consist of α and β subunits only, i.e., **α2β2 or α3β3.** However, the nicotinic acetylcholine receptor at the neuromuscular junction is a pentamer consisting of two α, one β, one γ, and one δ subunit, i.e., **α2βγδ (B)**.[2,3,4]

7. A – It contains four hydrophobic transmembrane proteins.

> The ligand binding site is located on the α subunit **(B is false)**, the transmembrane segment is the most highly conserved **(E is false)**, and the cytoplasmic loop connecting M3 and M4 is the least highly conserved **(C is false)**. Both the N and the C terminals are extracellular **(D is false)**. Response **A** is correct.[2,5]

8. B – 2

> Each nicotinic acetylcholine receptor complex has **two extracellular ace-tylcholine binding sites (B)** that are primarily composed of six amino acids located on the α subunits.[2,6]

9. C – Both
10. A – α subunit of GABA$_A$ receptor

> The GABA$_A$ receptor functions as a chloride ion channel and is activated by multiple ligands including benzodiazepines, barbiturates, and zolpidem. The binding site for GABA on the GABA$_A$ receptor is located between the **α and β subunits (C)**. The binding site for benzodiazepines is located between the **α and gamma subunits (A)**.[4]

11. B – Glutamate receptor
12. C – Glycine receptor
13. C – Glycine receptor
14. A – GABA receptor
15. B – Glutamate receptor
16. B – Glutamate receptor

> **GABA receptors (A)** have been characterized as the site of action of benzodi-azepines. Ligand-gated **glutamate receptors (B)** can be divided into NMDA and non-NMDA receptors. The *N*-methyl-D-aspartate (NMDA) receptor is voltage regulated in that the open channel is occluded at normal resting po-tential by Mg^{2+}. Depolarization drives Mg^{2+} out of the cell, allowing other ions to pass. High concentrations of glutamate may induce neuronal cell death via activation of NMDA and AMPA (a non-NMDA **glutamate receptor [B]**), allowing calcium influx into the cell. Glycine receptors share many features of the GABA$_A$ receptor. Both function as ligand-gated chloride ion channels and are present throughout the brainstem and spinal cord. The **glycine receptor (C)** is antagonized by strychnine. Nicotinic acetylcholine receptors function as cation-selective ion channels. **Nicotinic acetylcholine receptors (D)** are pres-ent at the neuromuscular junction and at the preganglionic terminals of sym-pathetic and parasympathetic fibers. **Serotonin receptors (E)** can be found at multiple sites and are prominent in the dorsal raphe nucleus.[5]

17. B – NMDA receptor only
18. E – A, B, and C
19. E – A, B, and C
20. B – NMDA receptor only
21. B – NMDA receptor only

> The ligand-gated glutamate receptors can be grouped into *N*-methyl-D-aspartate (NMDA) receptors (B)** and non-NMDA receptors, all of which in-crease cation conductance when activated. The non-NMDA receptors include the **α-amino-3-hydroxy-5-methyl-4-isoxazoleproprionic acid (AMPA) receptor (C)** and the **kainic acid (A) receptor**. The **NMDA receptor (B)** can be blocked by magnesium at resting membrane potentials and is therefore both ligand and voltage gated. **NMDA receptors (B)** are particularly permeable to

calcium ions, participate in long-term potentiation, and are thought to be important for neuronal plasticity, learning, and memory.[4,5]

22. B – One quanta contains 10,000 molecules of Ach

Quanta refers to the acetycholine quantity of one synaptic vesicle and has been estimated in the range of 1,000 to 50,000 molecules of Ach per vesicle (per quanta).[5]

23. E – All of the above

Pre-proopiomelanocortin (POMC) is an opioid precursor peptide along with pre-proenkephalin and pre-prodynorphin. The major opioid peptide derived from POMC is **β-endorphin**. POMC is also converted into the nonopioid peptides **adrenocorticotropic hormone (ACTH)**, **melanocyte-stimulating hormone (α-MSH)**, and **β-lipotropin**.[5]

24. A – I, II, III (active transport, binding to cytosolic proteins, and transport into intracellular calcium storage vesicles)

Removal of calcium ions from the cytosol in a presynaptic nerve terminal following an action potential is thought to occur by **active transport, binding to cytosolic proteins, and transport into intracellular calcium storage vesicles**. Reversal of flow through voltage-gated channels is not a mechanism of removal of Ca^{2+} from the cytosol.[5]

25. E – The decreased concentration of cGMP results in depolarization of the plasma membrane (false)

In phototransduction, a photon of light leads to the **isomerization of 11-*cis*-retinal to an all-*trans* form, activating rhodopsin (D). Activated rhodopsin then stimulates a G-protein-coupled receptor, transducin (A), activating a cyclic GMP-specific phosphodiesterase (PDE [B])**. The decreased cGMP level (caused by increased cGMP PDE) leads to a **decreased Na conductance by cGMP-gated ion channels (C)** leading to hyperpolarization of the membrane. In summary, **light leads to hyperpolarization of the cell membrane via reduced levels of cGMP (E is false)**.[5]

26. A – Each G protein is regulated by only one type of receptor (false)

G proteins bind to the cytoplasmic face of a given receptor; **each G protein may be regulated by separate receptors (A is false)**. Agonists promote the **binding of GTP to the α subunit (C)**, which can then activate a **variety of effector proteins (B)**. The G protein remains active until GTP is hydrolyzed to GDP. The β and γ subunits help to **anchor the G protein to the membrane (D)**, **participate in modulation of GDP/GTP exchange (E)**, and confer localization via myristolization.[2,5]

27. C – Cyclic adenosine monophosphate (cAMP)
28. D – Cyclic guanine monophosphate (cGMP)
29. F – 1,2-diacylglycerol (DAG) and inositol-1,4,5-trisphosphate (IP3)
30. B – 1,2-diacylglycerol (DAG)

31. A – Calcium
32. D – Cyclic guanine monophosphate (cGMP)
33. E – Inositol-1,4,5-trisphosphate (IP3)

> Cytosolic **calcium (A)** levels are regulated by several different factors, and **calcium (A)** may exert its influence via multiple mechanisms—calcium is the only choice listed, however, that binds to calmodulin. G_q activates phospholipase C which hydrolyzes phosphatidylinositol-4,5-bisphosphate to **inositol-1,4,5-trisphosphate (IP3 [E])** and **diacylglycerol (DAG [B])**. **IP3 (E)** binds to receptors on the endoplasmic reticulum that cause a transient increase in cytosolic calcium concentrations. **DAG (B)** binds protein kinase C (PKC), lowering PKC's requirement for activation by calcium. **Cyclic AMP (cAMP [C])** is generated by adenylyl cyclase, stimulated by G_s, and inhibited by G_i. D_1 receptors are an example of a receptor that uses **cAMP (C)** as a second messenger. Nitric oxide generates **cyclic GMP (cGMP [D])** via activation of soluble guanylyl cyclase. Photoreception utilizes **cGMP (D)** as a second messenger. Recall that light leads to hyperpolarization of the cell membrane via reduced levels of **cGMP (D)**.[5]

34. E – Utilizes two molecules of ATP for every three Na⁺ ions transported (false)

> The sodium potassium ATPase contributes to the **resting potential of the cell (A)**; **hyperpolarizing the membrane (B)** by pumping **three Na⁺ ions into the cell for every two K⁺ ions it transports out of the cell (D)**. This action generates both a chemical and an **electrical gradient (C)** across the cell membrane. The Na⁺/K⁺ pump uses **one molecule** of **adenosine triphosphate (ATP)** for every **three Na⁺ ions transported (E is false)**.[5]

35. B – Chloride permeability increases during depolarization (false)

> An action potential consists of two phases, the first of which is due to an increased permeability to Na caused by the **opening of voltage-gated Na channels (A)**. Thus there is rapid depolarization of the cell due to sodium influx. The second phase is due to **fast activation of Na channels (D)** and delayed opening of K channels that **allow K to leave the cell and terminate depolarization (C, E)**. Chloride permeability does not change during the action potential **(B is false)**.[5]

36. B – High transmembrane resistance, low internal resistance, and low membrane capacitance

> The velocity of an action potential increases with **high transmembrane resistance, low internal resistance, and low membrane capacitance (B)**. The conduction velocity is dependent on the diameter of the axon and myelination status. Increased axonal diameter leads to lower internal resistance and higher conduction velocities. Myelination leads to increased velocities via increased transmembrane resistance and decreased membrane capacitance, and therefore higher conduction velocities.[7]

37. D – It increases transmembrane resistance and decreases membrane capacitance.

> Myelination increases transmembrane resistance and decreases membrane capacitance, leading to increased conduction velocities.[6]

38. A – End-plate potential
39. B – Miniature end-plate potential
40. D – Neither

> **End-plate potential (A)** refers to the depolarizing process that occurs at the neuromuscular junction, triggering a muscle action potential, and therefore leading to muscle contraction. **Miniature end-plate potentials (B)** result from random release of quanta of acetylcholine causing minor regional membrane depolarizations (excitatory end-plate potentials) but do not reach the threshold necessary to produce an action potential. Action potentials are an all-or-nothing phenomenon **(D)**.[5]

41. B – Cl⁻ or K⁺

> Localized depolarizations of the cell membrane are usually due to increased **Na⁺ permeability (C)** and are called excitatory postsynaptic potentials (EPSPs). The summation of multiple EPSPs can cause an action potential to occur if the depolarization reaches threshold. This effect can be blocked by inhibitory postsynaptic potentials (IPSPs) that represent regional hyperpolarization mediated by increased permeability to **Cl⁻ or K⁺ ions (B)**.[5]

42. A – Dynamin does not use ATP.

> Dynamin uses **GTP as an energy source (A)**. Dynein is the motor protein for retrograde fast axonal transport **(B and E are false)**. Slow axonal transport occurs at several millimeters per day **(E is false)**; fast axonal transport occurs at 200 to 400 mm/day and utilizes microtubules **(C is false)**.[2,6]

43. C – Both
44. A – Golgi tendon organ
45. A – Golgi tendon organ
46. B – Muscle spindle
47. B – Muscle spindle
48. B – Muscle spindle
49. C – Both
50. B – Muscle spindle
51. D – Neither
52. B – Muscle spindle

> Both **Golgi tendon organs (A)** and **muscle spindles (B)** are proprioceptive receptors that are activated by passive stretch and are innervated by group I (large myelinated) fibers. **Golgi tendon organs (A)** are arranged in series with the muscle in the tendon and are activated maximally by muscle contraction. **Muscle spindles (B)** are arranged in parallel with the muscle fibers and consist of a dynamic nuclear bag, static nuclear bag, and nuclear chain fibers. Muscle spindles are sensitive to muscle stretch and length. Motor innervation to the muscle spindle via gamma motor neurons allows for the length of the muscle spindle to change its sensitivity to length and velocity of length change.[6,8]

193

53. C –   It is reduced by destruction of the anterior lobe of the cerebellum (false)

Decerebrate rigidity, or extensor posturing, results from tonic activity of the **lateral vestibular and pontine reticular nuclei (A)** promoting unopposed extensor tone of the upper and lower extremities, and may be induced **by transection between the colliculi (D)**. Decerebrate rigidity is associated with **increased gamma motor neuron activity (E)** and may be **reduced by sectioning of the dorsal roots (B)**. Destruction of the anterior lobe of the cerebellum releases the cells of origin of the lateral vestibular tract from inhibition by Purkinje's cells, thereby facilitating extensor motor neurons (**C is false**).[3,8]

54. C –   F response
55. F –   Stretch reflex
56. B –   Flexion reflex
57. D –   H response
58. E –   M response
59. A –   Clasp-knife response

The **H reflex (Hoffman's [D])** is the electrical equivalent of the tendon reflex circuit and represents the activation of a muscle contraction with submaximal stimulation insufficient to illicit a direct motor response—the response is mediated by the activation of muscle spindles and involves both the dorsal and ventral horns. The **H reflex (D)** is particularly useful in the diagnosis of S1 radiculopathy. The **F wave (C)** is evoked by supramaximal stimulus of a mixed motor-sensory nerve and consists of a small muscle action potential recorded after the direct motor response. The **F wave** results from antidromic impulses traveling up the motor nerve to the anterior horn causing an orthodromic response recorded in distal muscle. A normal **F wave** and absent **H reflex** occur in diseases of sensory nerves and roots. The **M wave (E)** is the direct motor response caused by stimulation of a motor nerve. A clasp-knife response consists of the following: if muscles are briskly stretched, the limb moves freely for a short distance followed by rapid resistance—with increasing passive stretch, the resistance disappears. The **spinal flexion (B)** reflexes result in flexion across multiple joints to withdraw from painful stimuli and may be exaggerated in states of spasticity. The **stretch reflex (F)** is the familiar myotactic reflex (tendon jerk) as occurs with tapping on the knee with a hammer. The **stretch reflex** occurs due to the activation of the muscle spindle and nuclear bag fibers causing reflex contraction of skeletal muscle fibers via a monosynaptic pathway—the stretch reflex has both a phasic and tonic component.[3,8,9]

60. B –   Parasympathetic fibers from S2 to S4

The detrusor muscle of the bladder is innervated by **parasympathetic fibers from the S2-S4 (B)** nerve roots.[9]

61. C – Terminal degeneration leads to loss of presynaptic terminals.

Chromatolysis is associated with **increased protein synthesis (A is false)**. Retraction bulbs, from the buildup of transported materials, occur at **both the proximal and the distal ends of the cut nerve (B is false)**. Wallerian degeneration **begins in the distal end of the axon ~1 week after initial degenerative changes begin in the axon terminal (D and E are false)**. Terminal degeneration does lead to the **loss of presynaptic terminals (C)**.[8]

62. B – I, III (carbon dioxide and volatile anesthetic agents)

Carbon dioxide and **volatile anesthetic agents** increase cerebrospinal fluid (CSF) production, whereas **carbonic anhydrase inhibitors** and **norepinephrine** inhibit CSF production.[10]

63. D – Glycine

Renshaw cells are inhibitory interneurons located in the ventral horn and are responsible for a negative feedback reflex called recurrent inhibition. Renshaw cells use glycine as their principle neurotransmitter.[6]

64. A – Wave I
65. B – Wave II
66. E – Wave V
67. D – Wave IV
68. C – Wave III

Stimulation of the cochlear nerve by clicks delivered to the ear causes the appearance of seven waves as recorded by scalp electrodes—brainstem auditory evoked responses (BAERs). **Wave I** represents activation of the auditory nerve. **Wave II** represents activation of the cochlear nucleus. **Wave III** represents activation of the superior olivary nucleus. **Wave IV** represents activation of the lateral lemniscus. **Wave V** represents activation of the inferior colliculus. **Wave VI** corresponds to the medial geniculate nucleus. **Wave VII** corresponds to the auditory radiations.[9]

69. B – N11
70. A – Erb's point
71. C – N13/P13
72. A – Erb's point

Somatosensory evoked potentials (SSEPs) involve the application of 5-per-second transcutaneous stimuli to the median, peroneal, and tibial nerves, and recording the evoked potentials as they pass the brachial plexus 2–3 cm above the clavicle **(Erb's point [A])**, over the C2 vertebra, and over the contralateral parietal cortex. A delay between the peripheral stimulus and **Erb's point (A)** suggests a peripheral lesion. Absence or delay in **N11 (B)** implies cervical cord disease. The summated wave that is recorded at the cervicomedullary junction is **N13/P13 (C)**. The cortical potential recorded at the cortex from median nerve stimulation is **N19/P22 (D and E)**. The cortical wave after tibial or peroneal stimulation is N/P 37.[9]

73. C – 23 mL/100 g/min
74. E – 8 mL/100 g/min
75. B – 55 mL/100 g/min

Normal cerebral blood flow is **55 mL/100 g/min (B)**. Flow reduction below **8–10 mL/100 g/min (E)** results in irreversible cerebral infarction. Functional impairment occurs at a cerebral blood flow of **23 mL/100 g/min (C)**. The biochemical abnormalities, including depletion of ATP and creatine phosphate and increase of K^+ level (from injured cells), can be reversed if adequate blood flow is restored in a timely fashion.[9]

76. C – Granule cells
77. B – Golgi cells
78. C – Granule cells
79. C – Granule cells
80. D – Purkinje cells
81. D – Purkinje cells
82. A – Basket cells
83. C – Granule cells

The cerebellar cortex consists of three layers that contain five cell types. The molecular layer (outermost) is composed of the axons of the **granule cells (C)** (parallel fibers), **stellate (E)** and **basket cells (A)** (interneurons), and dendrites of the underlying **Purkinje cells (D)**. The Purkinje cell layer (middle) contains the cell bodies of the Purkinje neurons. They are the sole output of the cerebellar cortex and are inhibitory. The granular (innermost) layer contains numerous **granule cells (C, excitatory; utilize glutamate)**, a few **Golgi cells (B)**, and glomeruli (where cells in the granular layer form complex synaptic contacts with the incoming mossy fibers). Afferents to the cortex terminate either in the granule cell layer as mossy fibers or on the dendrites of Purkinje cells as climbing fibers. Both mossy and climbing fiber inputs are excitatory to both the deep cerebellar nuclei and the cortex. **Stellate (E)** and **basket cells (A)** directly inhibit **Purkinje (D)** and **Golgi cells (B)**, and Golgi cells inhibit **granule cells (C)**.[8]

84. A – The utricular macule is oriented horizontally and the saccular macule is oriented vertically.

When the head is upright, the utricular macule is oriented in the horizontal plane and can be activated by linear forces in the horizontal plane. The saccular macule is oriented in the vertical plane and can be stimulated by linear forces in the vertical plane **(A is correct)**.[7]

85. D – Aδ fibers

Nociception is mediated primarily by lightly myelinated free nerve endings of type **Aδ fibers (D)** or unmyelinated **C fibers (E)**. The sensation of sharp pain is mediated by **Aδ fibers (D)**. **C fibers (E)** relay information regarding mechanical, thermal, or chemical stimuli.[7]

86. D – The fast EPSP is mediated by nicotinic ACh receptors.

Unlike the ACh receptors at the neuromuscular junction, the ACh receptors in autonomic ganglia contain only two types of subunits **(A is false)**. The fast excitatory postsynaptic potential (EPSP) is mediated by nicotinic ACh receptors **(D is true)**, the slow EPSP is mediated by muscarinic receptors opening Na^+ and Ca^{2+} channels and closing K^+ channels **(B is false)**, and the slow inhibitory postsynaptic potential (IPSP) is mediated by muscarinic receptors that open K^+ channels **(C is false)**. A variety of peptides that appear to be modulatory in action may be co-released with Ach **(E is false)**.[8]

87. A – Increased postganglionic sympathetic activity results in bladder wall contraction (false)

Increased sympathetic activity results in bladder wall relaxation **(A is false)**. The other responses are true regarding innervation of the urinary system. Increased postganglionic sympathetic activity results in α-adrenergic inhibition of parasympathetics in the pelvic ganglion **(B)**, motor neurons in the ventral horn of the sacral spinal cord innervate the external sphincter **(C)**, parasympathetic activity promotes bladder emptying **(D)**, and the internal sphincter is innervated by sympathetic fibers **(E)**.[7]

88. B – I, III (pterygopalatine ganglion, submandibular ganglion)

Fibers from the superior salivatory nucleus travel with the facial nerve reaching either the pterygopalatine ganglion via the GSPN and vidian nerve or the submandibular ganglion via the chorda tympani nerve. The geniculate ganglion contains the cell bodies of pseudounipolar neurons carrying afferent information in the facial nerve. The trigeminal ganglion houses the cell bodies of pseudounipolar neurons carrying afferent information in the trigeminal nerve.[7]

89. B – II and III

Ipsilateral cortico-cortical association fibers arise from cells in cortical **layers II and III**. Cells that give rise to commissural fibers that interconnect homologous cortical areas via the corpus callosum are found in **layer III** of the cerebral cortex (the external pyramidal layer). **Layer I** is the plexiform molecular layer and consists mainly of nerve cell processes. **Layer II** is the external granular layer comprised mostly of small granule cells and projects primarily to local or distant cortical areas as association fibers. **Layer IV**, the internal granular layer, is important for afferent signaling and is thicker in the primary sensory area. **Layer V**, the internal pyramidal layer, is the source of the majority of output fibers for the cerebral cortex. **Layer VI** is the fusiform layer and lies adjacent to underlying white matter and consists primarily of association neurons.[7]

90. C – EPSP decreases and IPSP increases

As the membrane of a motor neuron becomes increasingly depolarized, excitatory postsynaptic potentials decrease while inhibitory postsynaptic potentials increase. **Choice C is correct.**[8]

91. B – They facilitate Ia inhibitory neurons that act on antagonist motor neurons (false)

> Renshaw cells are located in the anterior horn and participate in a negative feedback loop to the motor neurons (**A**). They receive input from descending pathways (**E**), make divergent connections to motor neurons (**D**), and inhibit motor neurons that inhibit synergistic muscles (**C**). During development, Renshaw cells receive input from Ia afferents, but they project to α motor neurons (**B is false**).[3,6,8]

92. B – Lateral vestibular nucleus
93. D – Superior vestibular nucleus
94. B – Lateral vestibular nucleus
95. A – Inferior vestibular nucleus
96. B – Lateral vestibular nucleus

> Part of the **lateral vestibulospinal nucleus (Deiters' nucleus [B])** receives direct inhibitory input from Purkinje cells in the cerebellar vermis. Decerebrate rigidity is exacerbated if the portion of the cerebellum connected to **Deiters' nucleus (B)** is interrupted because of removal of this inhibitory action. The **lateral vestibulospinal tract (B)** has a facilitatory effect on both α and γ neurons that innervate muscles in the limbs; this tonic excitation of the extensors of the leg and the flexors of the arm helps in the maintenance of posture. The **superior and medial vestibular nuclei (D)** receive sensory input from the semicircular canals via the vestibular nerve and project to the medial longitudinal fasciculus and medial vestibulospinal tract to mediate reflexes of both ocular and head movements in response to vestibular stimuli. The **inferior vestibular nucleus (A)** receives afferents from the semicircular canals and utricle and sends its projections to the reticular formation and cerebellum, acting as an integration center for the vestibular labyrinth and cerebellum.[7,8]

97. C – Initiation of N-linked glycosylation

> The Golgi apparatus serves two major functions for the processing of membrane proteins: sorting and targeting of proteins, and post-translational modifications—particularly of oligosaccharide chains that have already been added in the rough endoplasmic reticulum. (**The initial steps of N-linked glycosylation take place in the endoplasmic reticulum; C is false.**) The other choices listed take place in the Golgi apparatus: **attachment of fatty acids (A)**, **formation of O-linked sugars (B)**, **sugar phosphorylation (D)**, and **sulfation of tyrosine residues (E)**.[2,6]

98. A – Binds to the ACh receptor
99. G – Prevents presynaptic release of quanta of ACh
100. F – Inhibits GTP hydrolysis
101. B – Blocks reuptake of dopamine
102. E – Depletes norepinephrine from vesicles
103. C – Blocks voltage-gated K^+ channels

104. D – Blocks voltage-gated Na$^+$ channels

α-**Bungarotoxin (A)** is a neurotoxin found in snake venom that is selective for the nicotinic acetylcholine receptor at the muscle end-plate. **Botulinum toxin (G)** blocks the release of acetylcholine quanta at the presynaptic membrane. **Cholera toxin (F)** inhibits GTP hydrolysis leading to constitutive activity of adenylyl cyclase and increased intracellular cAMP levels. **Cocaine (B)** acts on the dopamine transporter (DAT) inhibiting dopamine reuptake. **Reserpine (E)** interacts with adrenergic storage vesicles and inhibits their capacity to concentrate and store norepinephrine and dopamine. **Tetraethylammonium (C)** is an ammonium salt similar to hexamethonium that functions as a "nicotine paralyzing" ganglion blocker, acting primarily via blockade of voltage-gated K$^+$ channels. **Tetrodotoxin (D)** is a fish toxin that blocks Na$^+$ channels in excitable cells.[2,5,8]

105. A – The electrical force equals the chemical force

At the equilibrium potential, the chemical and electrical forces are equal, but opposite **(A)**. There is no *net* movement of K ions across the membrane **(D is false)**. Neither the net chemical nor the net electrical force equal zero at the equilibrium potential of potassium **(B and C are false)**.[2,11]

106. D – The βγ subunit stabilizes the binding of GTP (false)

Upon binding of a ligand to a G-protein-coupled receptor, GDP on the α subunit is converted to GTP and the G protein dissociates from the receptor. The α and βγ subunits then dissociate **(the α subunit's affinity for the βγ subunit decreases [E])**. Both subunits are then free to exert their effects on downstream effectors, including the inhibition of other G proteins in the membrane **(A)**. The α subunit then catalyzes hydrolysis of GTP to GDP, promoting reassembly of the trimer and receptor inactivation **(B)**. At rest, the βγ subunit inhibits activation by both stabilizing the binding of GDP **(C)** and inhibiting the binding of GTP **(D is false)**.[2,11]

107. C – Not reversed by anticholinesterase agents

Succinylcholine and decamethonium cause depolarizing neuromuscular blockade **(B and D are false)**. The effect is not reversed by anticholinesterase agents **(C)** and is amplified by decreased muscle temperature **(A is false)**. Succinylcholine is resistant to the action of acetylcholinesterase **(C is true)**.[5]

108. C – Area 3a
109. B – Area 2
110. D – Area 3b
111. A – Area 1

The primary somatosensory area consists of Brodmann's areas 1, 2, and 3. **Area 1 (A)** receives input from rapidly adapting receptors in the skin. **Area 2 (B)** deals with pressure and joint position in deep tissues. **Area 3a (C)** receives muscle, tendon, and joint stretch receptors. **Area 3b (D)** receives input from both slowly and rapidly adapting receptors in the skin.[3,8]

112. A – Proprioception from the leg is relayed in the dorsal columns (false)

Proprioception from the leg is relayed in the lateral column by axons of neurons in Clarke's column (**A is false**). The other responses regarding the dorsal column medial lemniscal system are true. In addition to sending axons to the primary somatic sensory cortex (SI **[C]**), thalamic neurons send a sparse projection to the secondary somatic sensory cortex (SII **[D]**). Touch and vibration sense from the arm are relayed in the dorsal columns (**E**). Second-order neurons cross the midline in the medial lemniscus (**B**).[8]

113. D – Vermis (fastigial nucleus)
114. A – Cerebellar hemisphere, intermediate part (interposed nuclei)
115. B – Cerebellar hemisphere, lateral part (dentate nuclei)
116. C – Flocculonodular (lateral vestibular nucleus)
117. D – Vermis (fastigial nucleus)
118. E – None of the above
119. D – Vermis (fastigial nucleus)
120. B – Cerebellar hemisphere, lateral part (dentate nuclei)
121. B – Cerebellar hemisphere, lateral part (dentate nuclei)

The cells of the interposed nuclei are associated with the paravermal cortex and spinocerebellum, which contributes to posture, muscle tone, and muscle activity of the trunk and limbs during stereotyped activities—injuries to the **interposed nuclei and associated cortex (A)** may lead to appendicular ataxia. The cells of the dentate nucleus are associated with the lateral cerebellar cortex and cerebrocerebellum, which participate in planning and coordination of skilled movement. Lesions to the **dentate nucleus and associated cortex (B)** can result in terminal tremor, decomposition of multijoint movements, and delay in initiating movements. Lesions to **the flocculonodular lobe and lateral vestibular nucleus (C)** may lead to nystagmus; generally, the flocculonodular lobe is involved in balance, posture, and the coordination of head and neck movements via its reciprocal connections with the vestibular system. The vermis is part of the spinocerebellum and is largely responsible for the maintenance and coordination of axial and girdle musculature and the fastigial nucleus is associated with the vestibulocerebellum. Injuries to the **vermis and fastigial nucleus (D)** may lead to truncal ataxia, scanning speech, and hypotonia. Lesions to the cerebellum are not known to cause hypertonia (**E**).[7,8]

122. A – Arginine

Nitric oxide production in neurons is from ʟ-**arginine (A)** and molecular oxygen by nitric oxide synthetase acting in conjunction with the cofactor, reduced nicotinamide adenine dinucleotide phosphate (NADPH), and Ca^{2+} ions. The **arginine (A)** is converted to **citrulline (B)**.[5]

123. E – Serotonin

The pineal gland synthesizes melatonin from **serotonin (E)** by the action of two enzymes sensitive to variations of diurnal light. The rhythmic fluctuations in melatonin synthesis are directly related to the daily light cycle.[10]

124. C – Both
125. B – Nicotinic receptor
126. C – Both
127. B – Nicotinic receptor
128. A – Muscarinic receptor

> The nicotinic and muscarinic receptors **both (C)** bind acetylcholine and are found in sympathetic neurons, whereas the directly gated receptors in skeletal muscle are **nicotinic (B)**. Hexamethonium selectively blocks **nicotinic ACh receptors (B)**. **Muscarinic receptors (A)** activate second messenger systems via G proteins, whereas nicotinic receptors are ligand-gated ion channels.[4,8]

129. D – Na⁺ and K⁺ channels

> The excitatory postsynaptic potential in spinal motor neurons is mediated by the action of acetylcholine on the acetylcholine receptor (a nonselective cation channel), which increases membrane permeability to **both Na⁺ and K⁺ (D)**.[4,11]

130. E – All of the above

> Increased mean arterial pressure leads to increased stretch across the baroreceptors located in the carotid sinus (carried to the brainstem with the glossopharyngeal nerve) leading to reflex vasodilation and bradycardia. These effects are mediated by decreased sympathetic tone and increased vagal tone, which leads to a decrease in heart rate and cardiac contractility, as well as systemic vasodilation, lowering systemic vascular resistance as well as blood pressure.[8,11]

131. B – Thin filaments
132. A – Thick filaments
133. B – Thin filaments
134. B – Thin filaments
135. A – Thick filaments
136. C – Both
137. B – Thin filaments

> **Thin filaments (B)** consist of actin, tropomyosin, and troponin and are attached to the Z disks. **Thick filaments (A)** are composed of multiple myosin molecules and bind ADP during rest. A sarcomere is the building block of a myofibril and extends from one Z disk to the next. A sarcomere is composed of **both (C) thick and thin filaments**.[8,11]

138. B – Rotation of myosin heads pulls thin filaments toward the center of the sarcomere.

> During skeletal muscle contraction, calcium binds to troponin **(A is false)**. Both the association and detachment of cross bridges require ATP **(not GTP; C and D are false)**. During relaxation, Ca²⁺ is actively pumped out of the intracellular space and back into the sarcoplasmic reticulum **(E is false)**.[8,11]

139. B – −65 mV

> The resting potential of a neuron is approximately **−65 mV (B)**. The other responses are incorrect.[8]

140. A – Alcohol

> Antidiuretic hormone, or arginine vasopressin, is secreted by the posterior pituitary gland and inhibits renal excretion of free water. **Increased plasma osmolality (E)** stimulates osmoreceptor cells in the hypothalamus, which leads to the release of ADH. Volume contraction, or **decreased blood volume (C)**, promotes ADH release via three mechanisms: (1) At a fixed osmolality, volume contraction increases the rate of ADH release—during a low-volume state, a low plasma osmolality that would normally inhibit the release of ADH would allow ADH secretion to continue. (2) Low left atrial pressure decreases the firing of vagal afferents, leading to increased ADH secretion. (3) Low circulating blood volume leads to renin production by the juxtaglomerular apparatus in the kidneys. Renin is converted to **angiotensin II (B)**, which acts on the subfornical organ and organum vasculosum of the lamina terminalis to stimulate ADH release. Pain and **nausea (D)** tend to promote ADH secretion. **Alcohol (A)** inhibits the release of ADH from the posterior pituitary gland.[5,8,11]

141. D – The enzymes that catalyze the steps in its synthesis are cytoplasmic (false)

> The enzymes that catalyze the synthesis of the low-molecular-weight transmitters are usually cytoplasmic (dopamine-β-hydroxylase is an exception), but this is not a criterion that must be fulfilled for a chemical to be considered a transmitter **(D is false)**.[8]

142. E – Vasoactive intestinal polypeptide (VIP) (false)

> **VIP (E)** is considered a neuroactive peptide, not a neurotransmitter. The other choices listed are considered to be neurotransmitters: **epinephrine (A), glycine (B), histamine (C),** and **serotonin (D)**.[8,11]

143. E – Sweat glands

> In general, postganglionic sympathetic neurons release norepinephrine. **Sweat glands (E)** are an exception to this rule, however. **Sweat glands** are innervated by sympathetic neurons that release acetylcholine and act via muscarinic receptors. The **sweat glands** are innervated by the sympathetic system only.[8,11]

144. B – Their activity is increased after lesions of the spinocerebellum (false)

> Upon stimulation of extrafusal muscle fibers innervated by α motor neurons, the muscle spindles (intrafusal fibers) would have a tendency to go slack, which would make them insensitive to further changes in length. γ motor neurons **innervate intrafusal fibers (C)**, causing intrafusal fibers to contract to sense ongoing **changes in length of the muscle (A)**. The activity of γ motor neurons is profoundly **reduced by lesions in the cerebellum (B is false)**.[8,11]

145. C – II, IV (norepinephrine and serotonin)

Descending **serotonergic** pathways (from rostroventral medullary neurons) and **noradrenergic** pathways (from the pons) are important links in the supraspinal modulation of nociceptive transmission.[7,8]

146. B – I, III (retinal ganglion cells and lateral geniculate cells)

Cells of the **retina** and **lateral geniculate nucleus** have concentric receptive fields that fall into two classes: on-center or off-center. Simple cells of the visual cortex have rectangular receptive fields. The receptive field of a complex cell in the primary visual cortex has no clearly distinct excitatory or inhibitory zones. Orientation but not position of the light stimulus is important.[8]

147. E – Ruffini's corpuscles
148. B – Meissner's corpuscles
149. C – Merkel's receptors
150. D – Pacinian corpuscles
151. A – Free nerve endings

Meissner's corpuscles (B) and **Merkel's receptors (C)** are both found superficially in the dermal papillae and have small receptive fields. **Pacinian (D)** and **Ruffini's (E)** corpuscles are found in the deeper subcutaneous tissue and have large receptive fields. Both **Merkel's receptors (C)** and **Ruffini's corpuscles (E)** are slowly adapting and subserve pressure sensation. **Pacinian corpuscles (D)** are more sensitive to low- than high-frequency stimuli and transmit flutter. Pain sensation is transmitted by **free nerve endings (A)**.[8,11]

152. C – Anti-glutamic acid decarboxylase

The diagnosis in the case is "stiff-man" or "stiff-person" syndrome. Most cases of this disorder show circulating autoantibodies against **glutamic acid decarboxylase (C)**, which is the enzyme responsible for synthesizing GABA. The stiff-person syndrome can occur rarely as a paraneoplastic syndrome in association with breast cancer; in those cases, it is associated with an **anti-amphiphysin (A)** or an **anti-gephyrin (B)** autoantibody. The **anti-Yo (D)** antibody occurs with ovarian, lung, and Hodgkin tumors and causes cerebellar degeneration. The **anti-Ri (E)** antibody is responsible for the opsoclonus-myoclonus-ataxia seen with some breast and small-cell lung cancers.[9]

153. D – Mutation affecting the RAS signal-transduction pathway

This young patient presenting with an optic tract glioma may carry a diagnosis of neurofibromatosis type 1 (NF1). NF1 is associated with neurofibromas, optic nerve and tract gliomas, pigmented nodules of the iris, and hyperpigmented cutaneous macules. The NF1 gene is located on chromosome 17 and encodes the protein neurofibromin. **Neurofibromin is thought to be a tumor suppressor gene (B is false)** that has some structural homology to the **RAS superfamily of GTPases.** Therefore, **choice D is correct.** Neurofibromatosis type 2 is associated with **bilateral vestibular schwannomas (A)** and is caused by a **mutation on chromosome 22 (C).** Tuberous sclerosis is associated with mutations of the **hamartin gene on chromosome 9 (E).**[12]

154. B – G_1/S

The **G_1/S transition (B)** represents the point of no return in the cell cycle. At this point, DNA is checked for accuracy prior to entering the S phase. If DNA repair is not possible, apoptotic mechanisms are activated. Another checkpoint exists at the **G_2/M transition (D)**, which is particularly important for cells exposed to ionizing radiation.[12]

155. C – MIB1 labels cells proliferating in multiple stages of the cell cycle

Traditional H&E staining techniques rely on the identification of mitoses for the detection of proliferating cells. The key advantage of MIB1 labeling is the **ability to detect proliferating cells in multiple stages of the cell cycle (C)**, even those not currently in the M phase of the cell cycle. MIB1 labeling does add data that standard techniques cannot provide, so **choice B is incorrect**. Mitoses are typically counted on the H&E preparation, and while cells undergoing mitosis are positive for MIB1, **choice D is not the best answer**. While MIB1 labeling may be useful in determining the proliferative index of a tumor, it is **not a part of the WHO criteria for the grading of fibrillary astrocytomas (A and E)**.[13]

156. A – Value is higher in CSF than plasma.
157. B – Value is higher in plasma than CSF.
158. A – Value is higher in CSF than plasma.
159. B – Value is higher in plasma than CSF.
160. C – Value is equal in plasma and CSF.
161. B – Value is higher in plasma than CSF.
162. C – Value is equal in plasma and CSF.
163. B – Value is higher in plasma than CSF.

CSF contains a higher concentration of chloride than the blood plasma. Beta-2 transferrin is a component that is unique to CSF and can be helpful in the diagnosis of CSF leak **(A)**. Osmolality and sodium concentration are equal between CSF and plasma **(C)**. The concentrations of potassium, calcium, uric acid, and glucose are lower in CSF than in plasma **(B)**.[3]

164. C – Increased acetylcholine transferase activity (false)

Huntington's disease is a fatal, autosomal dominant, **progressive choreoathetosis (D)** that involves a **trinucleotide CAG (E)** repeat on **chromosome 4 (B)**. Brain imaging reveals **atrophy of the caudate heads (A)** with a characteristic appearance of hydrocephalus ex vacuo. While the pathophysiology is not well understood, there is believed to be decreased acetylcholine transferase activity in patients with Huntington's disease **(C is false)**.[3,12]

165. D – +61 mV

The equilibrium potential is the membrane potential at which no net diffusion of an ion occurs because of balanced electrical and chemical gradients. The resting membrane potential for sodium is **+61 mV (D)**, potassium is **−94 mV (A)**, chloride is **−86 mV (C)**, and calcium is **+267 mV (E)**. The resting membrane potential of large, myelinated peripheral nerves is approximately **−90 mV (B)**. The resting membrane potential is determined largely by the equilibrium potential of potassium (−94 mV) because potassium is 100 times more permeable than sodium.[3]

166. A – Methylation of the *MGMT* gene's promoter region upregulates MGMT gene expression

The O[6]-methylguanine-DNA methyltransferase *(MGMT)* gene codes for a **DNA repair protein (D)** that represents an **important mechanism for chemotherapy resistance (E)** in glioblastoma. Methylation of the gene's promoter region leads to **silencing of the *MGMT* gene (A is false)**. *MGMT* methylation is an **independent predictor of improved survival (B)** as well as a **predictor of survival benefit from temozolomide (C)** in patients with glioblastoma.[3]

167. A – < 4 minutes
168. C – 40 minutes
169. D – 80 minutes
170. E – Infinite
171. E – Infinite

Normal cerebral blood flow (CBF) is **50–55 mL/100 g/min (E)**. Cells can compensate at a CBF of **18 mL/100 g/min indefinitely (E)**. CBF in the ischemic penumbra is thought to be 8–23 mL/100 g/min. At **less than 8 mL/100 g/min, there is rapid cell death from ion pump failure (A)**. At 10 mL/100 g/min, cell death occurs after approximately **40 minutes (C)**. At 15 mL/100 g/min cell death occurs after **80 minute (D)**.[3]

172. C – Anti-Ma
173. E – Anti-Yo
174. B – Anti-Hu
175. D – Anti-Ri
176. A – Anti-glutamic acid decarboxylase

Limbic encephalitis is a subacute encephalitis that typically involves the mesial temporal lobes, cingulate gyri, and insula. Limbic encephalitis is associated with testicular cancer, lung cancer, and **anti-Ma (C)** antibodies. **Anti-Yo (E)** antibodies are associated with ovarian and breast cancer and lead to cerebellar degeneration. **Anti-Hu (B)** antibodies are associated with oat cell pulmonary carcinoma and lymphoma and are associated with sensory neuropathy, encephalitis, and cerebellar degeneration. **Anti-Ri (D)** antibodies are associated with breast cancer and lead to opsoclonus. Stiff-man syndrome is associated with antibodies to **glutamic acid decarboxylase (A)** in > 60% of cases.[3]

References

1. Winn HR, ed. Neurological Surgery, 5th ed. Philadelphia, PA: W.B. Saunders; 2003
2. Hall ZW, ed. An Introduction to Molecular Neurobiology. Sunderland, MA: Sinauer Associates, Inc.; 1992
3. Citow JS, Macdonald RL, Refai D, eds. Comprehensive Neurosurgery Board Review. New York: Thieme Medical Publishers; 2009
4. Katzung BG, ed. Basic and Clinical Pharmacology, 9th ed. New York: McGraw-Hill; 2004.
5. Brunton LL, Lazo JS, Parker KL, eds. Goodman & Gilman's the Pharmacological Basis of Therapeutics, 11th ed. New York: McGraw-Hill; 2006
6. Squire LR, Berg D, Bloom FE, du Lac S, Ghosh A, Spitzer NC, eds. Fundamental Neuroscience, 4th ed. New York: Elsevier; 2013
7. Patestas MA, Gartner LP, eds. Textbook of Neuroanatomy. Malden, MA: Blackwell Publishing; 2006
8. Kandel ER, Schwartz JH, Jessel TM, eds. Principles of Neural Science, 4th ed. New York: McGraw-Hill; 2000
9. Ropper AH, Brown RH, eds. Principles of Neurology, 8th ed. New York: McGraw-Hill; 2005
10. Carpenter MB. Core Text of Neuroanatomy, 4th ed. Baltimore, MD: Williams & Wilkins; 1991
11. Boron WF, Boulparp EL, eds. Medical Physiology. A Cellular and Molecular Approach. Philadelphia, PA: Elsevier; 2005
12. Kumar VK, Abbas AK, Fausto N, eds. Robbins and Cotran: Pathologic Basis of Disease, 7th ed. Philadelphia, PA: Elsevier; 2005
13. Dabbs DJ, Thompson LDR. Diagnostic Immunohistochemistry: Theranostic and Genomic Applications. Philadelphia: W. B. Saunders; 2010

1. The organism most frequently identified in brain abscesses is
   A. *Bacteroides*
   B. *Candida*
   C. *Citrobacter*
   D. Microaerophilic *Streptococcus*
   E. *Staphylococcus*

⇨ For questions **2** to **9**, match the metal with the toxicity or description. Each response may be used once, more than once, or not at all.
   A. Arsenic
   B. Lead
   C. Mercury
   D. Manganese

2. Mees' transverse white lines on fingernails

3. Psychological dysfunction ("mad as a hatter")

4. Parkinson's symptoms

5. Red blood cell basophilic stippling

6. Brain levels increased by dimercaprol (BAL)

7. Symptoms improve with L-dopa

8. Increased urine coproporphyrin

9. Both penicillamine and BAL are used in treatment

⇨ For questions **10** to **14**, match the structure with the description. Each response may be used once, more than once, or not at all.
   A. Neurofibrillary tangles
   B. Neuritic plaques
   C. Both
   D. Neither

10. Intranuclear

11. Core composed of α protein

12. Contains paired helical filaments

13. Immunoreactive for τ protein

14. Revealed with silver stains

15. Most meningiomas express immunoreactivity for
    A. Cytokeratin
    B. Desmin
    C. Glial fibrillary acidic protein (GFAP)
    D. S-100 protein
    E. Vimentin

16. Each of the following is true of gangliogliomas *except*
    A. The astrocytes are GFAP positive
    B. The ganglion cells are synaptophysin positive
    C. They contain neuropeptides
    D. They are usually diffusely infiltrative
    E. They are most common in the temporal lobes

17. Which of the following is *not* associated with trisomy 13?
    A. Holoprosencephaly
    B. Hypertelorism
    C. Microcephaly
    D. Microphthalmia
    E. Polydactyly

18. Which of the following is *not* characteristic of ependymomas?
    A. Blepharoplasts in the basal cytoplasm
    B. Intermediate filaments that are immunohistochemically identical to glial filaments of astrocytes
    C. Perivascular pseudorosettes
    D. Surface microvilli
    E. True rosette formation

⇨ For questions **19** to **28**, match the vitamin with the description of its deficiency or toxicity. Each response may be used once, more than once, or not at all.
    A. Thiamine
    B. Niacin
    C. Vitamin B$_{12}$
    D. Vitamin A
    E. Vitamin D

19. Wernicke's encephalopathy

20. Korsakoff's psychosis

21. Pellagra

22. Beriberi

23. Seen in rice eaters

24. Seen in corn eaters

25. Rickets

26. Pernicious anemia

27. Subacute combined degeneration

28. Pseudotumor

29. Which of the following is *true* of lymphomas (non-Hodgkin's malignant lymphomas) of the central nervous system (CNS)?
    A. All exhibit a diffuse histologic pattern.
    B. Meningeal lesions are more common in primary lymphomas.
    C. Most are of T cell lineage.
    D. Parenchymal lesions are more common in secondary lymphomas.
    E. They are radioresistant.

30. Which of the following is *not* seen in Sturge-Weber syndrome?
    A. Cortical arteriovenous malformations
    B. Facial nevus
    C. Intracortical calcification
    D. Meningeal angioma
    E. Seizures

31. Each of the following is true of the cord pathology in pernicious anemia *except*
    A. Demyelination occurs
    B. Lumbar levels are most severely affected
    C. Lesions may occur in the medulla
    D. Vacuolar distention of myelin sheaths occurs
    E. Wallerian degeneration occurs

32. Which of the following is associated with progressive multifocal encephalopathy?
    A. Bacterial infection
    B. Demyelination
    C. Increased numbers of oligodendroglial cells
    D. Intense inflammatory infiltrate
    E. Shrunken oligodendroglial nuclei at the periphery of the lesion

33. Which of the following is associated with von Hippel-Lindau disease?
        I. Hepatic cysts
        II. Hemangioblastoma of the spinal cord
        III. Renal cysts
        IV. Renal cell carcinoma
    A. I, II, III
    B. I, III
    C. II, IV
    D. IV
    E. All of the above

▷ For questions **34** to **38**, match the tumor with the description. Each response may be used once, more than once, or not at all.

    A.   Neurofibroma

    B.   Schwannoma

    C.   Both

    D.   Neither

34. Antoni A areas

35. Antoni B areas

36. Verocay bodies

37. Axons are present between tumor cells

38. The plexiform type is strongly associated with neurofibromatosis type 1

39. Which one of the following cerebral metastases has the greatest tendency to hemorrhage?

    A.   Breast

    B.   Choriocarcinoma

    C.   Gastrointestinal (GI) tract

    D.   Ovarian

    E.   Prostate

▷ For questions **40** to **44**, match the time period after a cerebral infarct with the histologic appearance. Each response may be used once, more than once, or not at all.

    A.   12–24 hours

    B.   Days 1–2

    C.   Days 5–7

    D.   Days 10–20

    E.   More than 3 months

40. Lipid-laden macrophages first appear

41. Fibrillary astrocytes present at the periphery of the lesion

42. Gemistocytic astrocytes present at the periphery of the lesion

43. Polymorphonuclear infiltrate

44. Neuronal necrosis is first apparent

45. Hepatic failure is most closely associated with

    A.   Endothelial proliferation

    B.   Gliosis localized to the globus pallidus and hippocampus

    C.   Gliosis localized to the white matter

    D.   Alzheimer's type II astrocytes

    E.   Loss of oligodendroglial cells

46. Each of the following has been associated with central pontine myelinolysis *except*

    A.   Alcoholism

    B.   Severe burns

    C.   Rapid correction of hyponatremia

    D.   Serum hyperosmolarity

    E.   Vitamin A excess

47. Rosenthal fibers are associated with

    I.   Astrocytosis

    II.   Alexander's disease

    III. Pilocytic astrocytoma

    IV. Pick's disease

  A.   I, II, III

  B.   I, III

  C.   II, IV

  D.   IV

  E.   All of the above

48. Which of the following is *not* typically seen in neurofibromatosis type 2?

  A.   Acoustic neuromas

  B.   Café-au-lait spots

  C.   Cutaneous neurofibromatosis

  D.   Lisch nodules

  E.   Plexiform neurofibromas

49. Which of the following is *not* associated with hepatic encephalopathy?

  A.   Thiamine deficiency

  B.   Asterixis

  C.   Alzheimer's type II astrocytes

  D.   Increased serum ammonia

50. In amyotrophic lateral sclerosis, the cranial nerve nucleus that typically does *not* exhibit cell loss is

  A.   III

  B.   V

  C.   VII

  D.   IX

  E.   XII

51. Which of the following vascular malformations have no intervening brain parenchyma between blood vessels?

  A.   Arteriovenous malformations

  B.   Capillary telangiectasias

  C.   Cavernous malformations

  D.   Cryptic arteriovenous malformations

  E.   Venous angiomas

⇨ For questions **52** to **57**, match the sites of damage in the axonal transport apparatus with the toxin. Each response may be used once, more than once, or not at all.

  A.   Microtubules

  B.   Oxidative phosphorylation

  C.   Transcription

  D.   Translation

  E.   Turnaround transport

52. Diabetes

53. Vincristine

54. Mercury

55. Actinomycin D

56. Dinitrophenol

57. Vinblastine

58. Catecholamine production can occur in which of the following tumors?
A. Choriocarcinomas
B. Glomus jugulare tumors
C. Oligodendrogliomas
D. Pineocytomas
E. Pleomorphic xanthoastrocytomas

59. The viral inclusions seen in herpes simplex encephalitis are
A. Basophilic
B. Called Cowdry type B bodies
C. Found in neurons only
D. Intranuclear
E. Only evident several weeks after the infection

60. High levels of α-fetoprotein are associated with
A. Endodermal sinus tumors
B. Choriocarcinomas
C. Germinomas
D. Pineoblastomas
E. Teratomas

61. The most common sites of hypertensive hemorrhage, in decreasing order of frequency, are
A. Lobar, putamen, cerebellum, thalamus, pons
B. Putamen, lobar, thalamus, cerebellum, pons
C. Putamen, thalamus, pons, lobar, cerebellum
D. Thalamus, cerebellum, lobar, putamen, pons
E. Thalamus, lobar, putamen, cerebellum, pons

⇨ For questions **62** to **65**, match the source of the metastatic brain lesion to the description. Each response may be used once, more than once, or not at all.
A. Breast
B. Choriocarcinoma
C. Lung
D. Lymphoma
E. Prostate

62. Most common

63. Greatest tendency to hemorrhage

64. Meningeal involvement is most common.

65. Least propensity to involve the brain

⇨ For questions **66** to **69**, match the mechanism of action to the disease. Each response may be used once, more than once, or not at all.

    A.   Presynaptic inhibition at the neuromuscular junction
    B.   Inhibition of Renshaw cells
    C.   Postsynaptic inhibition

66.   Botulism

67.   Myasthenia gravis

68.   Eaton-Lambert syndrome

69.   Tetanus

70.   Tuberous sclerosis is most closely associated with
    A.   Acoustic neuromas
    B.   Cortical calcification
    C.   Giant-cell astrocytomas
    D.   Optic gliomas
    E.   Renal cysts

71.   High levels of human chorionic gonadotrophin are seen in
    A.   Choriocarcinoma
    B.   Embryonal carcinoma
    C.   Endodermal sinus tumor
    D.   Germinoma
    E.   Teratoma

72.   Cushing's disease is most often associated with a(n)
    A.   Acidophilic pituitary adenoma
    B.   Basophilic pituitary adenoma
    C.   Chromophobic pituitary adenoma
    D.   Ectopic source of adrenocorticotropic hormone (ACTH)
    E.   Nonfunctioning pituitary adenoma

⇨ For questions **73** to **83**, match the sphingolipidosis with the description. Each response may be used once, more than once, or not at all.
    A.   Fabry's disease
    B.   Gaucher's disease
    C.   Niemann-Pick disease
    D.   Sandhoff's disease
    E.   Tay-Sachs disease

73.   Sphingomyelinase deficiency

74.   Hexosaminidase A and B deficiency

75.   Glucocerebrosidase deficiency

76.   Hexosaminidase A deficiency only

77. α-galactosidase deficiency

78.   Abnormal accumulation of ceramide trihexosides

79.   Tay-Sachs and this disorder are forms of the GM2 gangliosidoses

80. Supranuclear paresis of vertical gaze is highly characteristic

81. Episodes of pain occur

82. X-linked recessive

83. Cherry-red spots are found in virtually all patients with Sandhoff's and this disorder

⇨ For questions **84** to **88**, match the mucopolysaccharidosis (MPS) with the description. Each response may be used only once.
  A. Hunter's syndrome (MPS II)
  B. Hurler's syndrome (MPS I H)
  C. Morquio's syndrome (MPS IV)
  D. Sanfilippo's syndrome (MPS III)
  E. Scheie's syndrome (MPS I S)

84. Deficiency of α-L-iduronidase

85. Characterized by severe skeletal deformities and ligamentous laxity

86. Heparan sulfate only is excreted in the urine

87. Deficiency of iduronate sulfatase; pebbling of the skin may occur; X-linked recessive

88. All forms of Morquio's and this disorder are characterized by normal intelligence

⇨ For questions **89** to **95**, match the leukodystrophy with the description. Each response may be used once, more than once, or not at all.
  A. Adrenoleukodystrophy
  B. Alexander's disease
  C. Canavan's disease
  D. Krabbe's disease
  E. Metachromatic leukodystrophy

89. Deficiency of galactocerebrosidase

90. Deficiency of peroxisomes

91. Rosenthal fibers are prominent

92. Deficiency of arylsulfatase

93. X-linked recessive inheritance

94. Accumulation of small quantities of psychosine, a highly toxic compound

95. Accumulation of long-chain fatty acids

96. Each of the following is characteristic of Wilson's disease *except*
  A. Alzheimer's type II astrocytes
  B. Atrophy and brownish discoloration of the globus pallidus and putamen
  C. Autosomal dominant trait
  D. Decreased serum ceruloplasmin
  E. Decreased serum copper

⇨ For questions **97** to **100**, match the description with the disease or syndrome.
   A.   Idiopathic Parkinson's disease
   B.   Shy-Drager syndrome
   C.   Both
   D.   Neither

97. Loss of cells in the zona compacta of the substantia nigra

98. Loss of cells in the intermediolateral horn cells

99. Lewy bodies present

100. Prominent loss of neurons in the putamen

101. The most common neurologic complication of acquired immunodeficiency syndrome (AIDS) is
   A.   Dementia
   B.   Inflammatory polymyositis
   C.   Lymphoma
   D.   Myelopathy
   E.   Toxoplasmosis

102. Each of the following lesions is characteristic of tuberous sclerosis *except*
   A.   Adenoma sebaceum
   B.   Renal cell carcinoma
   C.   Rhabdomyomas of the heart
   D.   Subependymal giant-cell astrocytoma
   E.   Subungual fibromas

103. Each of the following is seen in neurofibromatosis type 1 *except*
   A.   Axillary freckling
   B.   Café-au-lait macules
   C.   Neurofibromas of the iris
   D.   Optic gliomas
   E.   Sphenoid dysplasia

104. Each of the following is true of amyloid angiopathy *except*
   A.   Amyloid β protein is the major protein seen
   B.   Aneurysmal dilations are seen in involved vessels
   C.   It occurs primarily in vessels of deep nuclear structures of the brain
   D.   It occurs primarily in patients over 70 years of age
   E.   A yellow-green dichromism is seen under polarized light when the amyloid is stained with Congo red

105. Characteristic pathologic findings in Guillain-Barré syndrome include each of the following *except*
   A.   Increased cerebrospinal fluid (CSF) protein at 5 weeks after onset of illness
   B.   Lymphocytic pleocytosis in 90% of patients
   C.   Normal CSF pressures
   D.   Perivascular lymphocytic and inflammatory cell infiltrate
   E.   Perivenular and segmental demyelination

⇨ For questions **106** to **162**, match the figure with the most appropriate response.

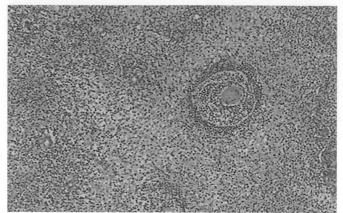

106.

    A. Rarely multiple
    B. Associated with immunosuppression in older men
    C. Associated with immunosuppression in younger men
    D. Resistant to steroids

107. Note inset at top right.

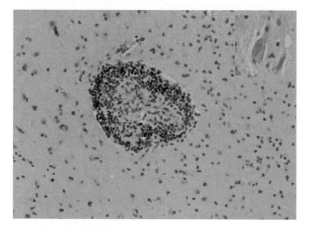

    A. Hirano bodies
    B. Inclusion bodies of herpes simplex virus-1 (HSV-1)
    C. Lewy bodies
    D. Pick bodies
    E. Rabies

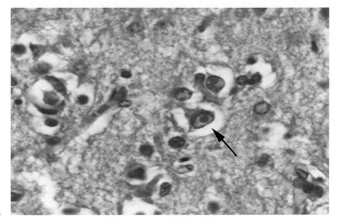

108.

A. Hirano bodies
B. Inclusion bodies of subacute sclerosing panencephalitis (SSPE)
C. Lewy bodies
D. Pick bodies
E. Rabies

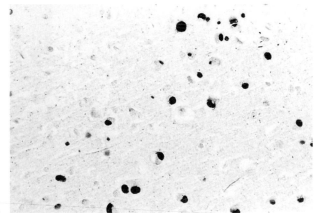

109.

A. Inclusion bodies of HSV-1
B. Lewy bodies
C. Pick bodies
D. Rabies
E. Inclusion bodies of SSPE

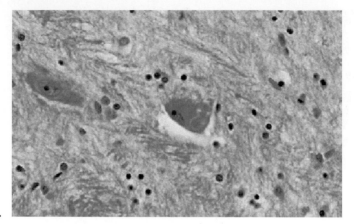

110.

    A.   Inclusion bodies of HSV-1
    B.   Lewy bodies
    C.   Pick bodies
    D.   Rabies
    E.   Inclusion bodies of SSPE

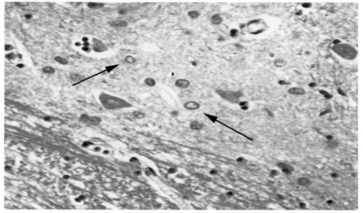

111.

    A.   Ganglioglioma
    B.   Hepatic encephalopathy
    C.   HSV-1
    D.   Parkinson's disease
    E.   Normal cortex

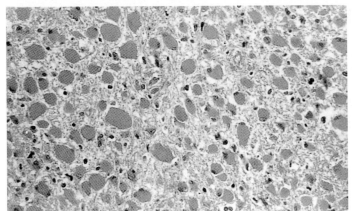

112.

A. Fibrillary astrocytoma
B. Gemistocytic astrocytoma
C. Glioblastoma multiforme
D. Hemangioblastoma
E. Oligodendroglioma

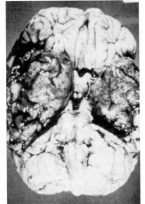

113.

A. Aneurysmal subarachnoid hemorrhage
B. Bacterial meningitis
C. Contusion
D. HSV-1
E. Subdural hematoma

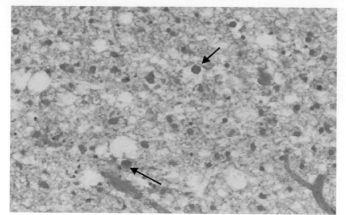

114.

    A.   AIDS encephalopathy
    B.   Giant-cell glioblastoma multiforme (GBM)
    C.   Hemangioblastoma
    D.   Creutzfeldt-Jakob disease
    E.   Progressive multifocal leukoencephalopathy

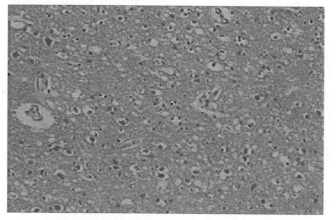

115.

    A.   AIDS encephalopathy
    B.   Giant-cell GBM
    C.   Hemangioblastoma
    D.   Creutzfeldt-Jakob disease
    E.   Progressive multifocal leukoencephalopathy

116. The patient in this photograph is most likely to have

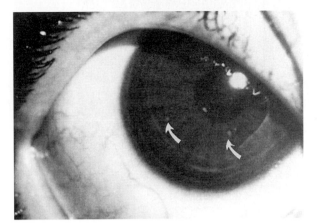

- **A.** Metastatic disease
- **B.** Neurofibromatosis type 1 (NF-1)
- **C.** NF-2
- **D.** Tuberous sclerosis
- **E.** von Hippel-Lindau disease

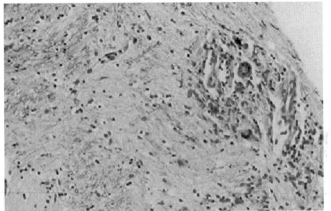

117.

- **A.** HIV encephalopathy
- **B.** Giant-cell GBM
- **C.** Hemangioblastoma
- **D.** Creutzfeldt-Jakob disease
- **E.** Progressive multifocal leukoencephalopathy

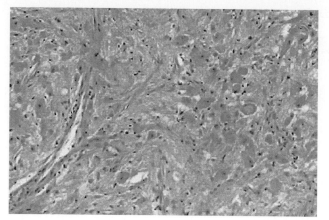

118.

    A.   Anaplastic astrocytoma
    B.   Ependymoma
    C.   Ganglioglioma
    D.   Meningioma
    E.   Oligodendroglioma

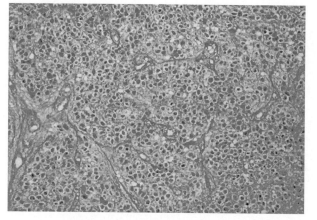

119.

    A.   Anaplastic astrocytoma
    B.   Meningioma
    C.   Normal pituitary gland
    D.   Oligodendroglioma
    E.   Pituitary adenoma

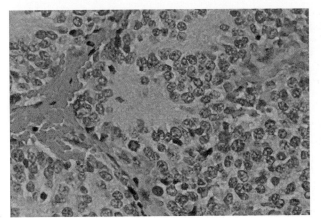

120.

A. Choroid plexus papilloma
B. Ependymoma
C. Medulloblastoma
D. Meningioma
E. Pituitary adenoma

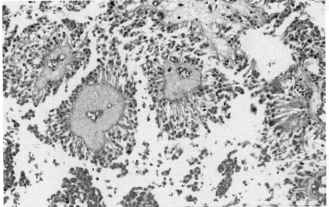

121.

A. Choroid plexus papilloma
B. Craniopharyngioma
C. Hemangioblastoma
D. Metastatic tumor
E. Myxopapillary ependymoma

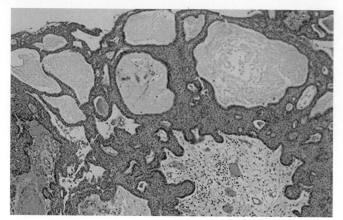

122.

    A.   Choroid plexus papilloma
    B.   Craniopharyngioma
    C.   Hemangioblastoma
    D.   Metastatic tumor
    E.   Myxopapillary ependymoma

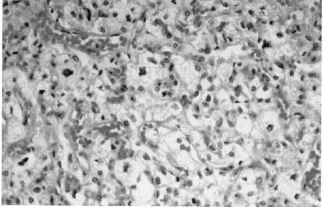

123.

    A.   Choroid plexus papilloma
    B.   Craniopharyngioma
    C.   Hemangioblastoma
    D.   Metastatic tumor
    E.   Myxopapillary ependymoma

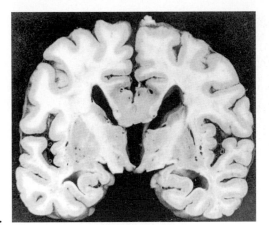

124.

    A.   Butterfly glioma
    B.   Carbon monoxide poisoning
    C.   Fat emboli
    D.   Lipoma
    E.   Lipofuscin deposition

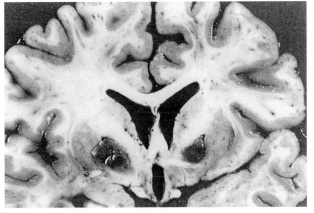

125.

    A.   Carbon monoxide poisoning
    B.   Fat emboli
    C.   Hallervorden-Spatz disease
    D.   Miliary tuberculosis
    E.   Wilson's disease

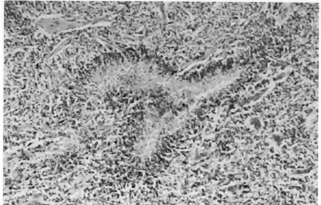

126.

    A.   Ependymoma
    B.   Glioblastoma
    C.   Medulloblastoma
    D.   Meningioma
    E.   Schwannoma

127. The patient in this photograph is most likely to have

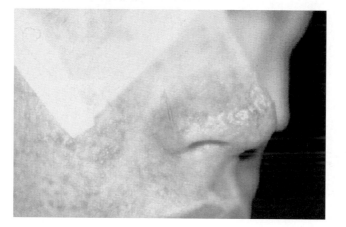

    A.   Metastatic disease
    B.   NF-1
    C.   NF-2
    D.   Tuberous sclerosis
    E.   von Hippel-Lindau disease

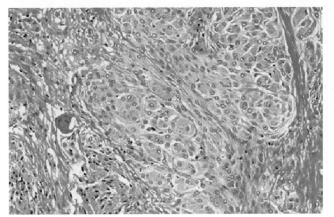

128.

A. Anaplastic astrocytoma
B. Medulloblastoma
C. Meningioma
D. Metastatic tumor
E. Oligodendroglioma

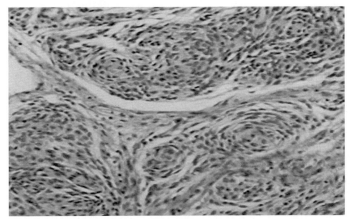

129.

A. Glioblastoma
B. Malignant peripheral nerve sheath tumor
C. Meningioma
D. Neurofibroma
E. Schwannoma

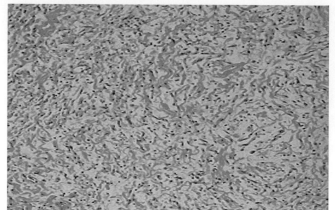

130.

    A. Glioblastoma
    B. Malignant peripheral nerve sheath tumor
    C. Meningioma
    D. Neurofibroma
    E. Schwannoma

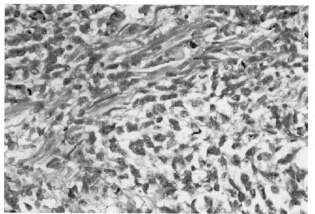

131.

    A. Glioblastoma
    B. Malignant peripheral nerve sheath tumor
    C. Meningioma
    D. Neurofibroma
    E. Schwannoma

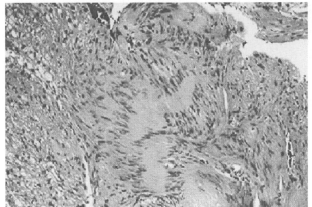

132.

    A.   Glioblastoma
    B.   Malignant peripheral nerve sheath tumor
    C.   Meningioma
    D.   Neurofibroma
    E.   Schwannoma

133. This lesion is associated with (the)

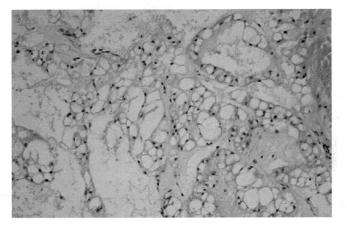

    A.   Filum terminale
    B.   Kidney
    C.   Notochord
    D.   Pituitary
    E.   von Hippel-Lindau disease

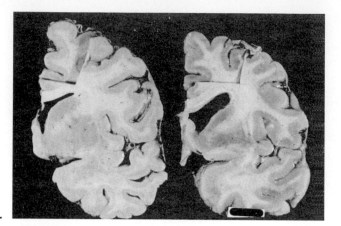

134.

    A.   Alzheimer's disease

    B.   HSV-1

    C.   Huntington's disease

    D.   Parkinson's disease

    E.   Pick's disease

135. Double arrows correspond to

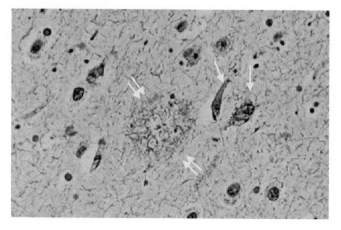

    A.   Bacterial meningitis

    B.   Candidiasis

    C.   Neuritic plaques

    D.   Neurofibrillary tangles

    E.   Pick bodies

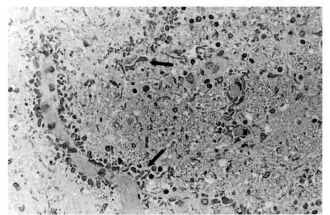

136.

    A.   Acute disseminated encephalomyelitis
    B.   Adrenoleukodystrophy
    C.   Alexander's disease
    D.   Krabbe's disease
    E.   Metachromatic leukodystrophy

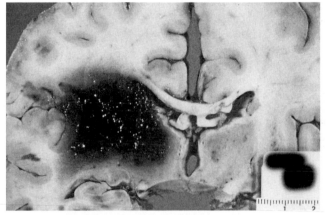

137.

    A.   Amyloid angiopathy
    B.   Duret's hemorrhage
    C.   Glioblastoma
    D.   Hypertensive hemorrhage
    E.   Melanoma

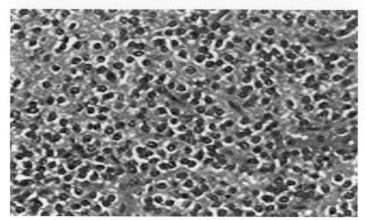

138.

    A.   Central neurocytoma
    B.   Colloid cysts
    C.   Glioblastoma
    D.   Hemangioblastoma
    E.   Schwannoma

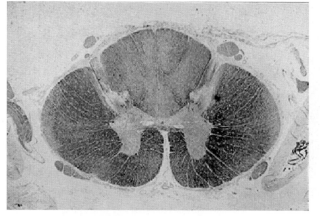

139.

    A.   Amyotrophic lateral sclerosis
    B.   Friedreich's ataxia
    C.   Multiple sclerosis
    D.   Radiation myelopathy
    E.   Subacute combined degeneration

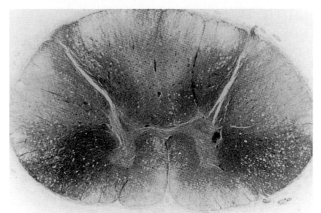

140.

A. Amyotrophic lateral sclerosis
B. Friedreich's ataxia
C. Multiple sclerosis
D. Radiation myelopathy
E. Subacute combined degeneration

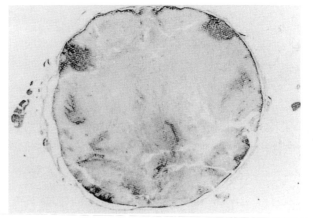

141.

A. Amyotrophic lateral sclerosis
B. Friedreich's ataxia
C. Multiple sclerosis
D. Radiation myelopathy
E. Subacute combined degeneration

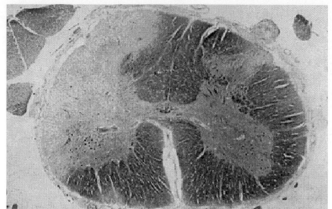

142.

 A. Amyotrophic lateral sclerosis
 B. Friedreich's ataxia
 C. Multiple sclerosis
 D. Radiation myelopathy
 E. Subacute combined degeneration

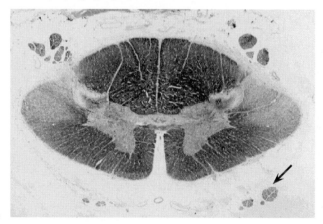

143.

 A. Amyotrophic lateral sclerosis
 B. Friedreich's ataxia
 C. Multiple sclerosis
 D. Radiation myelopathy
 E. Subacute combined degeneration

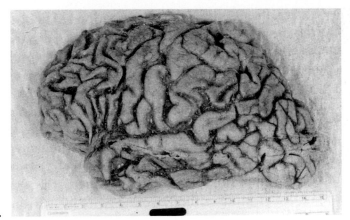

144.

    A. Gliomatosis cerebri
    B. Huntington's disease
    C. Krabbe's disease
    D. Multiple sclerosis
    E. Tuberous sclerosis

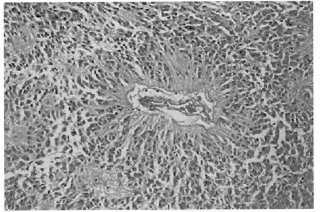

145.

    A. Choroid plexus papilloma
    B. Ependymoma
    C. Lymphoma
    D. Medulloblastoma
    E. Meningioma

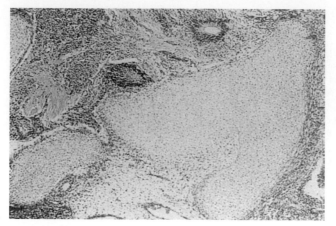

146.

    A. Chordoma
    B. Dermoid
    C. Metastatic tumor
    D. Myxopapillary ependymoma
    E. Teratoma

147. This patient is most likely to have

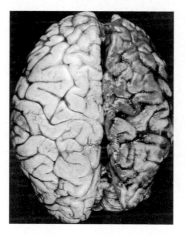

    A. Advanced age and lobar hemorrhages
    B. Alcoholism and prone to falls
    C. Port-wine nevus on the face
    D. Retinal hamartomas
    E. Subungual fibromas

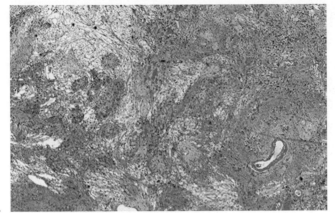

148.

    A. Acoustic neuroma
    B. Anaplastic astrocytoma
    C. Medulloblastoma
    D. Melanoma
    E. Meningioma

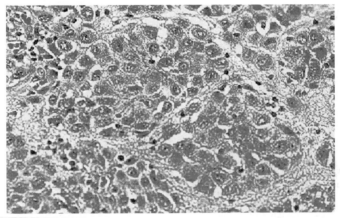

149.

    A. Carbon monoxide poisoning
    B. Cerebral contusions
    C. Herpes encephalitis
    D. Meningeal carcinomatosis
    E. Melanoma

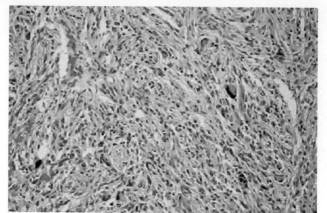

150.

    A.   Acoustic neuroma
    B.   Anaplastic astrocytoma
    C.   Medulloblastoma
    D.   Melanoma
    E.   Meningioma

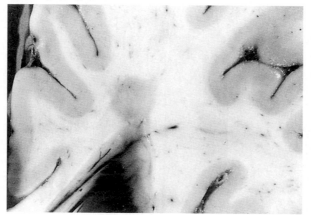

151.

    A.   Anaplastic astrocytoma
    B.   Infarct
    C.   Metachromatic leukodystrophy
    D.   Multiple sclerosis
    E.   Radiation necrosis

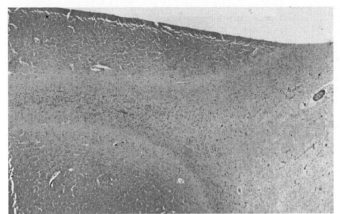

152.

A. Anaplastic astrocytoma
B. Infarct
C. Metachromatic leukodystrophy
D. Multiple sclerosis
E. Radiation necrosis

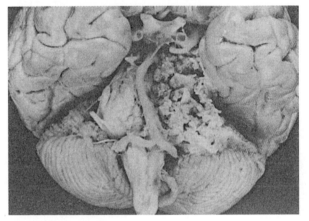

153.

A. Epidermoid
B. Lipoma
C. Metastatic tumor
D. Multiple sclerosis
E. Teratoma

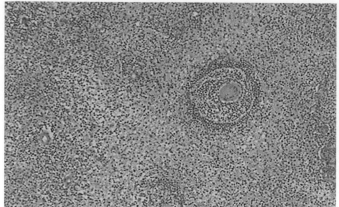

154.

- **A.** Astrocytoma
- **B.** Lymphoma
- **C.** Melanoma
- **D.** Oligodendroglioma
- **E.** Pituitary adenoma

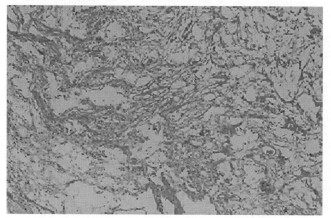

155.

- **A.** Meningioma
- **B.** Neurofibroma
- **C.** Pilocytic astrocytoma
- **D.** Pleomorphic xanthoastrocytoma
- **E.** Schwannoma

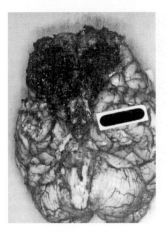

156.

   A.   Aneurysmal subarachnoid hemorrhage
   B.   Bacterial meningitis
   C.   Contusion
   D.   HSV-1
   E.   Subdural hematoma

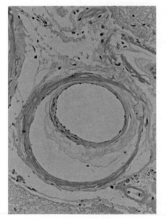

157.

   A.   Amyloid angiopathy
   B.   Arteriovenous malformation
   C.   Capillary telangiectasia
   D.   Embolism
   E.   Venous angioma

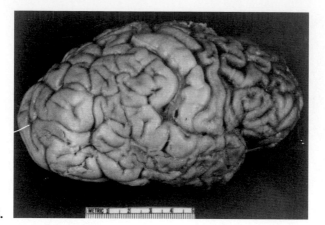

158.

A. Alzheimer's disease
B. Astrocytoma
C. Huntington's disease
D. Krabbe's disease
E. Pick's disease

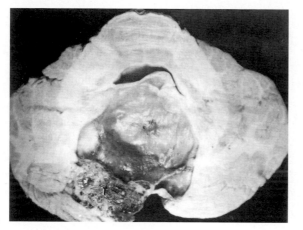

159.

A. Astrocytoma
B. Glioblastoma
C. Hemangioblastoma
D. Medulloblastoma
E. Metastasis

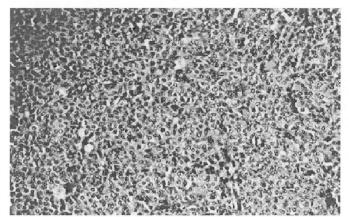

160.

   A. Astrocytoma
   B. Glioblastoma
   C. Neurofibroma
   D. Pituitary adenoma
   E. Schwannoma

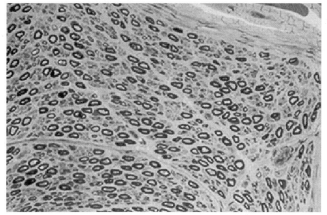

161.

   A. Dejerine-Sottas disease
   B. Krabbe's disease
   C. Metachromatic leukodystrophy
   D. Normal peripheral nerve
   E. Charcot-Marie-Tooth disease

162. The gross specimen seen here is most consistent with

A. Cysticercosis
B. Hemangioblastoma
C. Juvenile pilocytic astrocytoma
D. Renal cell carcinoma
E. Toxoplasmosis

⇨ For questions **163** to **168**, match the metal toxicity with the most appropriate feature or description. Each response may be used once, more than once, or not at all.
A. Arsenic toxicity
B. Lead toxicity
C. Manganese toxicity
D. Mercury toxicity

163. Encephalopathy, peripheral neuropathy, abdominal pain, nausea, vomiting, diarrhea, and shock

164. Malaise, transverse white lines, pigmentation and hyperkeratosis of the palms and soles

165. Irritability, seizures, abdominal pain, ataxia, coma, and increased ICP

166. Demyelinating motor polyneuropathy (wrist drop), anemia, gingival line

167. Psychological dysfunction, tremor, movement disorders, peripheral neuropathy, cerebellar signs

168. Parkinson's type symptoms and headache

169. Which of the following statements regarding primary CNS lymphoma is true?
    A. Herpes zoster virus has been implicated in the pathogenesis.
    B. It is often periventricular and brightly enhancing.
    C. Steroid therapy should be initiated immediately.
    D. It is typically of T cell lineage.
    E. It is an unlikely diagnosis in immunocompromised patients.

170. The photomicrograph seen here

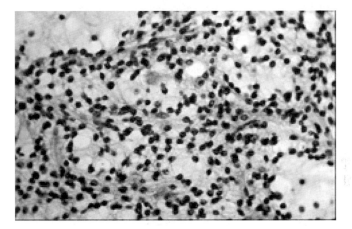

is most consistent with which of the following diagnoses?
    A. Central neurocytoma
    B. Dysembryoplastic neuroepithelial tumor
    C. Lymphoma
    D. Meningioma
    E. Schwannoma

171. Which of the following genetic abnormalities are usually observed in "primary" glioblastomas?
    A. Chromosome 10 deletions (PTEN)
    B. Epidermal growth factor receptor (EGFR) amplification
    C. p53 deletion
    D. None of the above
    E. All of the above
    F. A and B
    G. B and C

172. This photomicrograph

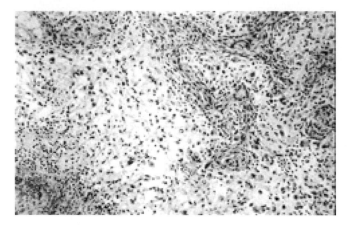

is an example of which of the following?
A. Chondrosarcoma
B. Chordoma
C. Glioblastoma
D. Gliosarcoma
E. Schwannoma

173. At least half of all meningiomas have deletions involving which of the following?
A. Chromosome 3
B. Chromosome 10
C. Chromosome 17
D. Chromosome 22
E. All of the above

174. Meningiomas tend to show immunopositivity for which of the following?
A. Epithelial membrane antigen (EMA)
B. Vimentin
C. Progesterone receptor
D. All of the above
E. None of the above

175. Which of the following is true regarding dementia pugilistica?
A. Diffuse deposits of β-amyloid are sometimes present.
B. Lewy bodies are prominent.
C. N-acetylaspartate content in the putamen and pallidum is increased.
D. The clinical syndrome is present in up to one-half of professional boxers.
E. There is a reduced incidence of cavum septum pellucidum in this disorder.

176. Which of the following features of medulloblastoma is associated with a worse prognosis?
A. Age < 3 years at diagnosis
B. Desmoplastic subtype on histology
C. Extensive nodularity on histology
D. Less than 1.5 cm² postoperative residual tumor
E. Nuclear positivity for β-catenin

177. Which of the following is true regarding the lesion seen here?

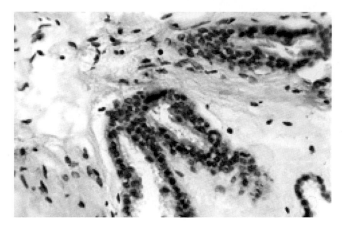

A. They are usually filled with keratin.
B. They tend to be dorsally located.
C. They tend to occur in the midline.
D. All of the above
E. None of the above

1.	D	27.	C
2.	A	28.	D
3.	C	29.	A
4.	D	30.	A
5.	B	31.	B
6.	C	32.	B
7.	D	33.	E
8.	B	34.	B
9.	B	35.	B
10.	D	36.	B
11.	D	37.	A
12.	C	38.	A
13.	A	39.	B
14.	C	40.	C
15.	E	41.	E
16.	D	42.	D
17.	B	43.	B
18.	A	44.	A
19.	A	45.	D
20.	A	46.	E
21.	B	47.	A
22.	A	48.	D
23.	A	49.	A
24.	B	50.	A
25.	E	51.	C
26.	C	52.	E

53.	A		92.	E
54.	D		93.	A
55.	C		94.	D
56.	B		95.	A
57.	A		96.	C
58.	B		97.	C
59.	D		98.	B
60.	A		99.	A
61.	B		100.	B
62.	C		101.	A
63.	B		102.	B
64.	D		103.	C
65.	E		104.	C
66.	A		105.	B
67.	C		106.	C
68.	A		107.	B
69.	B		108.	B
70.	C		109.	C
71.	A		110.	B
72.	B		111.	B
73.	C		112.	B
74.	D		113.	D
75.	B		114.	E
76.	E		115.	D
77.	A		116.	B
78.	A		117.	A
79.	D		118.	C
80.	C		119.	D
81.	A		120.	C
82.	A		121.	E
83.	E		122.	B
84.	B		123.	C
85.	C		124.	D
86.	D		125.	A
87.	A		126.	B
88.	E		127.	D
89.	D		128.	C
90.	A		129.	C
91.	B		130.	D

131. B
132. E
133. C
134. C
135. C
136. C
137. D
138. A
139. B
140. E
141. D
142. C
143. A
144. E
145. B
146. E
147. C
148. A
149. E
150. B
151. D
152. C
153. A
154. B

155. C
156. C
157. A
158. E
159. C
160. D
161. D
162. A
163. A
164. A
165. B
166. B
167. D
168. C
169. B
170. B
171. F
172. D
173. D
174. D
175. A
176. A
177. C

5C Neuropathology—Answers and Explanations

1. D – Microaerophilic *Streptococcus*

While brain abscesses tend to consist of mixed flora, microaerophilic and anaerobic streptococci are the most frequently identified organisms in brain abscesses.[1,2]

2. A – Arsenic
3. C – Mercury
4. D – Manganese
5. B – Lead
6. C – Mercury
7. D – Manganese
8. B – Lead
9. B – Lead

Arsenic toxicity (A) can be caused by insecticides. Chronic exposure to arsenic causes malaise, hyperkeratosis, and pigmentation of the palms and soles, as well as Mees' transverse white lines in the fingernails. Arsenic toxicity is treated with dimercaprol (BAL). **Lead poisoning (B)** causes encephalitis in children, but in adults causes a demyelinating motor polyneuropathy and anemia. **Lead toxicity** leads to basophilic stippling of the erythrocytes and increases excretion of urinary coproporphyrin. **Lead toxicity** can be treated with EDTA, BAL, and penicillamine. **Mercury (C)** can be found in contaminated fish and in felt hat dyes. **Mercury** poisoning may cause psychological dysfunction ("mad as a hatter") as well as cerebellar signs and renal tubular necrosis. Penicillamine is the treatment of choice for **mercury** toxicity; BAL increases brain levels of **mercury** and should be avoided. **Manganese toxicity (D)** primarily affects miners and is characterized by Parkinson's-type symptoms. Neuronal loss is observed in the basal ganglia, and symptoms generally respond to L-dopa.[3]

10. D – Neither
11. D – Neither
12. C – Both

13. A –   Neurofibrillary tangles

14. C –   Both

> **Neurofibrillary tangles (A)** and **neuritic plaques (B)** are both intracytoplasmic; both contain paired helical filaments and are revealed with silver stains. The central core of the **neuritic plaque (B)** is composed of β/A4, not α protein. The **neurofibrillary tangles (A)** are immunoreactive for τ protein.[1]

15. E –   Vimentin

> **Vimentin (E)** is an intermediate filament protein and is usually expressed by meningiomas. **Vimentin (E)** expression is not terribly useful in meningioma diagnosis, as the histopathologic differential diagnostic considerations include many other tumors that may also be vimentin positive such as carcinomas (positive for **cytokeratins [A]**), melanomas (positive for myelin A, HMB45, and **S-100 [D]**), gliomas (positive for **S-100 [D]**), and schwannomas (positive for **S-100 [D]**). Epithelial membrane antigen (EMA) is also expressed by the majority of meningiomas and is a reflection of their epithelial character. Metastatic carcinomas may also express EMA; however, EMA positivity helps to rule out schwannomas, melanomas, and hemangioblastomas. **GFAP (C)** staining is generally negative for meningiomas but has been reported in papillary meningiomas.[1,2]

16. D –   They are usually diffusely infiltrative (false)

> Gangliogliomas are usually well circumscribed and can be partially cystic **(D is false)**. The other responses regarding gangliogliomas are true: the astrocytes are GFAP positive **(A)**, the ganglion cells are synaptophysin positive **(B)**, they contain neuropeptides **(C)**, and they most commonly occur in the temporal lobes **(E)**.[1,2]

17. B –   Hypertelorism

> Trisomy 13, Patau's syndrome, is associated with hypotelorism, **holoprosencephaly (A)**, **microcephaly (C)**, **microphthalmia (D)**, cleft palate, **polydactyly (E)**, dextrocardia, and ocular abnormalities. Patients typically survive no more than 9 months. Hypotelorism, not **hypertelorism (B)**, is associated with trisomy 13.[3,4]

18. A –   Blepharoplasts in the basal cytoplasm

> Ependymomas are CNS neoplasms that resemble the structure of the brain's ependyma. The most definitive evidence of ependymoma is the presence of **true rosettes (E)**, also called "Flexner-Wintersteiner rosettes." Most ependymomas contain **perivascular pseudorosettes (C)** involving tumor cells surrounding an endothelial-lined lumen. Ependymomas tend to stain for **GFAP and vimentin (B)**, particularly in the perivascular pseudorosettes. On electron microscopy, extensive surface microvilli **(D)** forming both intra- and extracellular lumens can be seen. Blepharoplasts (ciliary basal bodies) are found in the apical, not basal, cytoplasm **(A is false)**.[1,2]

19. A –   Thiamine

20. A –   Thiamine

21. B – Niacin
22. A – Thiamine
23. A – Thiamine
24. B – Niacin
25. E – Vitamin D
26. C – Vitamin B$_{12}$
27. C – Vitamin B$_{12}$
28. D – Vitamin A

Diets heavy in corn lack tryptophan that is used to synthesize **niacin (B)**; niacin deficiency causes pellagra—dermatitis, diarrhea, and dementia. Diets heavy in refined rice are more likely to lack sufficient **thiamine (A)**. Thiamine deficiency is associated with Wernicke's encephalopathy and Korsakoff's psychosis, as seen in chronic alcoholism, and is also associated with beriberi—characterized by peripheral polyneuropathy, demyelination, and autonomic dysfunction. **Vitamin A (D)** toxicity may cause cerebral edema with a pseudotumor presentation. Pernicious anemia can lead to a **vitamin B$_{12}$ (C)** deficiency with megaloblastic anemia and subacute combined degeneration of the spinal cord. **Vitamin D deficiency (E)** causes rickets, which is associated with decreased parathyroid hormone and brittle bones.[3]

29. A – All exhibit a diffuse histologic pattern.

Meningeal infiltration is the most common lesion in secondary lymphomas **(B is false)**, and parenchymal lesions are the most common lesion in primary lymphomas **(D is false)**. Most are of B cell lineage and are radiosensitive **(C and E are false)**. Nodular lymphomas are not seen in the central nervous system (CNS); all show a diffuse histology **(A is true)**.[1,2]

30. A – Cortical arteriovenous malformations

Sturge-Weber syndrome is characterized by a usually unilateral **port-wine nevus (B)** that typically involves the orbit or upper eyelid, unilateral **meningeal angioma (D)**, **calcifications** confined to the second and third layers of **cerebral cortex (C)**, and **seizure activity (E)**. The abnormal meningeal vessels are typically veins and are not well-visualized on angiography—a feature that is not consistent with arteriovenous malformations. Arteriovenous malformations (AVMs) are not characteristic of the Sturge-Weber syndrome **(A)**.[5]

31. B – Lumbar levels are most severely affected (false)

The **demyelination (A)**, **spongiosis (D)**, and gliosis seen in vitamin B$_{12}$ deficiency are most common at lower cervical and thoracic levels **(B is false)**.[1]

32. B – Demyelination

Progressive multifocal leukoencephalopathy is caused by a **papovavirus (notably the JC virus; A is false)**. Lesions occur mainly in the white matter and consist of foci of myelin and oligodendroglial cell loss with minimal inflammatory infiltrate **(C and D are false)**. Hyperchromatic enlarged oligodendroglial nuclei are found at the margin of the lesions **(E is false)**. **Demyelination is present (B)**; some early cases were thought to represent atypical MS.[1,2]

33. E –   All of the above

> von Hippel-Lindau (VHL) disease is an autosomal dominant disorder linked to the VHL gene on chromosome 3—a tumor suppressor gene. The disease is associated with **hemangioblastomas of the brain and spinal cord (II)**, retinal hemangioblastomas, **renal cell carcinomas and renal cysts (III, IV)**, pheochromocytoma, pancreatic tumors and cysts, **hepatic cysts (I)**, and polycythemia vera.[5,6]

34. B –   Schwannoma
35. B –   Schwannoma
36. B –   Schwannoma
37. A –   Neurofibroma
38. A –   Neurofibroma

> **Schwannomas (B)** are characterized by a biphasic cellular pattern composed of compact spindle cells (Antoni A areas) and loosely arranged stellate cells (Antoni B areas). Also seen are Verocay bodies, which result from the palisading of elongated nuclei alternating with anuclear fibrillar material. **Neurofibromas (A)** incorporate the parent nerve and hence have axons in their midst. The plexiform type is considered pathognomonic for neurofibromatosis type 1.[1,2]

39. B –   Choriocarcinoma

> Of these choices, **choriocarcinoma (B)** has the greatest tendency to hemorrhage. Hemorrhage is also common in melanoma, renal cell carcinoma, **colorectal carcinoma (C)**, and lung carcinoma. Cancers of **breast origin (A)** are unlikely to hemorrhage.[1,2]

40. C –   Days 5–7
41. E –   More than 3 months
42. D –   Days 10–20
43. B –   Days 1–2
44. A –   12–24 hours

> Irreversible ischemic injury is evident at the cellular level within 6 hours with microvacuolization of the cells and cytoplasmic bulging. Neuronal necrosis becomes apparent within **12–24 hours (A)**. Polymorphonuclear (PMN) leukocytes begin to accumulate 24 hours after the insult and PMN accumulation peaks at **48 hours (B)**. Macrophages begin to arrive on day 3; by **day 5–7 (C)** lipid-laden macrophages become apparent. Between **days 10** and **20 (D)** gemistocytic astrocytes begin to appear at the periphery of the lesion, and enhancement begins to occur on contrasted images. Fibrillary astrocytes do not appear at the periphery of the lesion for **more than 3 months (E)**.[1,3]

45. D –   Alzheimer's type II astrocytes

> Acquired hepatocerebral degeneration is associated with gliosis with a predilection for the cortex **(C is false)**. It tends to spare the hippocampus, globus pallidus, and deep folia of the cerebellar cortex **(B is false)**. Widespread hyperplasia of protoplasmic astrocytes (Alzheimer's type II astrocytes) is visible in the deep layers of the cerebral and cerebellar cortex and in deep nuclear structures **(D)**.[5]

46. E – Vitamin A excess (false)

"The outstanding characteristic of CPM is its invariable association with some other serious, often life threatening disease." Central pontine myelinolysis is an acute demyelinating condition of the brainstem that has been attributed to rapid correction of hyponatremia. The disorder has been associated with **alcoholism (A)**, **severe burns (B)**, and **serum hyperosmolarity (D)**. The common pathway of all of these disease processes seems to involve either the rapid correction of **hyponatremia (C)** or severe **acute hyperosmolarity (D)** (as in burn victims). **Vitamin A** excess has not been associated with central pontine myelinolysis (**E is false**).[5]

47. A – I, II, and III: (astrocytosis, Alexander's disease, and pilocytic astrocytoma)

Rosenthal fibers, eosinophilic masses observed in astrocytic processes, are associated with **pilocytic astrocytomas (III, neoplastic)**, **astrocytosis (I)**, and **Alexander's disease (II, nonneoplastic)**. **Pick's disease (IV)** is associated with Pick bodies, which are round, intracytoplasmic eosinophilic inclusions that are positive with silver stains and with antibodies to tau.[1,2,3]

48. D – Lisch nodules

Neurofibromas (E) and **café-au-lait spots (B)** occur less commonly in neurofibromatosis type 2 (NF-2) than in NF-1. **Bilateral acoustic neuromas (A)** are the hallmark of NF-2. **Lisch nodules (D)** are rare in NF-2.[1,5]

49. A – Thiamine deficiency

Asterixis (B) can appear in a variety of metabolic encephalopathies but is most common in hepatic encephalopathy. The **serum ammonia (D)** level usually exceeds 200 mg/dL. The most striking neuropathologic finding in patients who die in a state of hepatic encephalopathy is the presence of a large amount of large protoplasmic astrocytes with glycogen-containing inclusions. These **Alzheimer's type II astrocytes (C)** can be found throughout the deep cerebral cortex, lenticular nuclei, thalamus, substantia nigra, cerebellar cortex, red, dentate, and pontine nuclei. Thiamine deficiency is not associated with hepatic encephalopathy.[5]

50. A – III

The motor nuclei of cranial nerves **V (B)**, **VII (C)**, **IX (D)**, and **XII (E)** as well as the motor cortex may be affected.[1]

51. C – Cavernous malformations

Cavernous malformations (cavernous hemangiomas [C]) are composed of large, thin-walled vessels without interposed brain parenchyma. Typically **AVMs (A and D)** traverse disordered brain tissue that lies between the abnormal vessels. **Capillary telangiectasias (B)** contain intervening brain parenchyma; so do **developmental venous anomalies (venous angiomas [E])**.[1,2,3]

52. E – Turnaround transport
53. A – Microtubules
54. D – Translation
55. C – Transcription
56. B – Oxidative phosphorylation
57. A – Microtubules

> This question focuses on causes of toxic neuropathies. Both vincristine and vinblastine interfere with **microtubule (A)** function, although through slightly different mechanisms. Dinitrophenol is thought to disrupt **oxidative phosphorylation (B)**. Actinomycin D is an antibiotic produced by streptomyces that is used in cancer therapy. Its phenoxazone ring intercolates with DNA and interferes with **DNA transcription (C)**. Mercury inactivates sulfhydryl groups of enzymes interfering with cellular metabolism and function—**translation (D)**, in particular. End-organ glycosylation may disrupt **turnaround transport (E)**, as seen in diabetes.[1,3,7]

58. B – Glomus jugulare tumors

> **Glomus jugulare tumors (B)** originate from foci of paraganglionic tissue around the jugular bulb (they are paragangliomas of the glomus jugulare). These invasive tumors contain neurosecretory granules similar to those in the carotid body. Some of them produce clinically detectable amounts of catecholamine. The most common paraganglioma is that of the adrenal gland and goes by another name: pheochromocytoma. None of the other options listed are known to secrete catecholamines.[2,8]

59. D – Intranuclear

> The viral inclusions of herpes simplex type 1 (Cowdry type A) are dense, intranuclear, eosinophilic bodies found in neurons, astrocytes, and oligodendrocytes. They are more likely to be found early in the course of the disease.[1]

60. A – Endodermal sinus tumors

> High levels of human chorionic gonadotrophin (HCG) are associated with **choriocarcinomas (B)**, and high levels of α-fetoprotein (AFP) are associated with **endodermal sinus tumors (yolk sac tumors [A])**. Fifteen percent of **germinomas (C)** may be associated with increased HCG. Embryonal carcinomas will show elevations in both AFP and HCG. **Teratomas (E)** may cause a rise in serum CEA levels.[1,3]

61. B – Putamen, lobar, thalamus, cerebellum, pons

> The most common sites of hypertensive cerebral hemorrhage are (1) putamen and internal capsule (50%); (2) lobar hemorrhages of the central white matter of the temporal, parietal, or frontal lobes; (3) thalamus; (4) cerebellar hemisphere; and (5) pons.[5]

62. C – Lung
63. B – Choriocarcinoma
64. D – Lymphoma

65. E – Prostate

> **Lung (C)** metastasis is the most common intracranial metastatic tumor. **Choriocarcinoma (B)** has the greatest propensity to hemorrhage. Secondary (metastatic) CNS **lymphoma (D)** tends to involve the meninges, while primary CNS lymphoma tends to involve the parenchyma. Of the options listed, **prostate (E)** has the lowest propensity to metastasize to brain.[1]

66. A – Presynaptic inhibition at the neuromuscular junction
67. C – Postsynaptic inhibition
68. A – Presynaptic inhibition at the neuromuscular junction
69. B – Inhibition of Renshaw cells

> Both botulism and Eaton-Lambert syndrome cause **presynaptic inhibition at the neuromuscular junction (A)**, albeit via different mechanisms. Botulinum toxin prevents binding of synaptic vesicles to the presynaptic membrane inhibiting acetylcholine release. Eaton-Lambert syndrome is caused by antibodies directed against voltage-gated calcium channels located at the presynaptic terminal; interference with these voltage-gated Ca^{2+} channels causes decreased release of ACh quanta, as synaptic vesicle binding is a calcium-dependent process. Tetanus toxin causes excitation of agonist and antagonist muscles by **inhibiting the release of glycine from Renshaw cells (B)** (similar to strychnine poisoning). Myasthenia gravis is caused by antibodies to acetycholine receptors located on the **postsynaptic end-plate (C)**.[3]

70. C – Giant-cell astrocytomas

> Tuberous sclerosis is an autosomal dominant condition localized to chromosomes 9 and 16 that is associated with a classic triad of mental retardation, seizures, and adenoma sebaceum. **Subependymal giant-cell astrocytomas (C)** are present in 15% of cases. **Acoustic neuromas (A)** are associated with NF-2. **Cortical calcifications (B)** are associated with Sturge-Weber syndrome. **Optic gliomas (D)** are associated with NF-1. **Renal cysts (E)** are associated with VHL disease.[1,3]

71. A – Choriocarcinoma

> High levels of human chorionic gonadotrophin (HCG) are associated with **choriocarcinomas (A)**, and high levels of α-fetoprotein (AFP) are associated with **endodermal sinus tumors (yolk sac tumors [C])**. Fifteen percent of **germinomas (D)** may be associated with increased HCG. **Embryonal carcinomas (B)** will show elevations in both AFP and HCG. **Teratomas (E)** may cause a rise in serum carcinoembryonic antigen levels.[1,3]

72. B – Basophilic pituitary adenoma

> Cushing's disease is hypercortisolemia caused by an ACTH-secreting pituitary tumor **(D is false)**. Cushing's syndrome is a hypercortisol state that may be due to a variety of causes. **Acidophilic (A)** pituitary cells may produce prolactin, growth hormone, or FSH/LH. **Basophilic (B)** pituitary cells may produce ACTH or TSH. Therefore, Cushing's disease, by definition, is most often associated with a **basophilic pituitary adenoma (B)**.[1,3]

73. C – Niemann-Pick disease
74. D – Sandhoff's disease
75. B – Gaucher's disease
76. E – Tay-Sachs disease
77. A – Fabry's disease
78. A – Fabry's disease
79. D – Sandhoff's disease
80. C – Niemann-Pick disease
81. A – Fabry's disease
82. A – Fabry's disease
83. E – Tay-Sachs disease

The five options listed are sphingolipidoses, lysosomal storage disorders that result in abnormal accumulation of lipids. All of the choices are inherited in an autosomal recessive fashion except for **Fabry's disease (A)**, which is X-linked recessive. **Tay-Sachs (E)** and **Sandhoff's disease (D)** are the two GM2 gangliosidoses, and both have cherry-red spots in the macula as a prominent feature. **Niemann-Pick disease (C)** is caused by sphingomyelinase deficiency with an accumulation of sphingomyelin and cholesterol. Supranuclear paresis of vertical gaze is highly characteristic of this disease. **Fabry's disease (A)** is caused by a deficiency of α-galactosidase with accumulation of ceramides. Painful dysesthesias are prominent in this disorder. **Gaucher's disease (B)** is caused by a glucocerebrosidase deficiency with accumulation of glucocerebrosides. **Sandhoff's disease (D)** is caused by hexosaminidase A and B deficiency with accumulation of GM2 gangliosides. **Tay-Sachs disease (E)** is caused by a deficiency of hexosaminidase A with accumulation of GM2 gangliosides.[1,3]

84. B – Hurler's syndrome
85. C – Morquio's syndrome
86. D – Sanfilippo's syndrome
87. A – Hunter's syndrome
88. E – Scheie's syndrome

The options listed are mucopolysaccharidoses (MPS), which produce lipid accumulation in the lysosomes of the gray matter and polysaccharide accumulation in connective tissue. All of these options are inherited in an autosomal recessive fashion, with the exception of **Hunter's syndrome (A)**, which is inherited in an X-linked recessive fashion. **Hunter's syndrome (A)** is caused by a deficiency of iduronidase sulfatase with heparan and dermatan excretion in the urine—skin pebbling and peripheral nerve entrapment are common. **Hurler's syndrome (B)** is caused by an α-L-iduronidase deficiency with heparan and dermatan sulfate excretion in the urine. **Scheie's syndrome (E)** is a milder form of Hurler's disease that is also caused by a deficiency of α-L-iduronidase. It is characterized by normal intelligence. **Morquio's syndrome (C)** is caused by β-galactosidase and galactose-6-sulfatase deficiency with keratin excretion in the urine. Ligamentous laxity, skeletal deformities, and atlantoaxial subluxation are characteristic. **Sanfilippo's syndrome (D)** is caused by sulfamidase deficiency with heparan excretion in the urine.[1,3]

89. D – Krabbe's disease
90. A – Adrenoleukodystrophy
91. B – Alexander's disease
92. E – Metachromatic leukodystrophy
93. A – Adrenoleukodystrophy
94. D – Krabbe's disease
95. A – Adrenoleukodystrophy

> The choices listed are leukodystrophies, a group of disorders involving enzyme deficiencies causing abnormal myelin synthesis, degradation, or maintenance. **Adrenoleukodystrophy (A)** is an X-linked recessive disorder resulting from abnormal lipid oxidation in peroxisomes leading to accumulation of long-chain fatty acids accompanied by adrenal insufficiency. **Alexander's disease (B)** is a sporadically inherited disease resulting from a defect in the *GFAP* gene. Psychomotor retardation and seizures are common, and Rosenthal fibers are present on histologic sections. **Canavan's disease (C)** is an autosomal recessive disorder caused by a deficiency of aspartoacylase with spongy vacuolization preferentially affecting subcortical U-fibers. **Krabbe's disease (D)** is an autosomal recessive disorder of the enzyme β-galactosidase with accumulation of galactocerebroside as well as psychosine, which is toxic for oligodendroglial cells. In Krabbe's disease, there is vacuolization of the white matter with sparing of subcortical U-fibers.[1,3]

96. C – Autosomal dominant trait (false)

> Wilson's disease is transmitted as an **autosomal recessive trait (C is false)**, and involves the *ATP7B* gene, which causes two disturbances of copper metabolism. There is reduced incorporation of copper into ceruloplasmin, and there is reduction in biliary excretion of copper. **Decreased serum copper levels (E)**, **decreased serum ceruloplasmin levels (D)**, and increased urinary excretion of copper are typical laboratory findings. **Cavitation and discoloration (B) of the lentiform nuclei** (hence, "hepatolenticular degeneration") are typical on pathologic examination. There is marked hyperplasia of protoplasmic astrocytes **(Alzheimer's type II astrocytes [A])** in both cortical and subcortical structures.[5]

97. C – Both
98. B – Shy-Drager syndrome
99. A – Idiopathic Parkinson's disease
100. B – Shy-Drager syndrome

> Both idiopathic **Parkinson's disease (A)** and the **Shy-Drager syndrome (a form of striatonigral degeneration [B])** are characterized by loss of cells in the zona compacta of the substantia nigra, but in **Shy-Drager syndrome (B)**, significant cell loss in the putamen and the intermediolateral column is also found. Lewy bodies are not found in the **Shy-Drager syndrome (B)**. Patients with this syndrome suffer from parkinsonian symptoms and orthostatic hypotension.[5]

101. A – Dementia

> **Dementia (A)**, characterized by cognitive dysfunction, behavioral disturbance, and motor impairment, occurs in one-third to two-thirds of patients with AIDS. **Myelopathy (D)** occurs in less than 10%, **inflammatory polymyositis (B)** in 20%, **toxoplasmosis (E)** in 10%, and **lymphoma (C)** in 5% of AIDS patients.[1,5]

102. B – Renal cell carcinoma

> The triad of **adenoma sebaceum (A)** (actually angiofibromas), epilepsy, and mental retardation characterizes tuberous sclerosis. Although benign tumors (angiomyolipomas) of the kidney and other organs are seen, **renal cell carcinomas (B)** are not (renal cell carcinoma is associated with VHL). **Rhabdomyomas of the heart (C)**, **subependymal giant-cell astrocytoma (D)**, and **subungual fibromas (E)** are all seen in tuberous sclerosis.[5]

103. C – Neurofibromas of the iris (false)

> Neurofibromatosis type 1 (NF of von Recklinghausen, peripheral or classic NF) is an autosomal dominant disorder localized to chromosome 17 (neurofibromin gene) characterized by areas of skin hyperpigmentation and cutaneous and subcutaneous neurofibromas. **Café-au-lait spots (B)** are present on the skin, and the presence of six or more > 1.5 cm lesions is indicative of the diagnosis. The presence of **axillary freckling (A)** in conjunction with café-au-lait macules is nearly pathognomonic of NF-1. NF-1 is also associated with the growth of multiple peripheral neurofibromas, bone cysts, scoliosis, **sphenoid dysplasia (E)**, and **optic glioma (D)** formation. The Lisch nodules of NF-1 represent hamartomas of the iris, not neurofibromas of the iris **(C is false)**.[5]

104. C – It occurs primarily in vessels of deep nuclear structures of the brain (false)

> Cerebral amyloid angiopathy is confined to intracranial arteries and arterioles in the leptomeninges and superficial cortex **(C is false)**. The other responses are true statements regarding amyloid angiopathy.[1]

105. B – Lymphocytic pleocytosis in 90% of patients (false)

> The CSF in Guillain-Barré syndrome is under **normal pressure (C)**, is **acellular in 90% of patients (B is false)**, and demonstrates an **increased protein level that peaks at 4 to 6 weeks after onset (A)**. Presence of a **perivascular lymphocytic inflammatory infiltrate (D)** and **perivenular and segmental demyelination (E)** are characteristic findings.[5]

106. C – Associated with immunosuppression in younger men

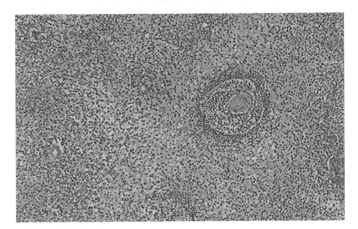

This is lymphoma with diffuse perivascular lymphocytic infiltration into the Virchow-Robin space around a blood vessel. Such lymphomas are **often multiple (A is false)**, **respond initially to steroids (D is false)**, but invariably recur, and are associated with **immunosuppression in younger men (C)**. They also occur in immunocompetent males over 60 years.[3]

107. B – Inclusion bodies of herpes simplex virus-1 (HSV-1)

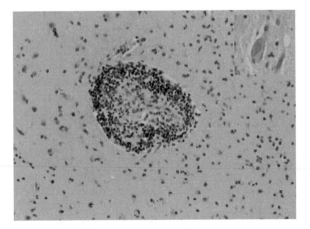

This hematoxylin and eosin H&E-stained section represents **HSV-1 encephalitis (B)** and shows lymphocytic perivascular cuffing on the main slide. The inset at the top right of the image shows a Cowdry type A body, the eosinophilic intranuclear inclusion with a surrounding halo typical for HSV-1.[3]

108. B – Inclusion bodies of SSPE

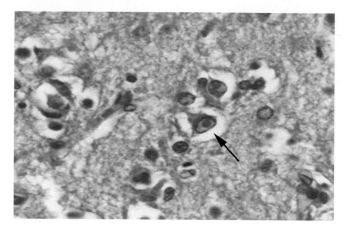

This H&E-stained section is an example of **subacute sclerosing panencephalitis (B)** as is seen sometimes following measles infection (1 in 1,000 cases). The inclusion bodies of HSV (dense, eosinophilic, and surrounded by a clear halo) and SSPE are intranuclear. The inclusion bodies seen in the other responses are intracytoplasmic. Smaller eosinophilic intracytoplasmic inclusions may also be seen in SSPE.[3]

109. C – Pick bodies

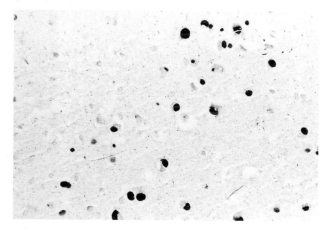

This silver stain shows an example of **Pick bodies (C)**, rounded intracytoplasmic masses. On H&E staining, it might be difficult to distinguish cortical Pick bodies from cortical **Lewy bodies (B)**, both of which would appear as round eosinophilic intracytoplasmic inclusions. Lewy bodies of the brainstem and nucleus basalis typically have a halo, which can help with the distinction. Pick bodies are marked with silver stains (Lewy bodies are not). Pick bodies are immunopositive with anti-tau antibodies.[2]

110. B – Lewy Bodies

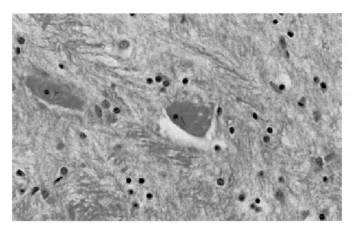

This is an H&E-stained section showing an example of a **Lewy body (neuronal intracytoplasmic inclusion with an eosinophilic core surrounded by a clear halo [B])**, which can be seen in the neurons of the substantia nigra in Parkinson's disease patients.[3]

111. B – Hepatic encephalopathy

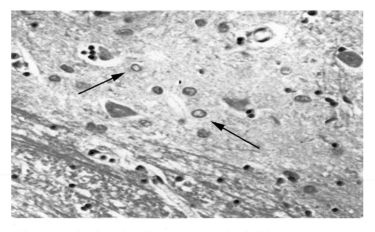

This H&E-stained section shows an example of Alzheimer's type II astrocytes, large vesicular nuclei, and little visible cytoplasm. These reactive protoplasmic astrocytes are found in **hepatic encephalopathy (B)** and Wilson's disease.[3]

112. B – Gemistocytic astrocytoma

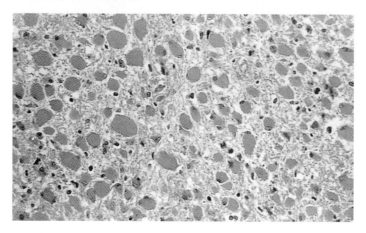

This H&E-stained section shows an example of a **gemistocytic astrocytoma (B)**. The cells of this variant of astrocytoma have prominent eosinophilic cytoplasm, short processes, and eccentric nuclei (comprised of gemistocytic astrocytes). Gemistocytic astrocytes can be seen in the setting of reactive gliosis, but the crowding and overlapping of cells in this slide support the diagnosis of neoplasm. Gemistocytic astrocytomas tend to behave more aggressively than other WHO grade II astrocytomas; for this reason, gemistocytic astrocytomas are sometimes graded WHO grade III because of gemistocytic features.[1,2]

113. D – HSV-1

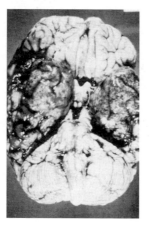

The hemorrhagic appearance of the medial temporal lobe is characteristic of **HSV-1 (D)**.[1,2]

114. E – Progressive multifocal leukoencephalopathy

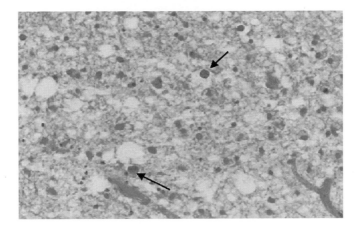

This H&E-stained section is an example of **progressive multifocal encephalopathy (E, associated with the JC virus and an immunocompromised state)**. Demyelination and oligodendroglial cell loss are seen. Residual oligodendroglial nuclei (arrows) are large and bizarre.[3]

115. D – Creutzfeldt-Jakob disease

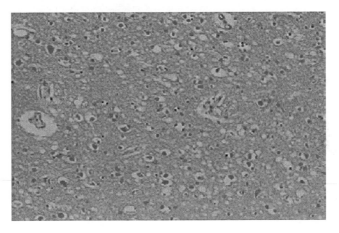

This is a representative H&E-stained section from a patient with **Creutzfeldt-Jakob disease (D)**, a prion disease causing vacuolization and spongiform changes.[3]

116. B – NF-1

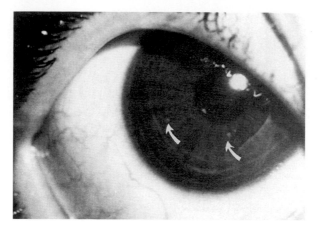

    | The iris hamartomas (Lisch nodules) of **NF-1 (B)** are seen in this photograph.[3]

117. A – HIV encephalopathy

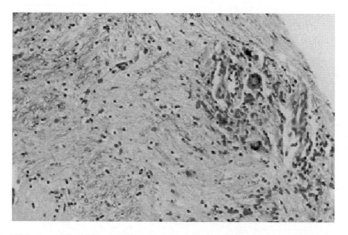

This Luxol fast blue H&E-stained section is an example of **HIV encephalopathy (A)**. Microglial nodules with foci of demyelination, neuronal loss, and reactive astrocytosis are typical. The characteristic multinucleated giant cell is seen here.[3]

118. C – Ganglioglioma

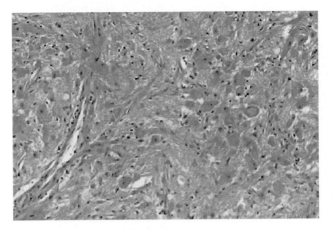

This is an H&E-stained section from a **ganglioglioma (C)**, which contains both neoplastic neurons and ganglion cells. The finding of abnormal ganglion cells (including binucleate forms) is key to the diagnosis of ganglioglioma.[3]

119. D – Oligodendroglioma

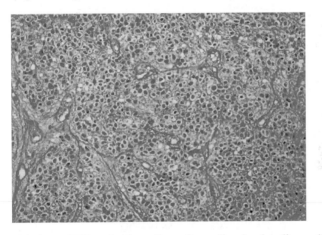

This is an H&E-stained section of an **oligodendroglioma (D)**. 1p and 19q co-deletions in these tumors are associated with improved progression-free and overall survival. A characteristic "chicken wire" vascular pattern and a monotonous "fried egg" nuclear array are seen.[3]

120. C – Medulloblastoma

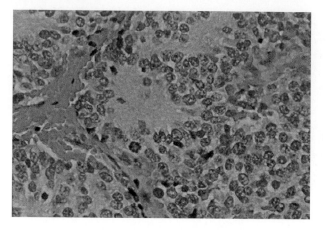

This H&E-stained sections shows dense, hyperchromatic cells that are radially arranged in Homer-Wright rosettes with central granulofibrillar material. These findings are most consistent with a primitive neuroectodermal tumor (**medulloblastoma [C]**), neuroblastoma, etc.).[3]

121. E – Myxopapillary ependymoma

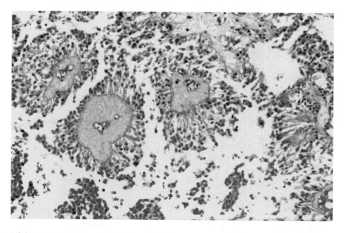

This H&E-stained section of a **myxopapillary ependymoma (E)** shows cohesive ependymal cells terminating around perivascular accumulations of mucinous material. Myxopapillary ependymomas tend to occur at the filum (conus medullaris).[3]

122. B – Craniopharyngioma

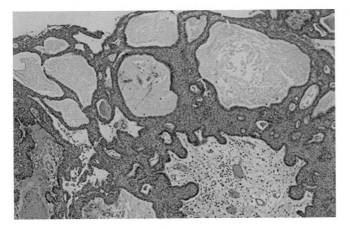

Question 122 shows an H&E-stained section from a **craniopharyngioma (B)** that demonstrates an adamantinomatous pattern with a basal layer of columnar cells separated by loosely arranged stellate cells. Palisading epithelial cells with keratinization and calcification are prominent. The papillary variant is more often seen in adults and contains papillae of well-differentiated squamous epithelium (not pictured here).[3]

123. C – Hemangioblastoma

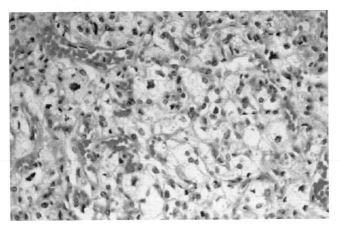

An H&E-stained section of **hemangioblastoma (C)** is pictured here. They are most commonly found in the posterior fossa, and 60% present as a cyst with a mural nodule. Multiple hemangioblastoma are associated with VHL. On H&E staining they are difficult to distinguish from renal cell carcinoma (particularly problematic in VHL patients who are at risk for renal cell carcinoma also). The diagnostic distinction can be made by immunohistochemistry. Vacuolated "stromal" cells in a complex capillary network are seen in this photomicrograph.[3]

124. D – Lipoma

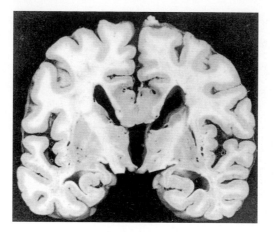

This gross anatomical specimen shows an example of a **lipoma (D)** of the corpus callosum.[3,9]

125. A – Carbon monoxide poisoning

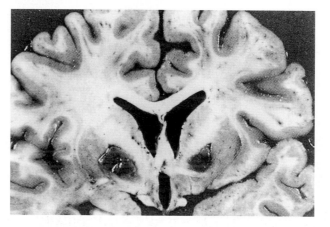

This gross anatomic specimen shows selective necrosis of the globus pallidus, most consistent with **carbon monoxide poisoning (A)**.[1,3]

126. B – Glioblastoma

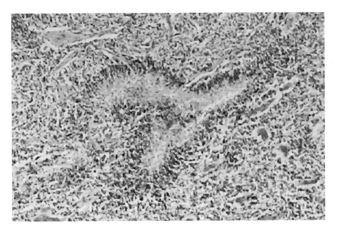

This is an H&E-stained section showing a section representative of **glioblastoma (B)**. Either microvascular proliferation or necrosis is required for an astrocytic tumor to qualify as glioblastoma (WHO grade IV). Necrosis with pseudopalisading is well illustrated in this photomicrograph.[3]

127. D – Tuberous sclerosis

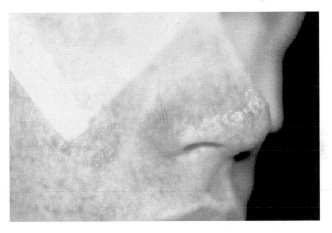

The adenoma sebaceum of **tuberous sclerosis (D)** is seen in this photograph. Tuberous sclerosis is an autosomal dominant condition linked to chromosomes 9 and 16 characterized by the classic triad of adenoma sebaceum, seizures, and mental retardation. Patients with tuberous sclerosis are prone to develop cortical tubers, subependymal giant cell astrocytomas, cardiac rhabdomyoma, retinal hamartoma, and renal angiomyolipoma.[3]

128. C – Meningioma

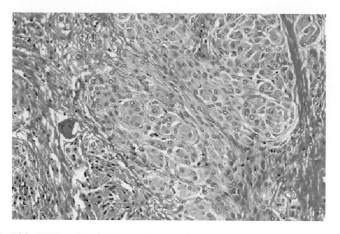

This H&E-stained photomicrograph is an example of a meningotheliomatous (syncytial) type of **meningioma (C)**. A psammoma body is noted as well.[3]

129. C – Meningioma

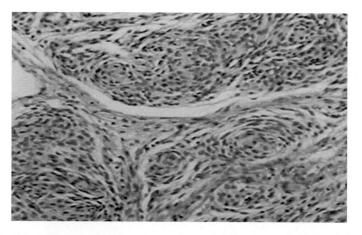

This H&E-stained section is another example of **meningioma (C)**. Note the prominent whorls.[3]

130. D – Neurofibroma

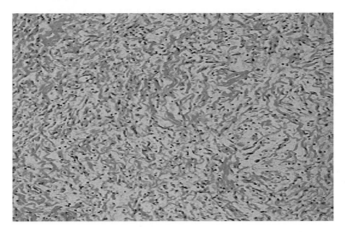

This is an H&E-stained section of a **neurofibroma (D)**. Bundles of elongated Schwann cells with characteristic wavy nuclei in a loose mucinous or collagenous matrix are features of the neurofibroma.[3]

131. B – Malignant peripheral nerve sheath tumor

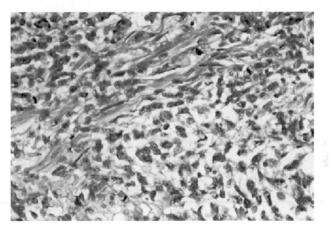

Malignant peripheral nerve sheath tumors (B) are composed of spindle cells in fascicles with occasional mitoses and foci of necrosis (H&E).[3]

132. E – Schwannoma

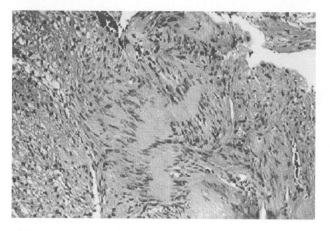

This H&E-stained section shows Verocay bodies, palisading elongated nuclei encircling anuclear fibrillary material, which are hallmarks of **schwannomas (E)**.[3]

133. C – Notochord

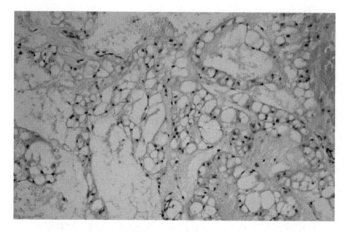

This H&E-stained section shows "physaliphorous" or "bubbly" cells surrounding pools of mucin, consistent with the diagnosis of chordoma. Chordomas are thought to arise from **notochord (C)** remnants, usually occurring in the clivus or sacrum.[3]

134. C – Huntington's disease

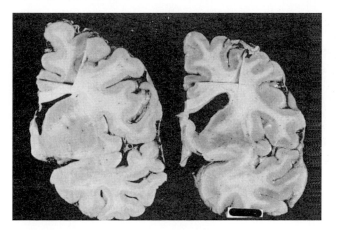

Huntington's disease (C) is an autosomal dominant hereditary movement disorder that localizes to chromosome 4 and involves a CAG trinucleotide repeat. The clinical syndrome involves choreiform movements of the trunk and upper limbs with subcortical dementia. Atrophy of the head of the caudate with "boxcar" ventricles is characteristic and can be seen in this gross pathologic specimen.[1,3]

135. C – Neuritic plaques

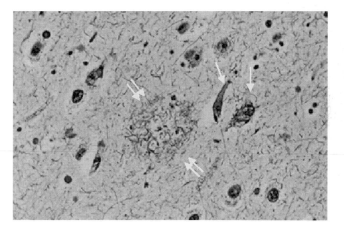

Neuritic ("senile") plaques (composed of degenerating nerve cell processes surrounding a central core of amyloid composed of β/A4 protein, double arrows **[C]**) and **neurofibrillary tangles (single arrows [D])** are seen (silver stain).[3]

136. C – Alexander's disease

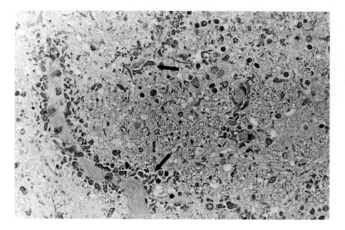

Alexander's disease (C) is one of the leukodystrophies and is caused by a defect in the GFAP gene leading to hemispheric demyelination and mitochondrial dysfunction. Numerous Rosenthal fibers (eosinophilic material in cell processes, likely from GFAP degradation products) in areas of astrocytosis are noted (H&E). Alexander's disease is an example of a nonneoplastic process where Rosenthal fibers may occur.[1,3]

137. D – Hypertensive hemorrhage

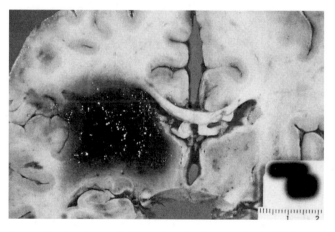

A massive basal ganglia **hypertensive hemorrhage (D)** is noted on this gross pathologic specimen.[1]

138. A – Central neurocytoma

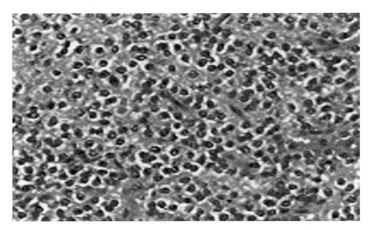

A dense array of uniform undifferentiated cells with small blue nuclei and perinuclear halos is found in **central neurocytomas (A)**. The findings are similar to oligodendrogliomas and can be difficult to differentiate on H&E staining. Central neurocytomas stain with synaptophysin and neuron-specific enolase (NSE).[3]

139. B – Friedreich's ataxia

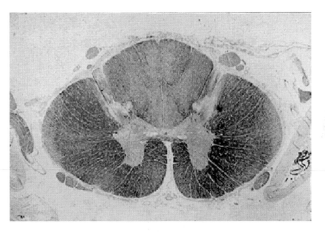

This Luxol fast blue stain shows demyelination of the posterior columns and ventral spinocerebellar tracts. Corticospinal tracts are also affected.[3]

140. E – Subacute combined degeneration

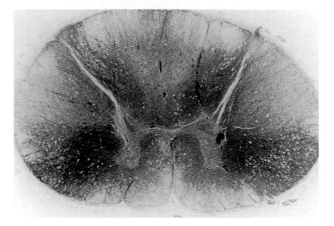

> This Luxol fast blue stain reveals a spongiform and gliotic appearance of the cord primarily affecting the posterior and lateral columns consistent with **subacute combined degeneration (E)**. Subacute combined degeneration occurs in the setting of vitamin B_{12} deficiency and leads to impaired proprioceptive sense and paraplegia.[3,9]

141. D – Radiation myelopathy

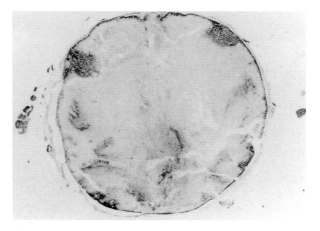

> There is an irregular area of coagulative necrosis involving both gray and white matter consistent with **radiation myelopathy (D)**.[3,9]

142. C – Multiple sclerosis

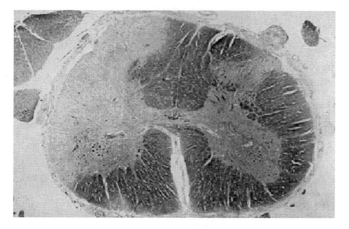

Well-defined plaques are seen involving both gray and white matter in this Luxol fast blue stained section. These findings support a diagnosis of **multiple sclerosis (C).**[3]

143. A – Amyotrophic lateral sclerosis

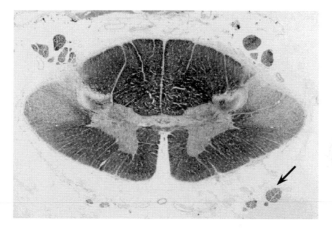

This photomicrograph of a Luxol fast blue stained section shows degeneration of the anterior horn and corticospinal tracts, consistent with **amyotrophic lateral sclerosis (A).**[3]

144. E – Tuberous sclerosis

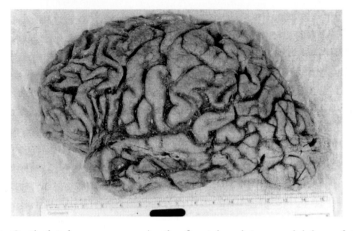

Cortical tubers are seen in the frontal and temporal lobes of this gross pathologic specimen as seen in > 95% of patients with **tuberous sclerosis (D)**. Tuberous sclerosis is an autosomal dominant condition linked to chromosomes 9 and 16 characterized by the classic triad of adenoma sebaceum, seizures, and mental retardation. Patients with tuberous sclerosis are prone to develop cortical tubers, subependymal giant cell astrocytomas, cardiac rhabdomyoma, retinal hamartoma, and renal angiomyolipoma.[1,3]

145. B – Ependymoma

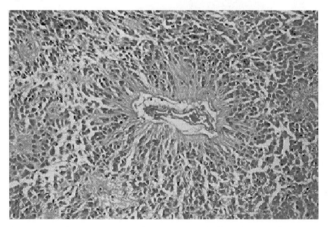

The histologic appearance of ependymomas is highly variable. A cellular variety with sheetlike growth of oval to polygonal cells arranged in a perivascular pseudorosette is illustrated (H&E). Ependymomas are CNS neoplasms that resemble the structure of the brain's ependyma. The most definitive evidence of ependymoma is the presence of true rosettes, also called "Flexner-Wintersteiner rosettes." Most ependymomas contain perivascular pseudorosettes involving tumor cells surrounding an endothelial-lined lumen (as seen here). Ependymomas tend to stain for GFAP and vimentin, particularly in the perivascular pseudorosettes. On electron microscopy extensive surface microvilli forming both intra- and extracellular lumens can be seen.[1,2,3]

146. E – Teratoma

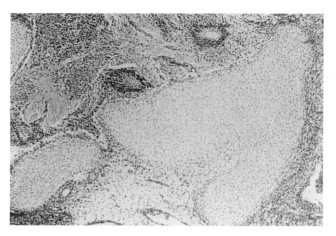

Teratomas are the most differentiated of the germ cell neoplasms and contain elements of all three germ layers: ectoderm, mesoderm, and endoderm. Cartilage, mucin-producing epithelium, and immature spindle cell stroma are all part of this immature **teratoma (E)**—a low-grade malignancy (H&E).[1,2]

147. C – Port-wine nevus on the face

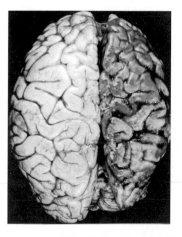

Atrophy of the hemisphere and leptomeningeal venous angioma are present in this specimen with Sturge-Weber syndrome. Sturge-Weber syndrome is characterized by a usually unilateral **port-wine nevus (C)** that typically involves the orbit or upper eyelid, unilateral meningeal angioma, calcifications confined to the second and third layers of cerebral cortex, and seizure activity. **Advanced age and lobar hemorrhage (A)** are associated with amyloid angiopathy. **Retinal hamartomas (D)** and **subungual fibromas (E)** are associated with tuberous sclerosis. **Choice B, alcoholism and prone to falls,** would be a better answer if the gross specimen showed cerebellar atrophy.[5,9]

148. A – Acoustic neuroma

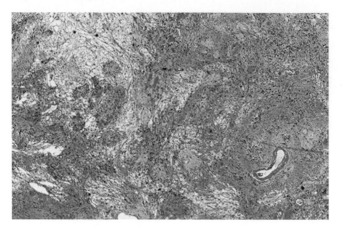

This low-power view (H&E) shows dense Antoni A areas (with compact spindle cells) and looser Antoni B areas (with stellate cells) consistent with acoustic neuroma (schwannoma).[3]

149. E – Melanoma

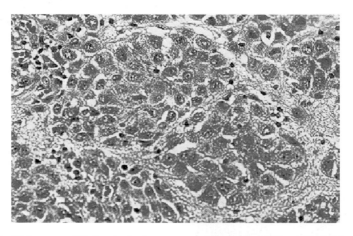

Melanoma (E) tends to be composed of cells with epitheloid or spindle cell configurations. Epitheloid cells with melanin inclusions are seen in this H&E-stained section, consistent with the diagnosis of melanoma. Primary CNS melanomas are more likely to be pigmented than metastatic melanomas, which tend to be amelanotic. Amelanotic metastatic melanomas may be difficult to distinguish from metastatic carcinoma, but this distinction can be made with immunohistochemical stains. The presence of ducts or glands rules out melanoma.[2,3]

150. B – Anaplastic astrocytoma

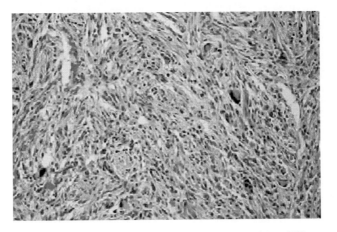

The **anaplastic astrocytoma (B, WHO grade III)** is a diffuse tumor with low to moderate cell density and moderate pleomorphism. There may be focal areas of increased cell density and increased pleomorphism; however, it must not contain areas of microvascular proliferation or necrosis (if either of these features are present, the diagnosis is glioblastoma—WHO grade IV). This H&E-stained section shows cellular pleomorphism, hypercellularity, and mitotic activity consistent with the diagnosis of anaplastic astrocytoma.[2,3]

151. D – Multiple sclerosis

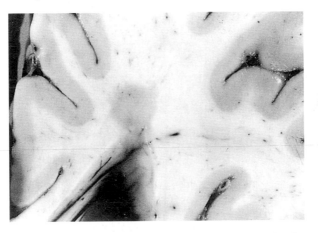

This gross anatomical specimen shows a periventricular demyelinating plaque. This finding is consistent with the diagnosis of **multiple sclerosis (D)**.[3]

152. C – Metachromatic leukodystrophy

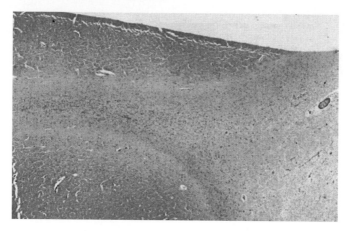

Metachromatic leukodystrophy (C) is caused by a deficiency of arylsulfatase A leading to the accumulation of sulfatides in lysosomes. Inheritance is autosomal recessive—it is the most common of the leukodystrophies. Large confluent areas of demyelination with U-fiber sparing are seen in the H&E-stained photomicrograph and are typical of metachromatic leukodystrophy.[3]

153. A – Epidermoid

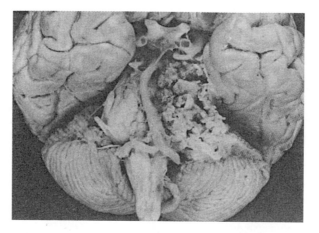

A large cerebellopontine angle **epidermoid (A)** with white flaky, keratinous debris is illustrated in this gross specimen. Epidermoid cysts consist of a cyst wall made up of stratified squamous epithelium without glandular structures. The cyst contains desquamated keratin. Dermoid cysts can be distinguished histopathologically from epidermoid cysts based on the presence of hair follicles, adnexal glands, and the beginnings of papillary dermis formation in dermoid cysts. Some authors argue that dermoid cysts may represent benign teratomas.[2,9]

154. B – Lymphoma

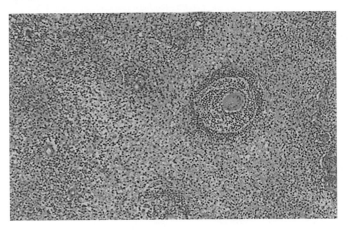

This is an example of **lymphoma (B)** with diffuse perivascular lymphocytic infiltration into the Virchow-Robin space around a blood vessel. Such lymphomas are often multiple, respond initially to steroids, but invariably recur, and are associated with immunosuppression in younger men. They also occur in immunocompetent males over age 60 years.[3]

155. C – Pilocytic astrocytoma

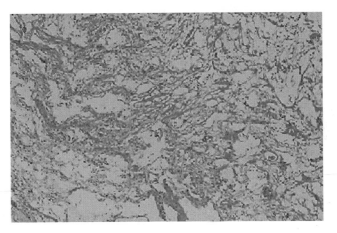

Compact fascicles of elongated cells and spongiform foci with stellate forms and microcystic change are noted in this example of **pilocytic astrocytoma (C)**.[3]

156. C – Contusion

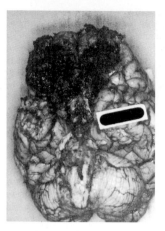

Extensive bilateral contrecoup contusions of the orbital surfaces and frontal poles are illustrated in this gross pathologic specimen.[1]

157. A – Amyloid angiopathy

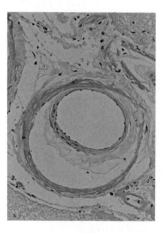

The arterioles of the leptomeninges and superficial cortex are dilated, and amorphous material infiltrates the wall in this H&E-stained section from a patient with **amyloid angiopathy (A)**.[3]

158. E – Pick's disease

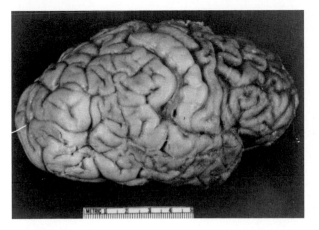

Pick's disease (E) is a form of cerebral degeneration characterized by atrophy of the frontal and temporal lobes involving both the gray and white matter (lobar atrophy). Selective atrophy of the frontal and temporal lobes consistent with Pick's disease is noted in this gross pathologic specimen. In **Alzheimer's disease (A)**, atrophy is more mild and diffuse. **Huntington's disease (C)** is associated with atrophy of the caudate.[1,5]

159. C – Hemangioblastoma

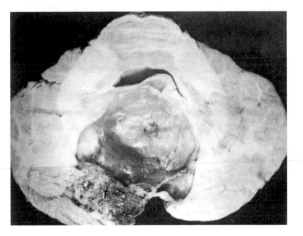

Hemangioblastoma **(C)** accounts for ~10% of posterior fossa tumors. The majority of hemangioblastomas are cystic with a mural nodule. In this gross specimen, a vascular mural nodule in the left cerebellar hemisphere and an associated cyst (midline) are consistent with the diagnosis of cerebellar hemangioblastoma.[3,9]

160. D – Pituitary adenoma

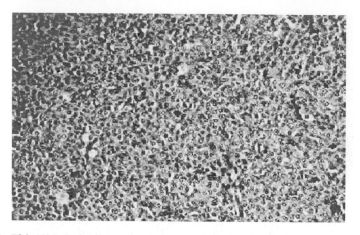

This H&E-stained section shows an example of a pituitary adenoma (**D**). The normal acinar, heterogeneous appearance of the pituitary is replaced by a diffuse sheet of polygonal cells.[2,3]

161. D – Normal peripheral nerve

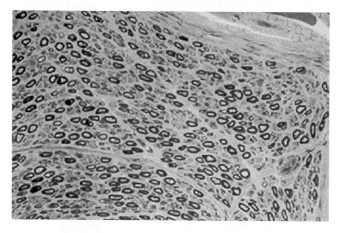

A section from normal sural nerve is illustrated.[3]

162. A – Cysticercosis

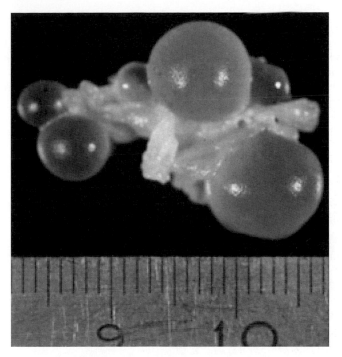

The lesion seen here is an example of cysticercosis **(A)**. This specimen was excised from the fourth ventricle. The other responses are incorrect.[2]

163. A – Arsenic toxicity (acute)
164. A – Arsenic toxicity (chronic)
165. B – Lead toxicity (in children)
166. B – Lead toxicity (in adults)
167. D – Mercury toxicity
168. C – Manganese toxicity

> **Arsenic toxicity (A)** is associated with insecticides and is manifested in its acute form by encephalopathy, peripheral neuropathy, abdominal pain, nausea, vomiting, diarrhea, and shock. Chronic **arsenic toxicity (A)** causes malaise, Mees' transverse white lines on the fingernails, and increased pigmentation and hyperkeratosis of the palms and soles. **Lead poisoning (B)** in children causes irritability, seizures, abdominal pain, ataxia, and coma. In adults, **lead poisoning (B)** causes a pure motor demyelinating polyneuropathy often associated with wrist drop, anemia, and a gingival lead line. **Manganese toxicity (C)** occurs in miners and causes Parkinson's type symptoms that typically respond to levodopa. Neuronal loss and gliosis are observed in the pallidum and striatum. **Mercury poisoning (D)** is associated with fish ingestion and exposure to felt hat dyes. Mercury poisoning leads to psychological dysfunction, tremor, movement disorders, peripheral neuropathy, and cerebellar signs.[3]

169. B – It is often periventricular and brightly enhancing.

> Primary CNS lymphoma is **usually of B cell origin (D is false)** and tends to occur in a **periventricular location (B)**. Primary CNS lymphoma is **more common in immunocompromised patients (E is false)**, and **Epstein-Barr virus has been implicated in the pathophysiology of the disease in immunocompromised patients (A is false)**. Generally, an effort is made to withhold steroid treatment until a tissue diagnosis is made, as steroids can **decrease the diagnostic yield of tissue biopsy (C is false)**.[10]

170. B – Dysembryoplastic neuroepithelial tumor

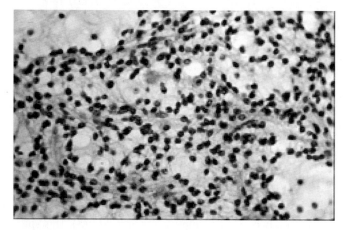

> This H&E-stained section is an example of **dysembryoplastic neuroepithelial tumor (B)**. Note the "floating neuron" in a microcyst surrounded by smaller neurocytic cells. The other answer choices are incorrect.[2]

171. F – A and B

> Primary glioblastomas are thought to arise de novo without any history of a prior known lower grade tumor. Primary glioblastomas tend to have normal **p53 genes (C)**, overexpression of the **epidermal growth factor receptor (EGFR [B])**, and partial deletions of chromosome 10 near the **phosphatase and tensin homologue (PTEN) gene (A)**. Secondary glioblastomas tend to lack overexpression of EGFR, but typically have a loss of heterozygosity of chromosome 17p leading to **decreased p53 (C)**.[2]

172. D – Gliosarcoma

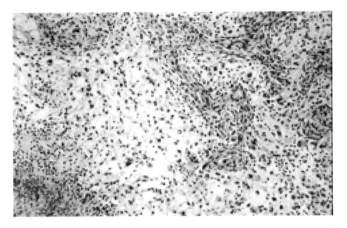

This H&E-stained photomicrograph shows an example of gliosarcoma (**D**) with a mosaic pattern of sarcomatous and gliomatous foci. Cells in the glial portion tend to be GFAP positive, while cells in the sarcomatous areas tend to be GFAP negative.[2]

173. D – Chromosome 22

At least half of all meningiomas have deletions or mutations involving chromosome 22 (**D**) involving the NF-2 gene. A wide variety of genetic aberrations have been described in meningiomas, but a reliable pattern has yet to be identified.

174. D – All of the above

Meningiomas tend to be strongly immunopositive for the intermediate filament protein **vimentin (B)**, which is a reflection of the mesenchymal character of meningiomas. This is not particularly useful diagnostically as other tumors in the differential are often vimentin positive, such as metastatic carcinoma, glioma, melanoma, schwannoma, and hemangioblastoma. The epithelial nature of meningiomas is reflected by their immunopositivity to **EMA (A)**, which helps to rule out schwannomas, melanomas, and hemangioblastomas. The vast majority of meningiomas show **progesterone receptor (C)** immunopositivity in their nuclei, but this tends not to be helpful diagnostically. The correct answer is **D, all of the above**.[2]

175. A – Diffuse deposits of β-amyloid are sometimes present.

> Dementia pugilistica, or "punch-drunk" encephalopathy, is a clinical syndrome characterized by dysarthric speech, slowness in thinking, and forgetfulness, along with slow, stiff movements and a wide-based gait. A large series found that the syndrome occurs in approximately **17% of professional boxers (D is false)**, although radiographic changes may occur in up to one-half of boxers. Radiographic findings include ventricular dilatation, sulcal widening, and an **increased incidence of cavum septum pellucidum (E is false)**. Diffuse deposition of β-amyloid (A) is a not uncommon finding in the brains of patients with dementia pugilistica. **Lewy bodies are not present, however (B is false)**. MRI spectroscopy reveals **decreased levels of *N*-acetylaspartate in the putamen and pallidum** that may be a result of neuronal loss in these regions **(C is false)**.[5]

176. A – Age < 3 years at diagnosis

> Medulloblastomas are the most common malignant brain tumor in children. High-risk patients are currently defined as children with **more than 1.5 cm² postoperative tumor residual (D)**, those **presenting at < 3 years of age (A)**, and those with metastases. **Desmoplastic medulloblastoma (B)** and **medulloblastoma with extensive nodularity (C)** are thought to have a better prognosis. Large-cell and anaplastic medulloblastoma are associated with a poor prognosis. **Nuclear positivity for β-catenin (E)** is a marker of Wnt pathway activation, which has been associated with a better prognosis. High expression of the *myc* and *erbB2* oncogenes is associated with worse outcomes.[10]

177. C – They tend to occur in the midline.

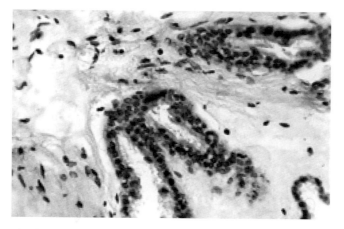

> The lesion seen here is an example of a neurenteric cyst. Neurenteric cysts likely represent developmental abnormalities involving entrapment of developing foregut tissue in the developing leptomeninges. They have a columnar epithelium that usually produces **a mucinous (PAS positive) material into the cyst lumen (A is false)**. Typically they occur **ventrally (B is false)**, in the **midline (C)**.[2]

References

1. Nelson JS, Mena H, Parisi JE, Schochet SS, eds. Principles and Practice of Neuropathology, 2nd ed. New York: Oxford University Press; 2003
2. Miller DC. Modern Surgical Neuropathology. New York: Cambridge University Press; 2009
3. Citow JS, Macdonald RL, Refai D, eds. Comprehensive Neurosurgery Board Review. New York: Thieme Medical Publishers; 2009
4. Friede R. Developmental Neuropathology, 2nd ed. New York: Springer-Verlag; 1989
5. Ropper AH, Brown RH. Principles of Neurology, 8th ed. New York: McGraw-Hill; 2005
6. Rowland LP, ed. Merritt's Textbook of Neurology, 9th ed. Baltimore, MD: Williams & Wilkins; 1995
7. Brunton LL, Lazo JS, Parker KL, eds. Goodman & Gilman's the Pharmacological Basis of Therapeutics, 11th ed. New York: McGraw-Hill; 2006
8. Burger PC, Scheithauer BW, Vogel FS. Surgical Pathology of the Nervous System and its Coverings, 4th ed. New York: Churchill Livingstone; 2002
9. Okazaki H. Fundamentals of Neuropathology: Morphologic Basis of Neurologic Disorders, 2nd ed. New York, Tokoyo: Igaku-Shoin; 1989
10. Quinones-Hinojosa A, ed. Schmidek & Sweet Operative Neurosurgical Techniques, 6th ed. Philadelphia, PA: Elsevier; 2012

6A Neuroradiology—Questions

1. Which of the following is a risk factor for clinically evident neurologic complications in the first 24 hours after cerebral angiography?
   - I. Age over 70 years
   - II. Duration of angiogram over 90 minutes
   - III. History of transient ischemic attack (TIA) or stroke
   - IV. History of systemic hypertension
   - **A.** I, II, III
   - **B.** I, III
   - **C.** II, IV
   - **D.** IV
   - **E.** All of the above

2. The most common nonneurologic complication of cerebral angiography via a femoral artery approach is
   - **A.** Angina
   - **B.** Allergic reaction
   - **C.** Hematoma
   - **D.** Myocardial infarction (MI)
   - **E.** Pseudoaneurysm

3. Branches of the meningohypophysial trunk include the
   - I. Tentorial artery
   - II. Inferior hypophysial artery
   - III. Dorsal meningeal artery
   - IV. Superior hypophysial artery
   - **A.** I, II, III
   - **B.** I, III
   - **C.** II, IV
   - **D.** IV
   - **E.** All of the above

⇨ For questions **4** to **6**, match the persistent anastomoses with the description. Each response may be used once, more than once, or not at all.

    A. Cervical intersegmental artery
    B. Proatlantal intersegmental artery
    C. Primitive hypoglossal artery
    D. Primitive otic artery
    E. Primitive trigeminal artery

4. The most common of the persistent anastomoses

5. Petrous internal carotid artery to the basilar artery

6. Proximal cavernous internal carotid artery to basilar artery

7. The precentral cerebellar vein usually drains into the
    A. Internal cerebral vein
    B. Lateral mesencephalic vein
    C. Posterior mesencephalic vein
    D. Straight sinus
    E. Vein of Galen

8. Anterior temporal lobe masses characteristically displace the
    A. Anterior choroidal artery laterally
    B. Anterior choroidal artery medially
    C. Anterior choroidal artery upward
    D. Posterior choroidal artery downward
    E. Posterior choroidal artery upward

⇨ For questions **9** to **14**, match the blood products with their appearance on magnetic resonance imaging (MRI). Each response may be used once, more than once, or not at all.

    A. Isointense on T1, isointense to hyperintense on T2
    B. Hyperintense on T1 and T2
    C. Hypointense on T1 and T2
    D. Isointense on T1, hypointense on T2
    E. Hyperintense on T1, hypointense on T2
    F. Hypointense on T1, hyperintense on T2

9. Oxyhemoglobin (0–24 hours)

10. Deoxyhemoglobin (1–3 days)

11. Intracellular methemoglobin (3–6 days)

12. Extracellular methemoglobin (6 days–2 months)

13. Nonparamagnetic heme pigments

14. Hemosiderin around periphery

⇨ For questions **15** to **23,** match the branch of the internal carotid artery with the statement that best describes it.

    A. Caroticotympanic artery
    B. Inferior hypophysial artery
    C. Inferolateral trunk
    D. Mandibulovidian artery
    E. McConnell's capsular vessels
    F. Tentorial artery

15. Potential supply to vascular tumors of the middle ear

16. Vestigial hyoid artery

17. Common supply to juvenile angiofibromas

18. Also called the artery of Bernasconi and Cassinari

19. Together with the inferior hypophysial artery, these vessels supply the pituitary gland

20. Together with the caroticotympanic artery, it is a branch of the petrous internal carotid artery

21. Anastomoses with the superior hypophysial artery

22. Remnant of the embryonic dorsal ophthalmic artery

23. Provides important branches to some of the cranial nerves

24. The correct order of the named segments of the anterior choroidal artery is
    A. Cisternal segment, plexal point, plexal segment
    B. Cisternal segment, plexal segment, plexal point
    C. Plexal point, cisternal segment, plexal segment
    D. Plexal point, plexal segment, cisternal segment
    E. Plexal segment, plexal point, cisternal segment

25. In the most common anatomic variation, the named branches of the proximal right subclavian artery from proximal to distal are
    A. Internal mammary artery, thyrocervical trunk, vertebral artery, costocervical trunk
    B. Internal mammary artery, vertebral artery, thyrocervical trunk, costocervical trunk
    C. Vertebral artery, internal mammary artery, costocervical trunk, thyrocervical trunk
    D. Vertebral artery, internal mammary artery, thyrocervical trunk, costocervical trunk
    E. Vertebral artery, thyrocervical trunk, internal mammary artery, costocervical trunk

26. The most common site of origin of the recurrent artery of Heubner is the
    A. A1 segment
    B. A2 segment
    C. Internal carotid artery
    D. M1 segment
    E. M2 segment

27. Intracranial hypotension related to leakage or removal of cerebrospinal fluid (CSF) is most closely associated with which magnetic resonance finding?
    A. Diffuse dural enhancement
    B. Ependymal enhancement
    C. Pneumocephalus
    D. Slitlike ventricles
    E. Ventriculomegaly

28. Which of the following imaging characteristics is *least* likely for pleomorphic xanthoastrocytoma?
    A. Calcification
    B. Cyst formation
    C. Multiple lesions
    D. Superficial location
    E. Temporal lobe location

29. Choroid plexus papillomas in children are most common in the
    A. Fourth ventricle
    B. Left lateral ventricle
    C. Right lateral ventricle
    D. Third ventricle

30. Choroid plexus papillomas in adults occur most commonly in the
    A. Fourth ventricle
    B. Left lateral ventricle
    C. Right lateral ventricle
    D. Third ventricle

31. Which of the following white matter lesions usually initially involves the parieto-occipital regions?
    A. Adrenoleukodystrophy
    B. Canavan's disease
    C. Metachromatic leukodystrophy
    D. Multiple sclerosis
    E. Schilder's disease

⇨ For questions **32** to **37**, match the description with the malformation.
    A. Chiari I malformation
    B. Chiari II malformation
    C. Both
    D. Neither

32. Caudal displacement of cerebellar tonsils

33. Beaking of the midbrain tectum is characteristic

34. A meningomyelocele is virtually always present

35. Medullary kinking is seen

36. Occipital or high cervical encephalocele is present

37. Usually presents in young adulthood

38. The term *bovine arch* refers to
    A. Bi-innominate arteries
    B. Left common carotid artery origin from the aortic arch
    C. Left common carotid artery origin from the right brachiocephalic trunk
    D. Right aortic arch
    E. Right subclavian artery distal to the left subclavian artery

39. The differential diagnosis of colpocephaly, or dilatation of the posterior portion of the lateral ventricles, includes
    I. Agenesis of the corpus callosum
    II. Leigh's disease
    III. Periventricular leukomalacia
    IV. Pantothenate kinase-associated neurodegeneration
    A. I, II, III
    B. I, III
    C. II, IV
    D. IV
    E. All of the above

40. Schizencephaly is essentially a
    A. Demyelinating illness
    B. Disease that first develops in the elderly
    C. Disorder of neuronal migration
    D. Neurodegenerative disorder
    E. Psychiatric disorder

41. The differential diagnosis of optic nerve thickening includes
    I. Optic nerve sheath meningioma
    II. Orbital pseudotumor
    III. Optic nerve glioma
    IV. Graves' disease
    A. I, II, III
    B. I, III
    C. II, IV
    D. IV
    E. All of the above

42. The most common primary benign tumor of the adult orbit is (a)
    A. Cavernous hemangioma
    B. Dermoid cyst
    C. Lymphangioma
    D. Optic nerve glioma
    E. Sarcoidosis

43. Which of the following is a branch of the ophthalmic artery?
    A. Anterior ethmoidal artery
    B. Posterior ethmoidal artery
    C. Both
    D. Neither

44. Which of the following sets of findings on a lumbar MRI scan performed immediately after contrast injection is most characteristic of a recurrent disk herniation and epidural fibrosis, respectively?

 A. A rim of enhancement in the recurrent disk, diffuse enhancement in the fibrosis

 B. A rim of enhancement in the fibrosis, diffuse enhancement in the recurrent disk

 C. A rim of enhancement in the recurrent disk, no enhancement in the fibrosis

 D. Diffuse enhancement in the recurrent disk, no enhancement in the fibrosis

 E. No enhancement of either the recurrent disk or fibrosis

45. Lesions in diffuse axonal injury are commonly found in the

 I. Corpus callosum

 II. Gray-white junction

 III. Rostral brainstem

 IV. Temporal lobe

 A. I, II, III

 B. I, III

 C. II, IV

 D. IV

 E. All of the above

46. Acute subarachnoid hemorrhage is more difficult to diagnose on T1- and T2-weighted MRI sequences than on computed tomography (CT) because

 A. Extracellular methemoglobin is isointense on T1 and T2

 B. Hemosiderin is isointense on T1 and T2

 C. Most radiologists are not familiar with the appearance of acute subarachnoid hemorrhage on MRI

 D. The high oxygen tension in the subarachnoid space prevents conversion of oxyhemoglobin to deoxyhemoglobin

 E. The low oxygen tension in the subarachnoid space prevents conversion of deoxyhemoglobin to oxyhemoglobin

47. Which of the following is *true* of the choroidal blush?

 A. It is an indicator of the choroidal plexus in the lateral ventricle.

 B. It is best seen on the anteroposterior projection.

 C. It is from the posterior ethmoidal branches of the ophthalmic artery.

 D. Its configuration is usually a thin, dense crescent.

 E. Its presence usually indicates an elevated intraocular pressure.

⇨ For questions **48** to **109**, match the figure with the most appropriate response.

48. The most likely etiology of this neonate's pathology is

- **A.** Astrocytoma
- **B.** Metastatic tumor
- **C.** *Staphylococcus aureus*
- **D.** *Citrobacter*

⇨ For questions **49** to **54**, identify the lesions.

- **A.** Eosinophilic granuloma
- **B.** Epidermoid cyst
- **C.** Fibrous dysplasia
- **D.** Hemangioma
- **E.** Multiple myeloma
- **F.** Osteoma

49.

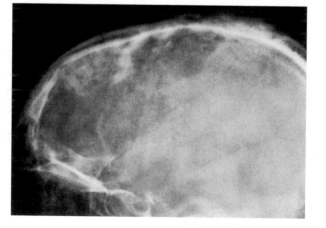

50.

51.

52.

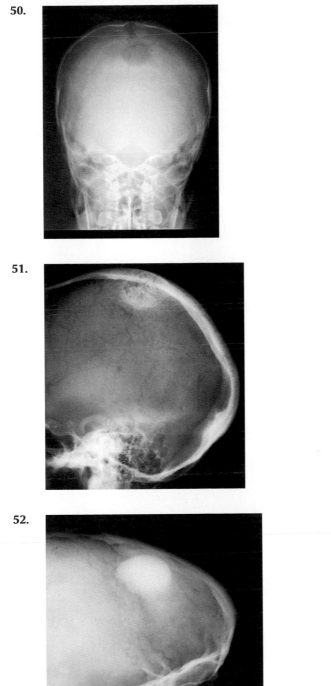

53.

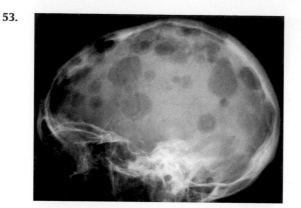

54.

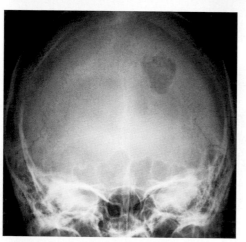

55.

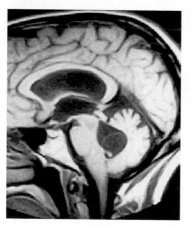

A. Hemangioblastoma
B. Juvenile pilocytic astrocytoma
C. Cysticercosis
D. Medulloblastoma

56.

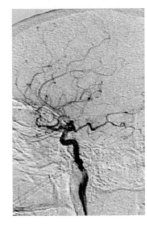

    A.   Fetal origin of the posterior cerebral artery
    B.   Moyamoya disease
    C.   Persistent acoustic artery
    D.   Persistent hypoglossal artery
    E.   Persistent trigeminal artery

57.

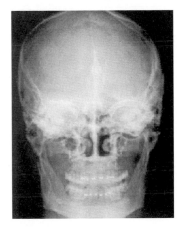

    A.   Corpus callosum lipoma
    B.   Craniopharyngioma
    C.   Giant aneurysm
    D.   Glioblastoma multiforme
    E.   Growing skull fracture

58.

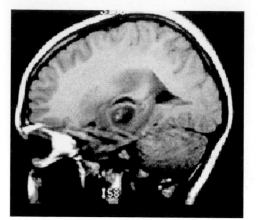

    A.   Cysticercosis
    B.   Infarct
    C.   Low-grade astrocytoma
    D.   Mycotic aneurysm
    E.   Neurocytoma

59.

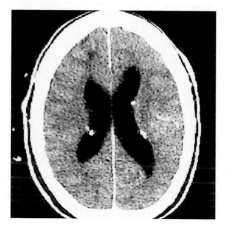

    A.   Multifocal glioblastoma multiforme (GBM)
    B.   Multiple sclerosis
    C.   Metastatic carcinoma
    D.   Neurocytoma
    E.   Tuberous sclerosis

60.

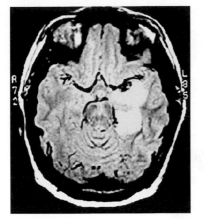

- **A.** Ganglioglioma
- **B.** *S. aureus*
- **C.** Herpes simplex virus
- **D.** Lymphoma

61.

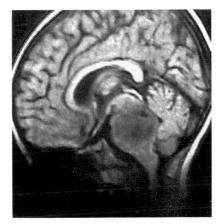

- **A.** Aqueductal stenosis
- **B.** Brainstem astrocytoma
- **C.** Chiari malformation
- **D.** Pituitary tumor
- **E.** Polymicrogyria

62. This patient is most likely to present with

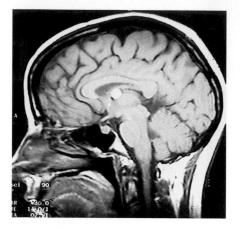

A. Congestive heart failure
B. Fever and chills
C. Headaches
D. Hemiparesis
E. Subarachnoid hemorrhage

63.

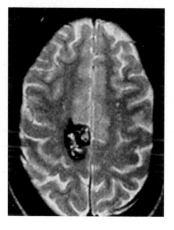

A. Arteriovenous malformation (AVM)
B. Cavernous hemangioma
C. GBM
D. Metastatic carcinoma
E. Tuberculoma

64.

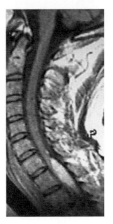

A. Astrocytoma
B. Chiari malformation
C. Diskitis
D. Metastatic disease
E. Syringomyelia

65. Associated with all but

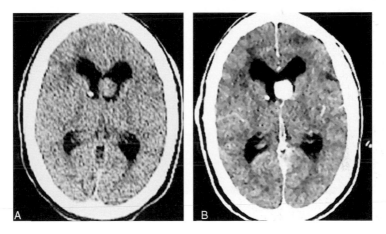

A. Renal cell carcinoma
B. Ash-leaf macules
C. Shagreen patches
D. Cardiac rhabdomyoma

66.

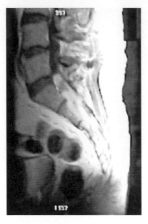

A. Astrocytoma
B. Ependymoma
C. Meningioma
D. Myelomeningocele
E. Tuberculosis

67.

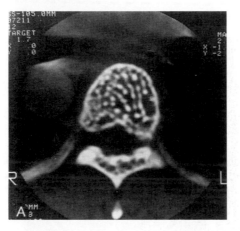

A. Aneurysmal bone cyst
B. Hemangioma
C. Metastatic disease
D. Osteomyelitis
E. Radiation change

68. The most appropriate treatment for a patient with multiple ischemic events and the accompanying angiogram is

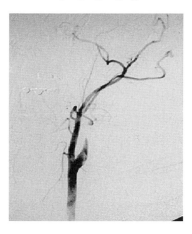

- **A.** Carotid endarterectomy
- **B.** Encephalomyosynangiosis
- **C.** Heparinization
- **D.** Superficial temporal artery to middle cerebral artery bypass
- **E.** No treatment

69.

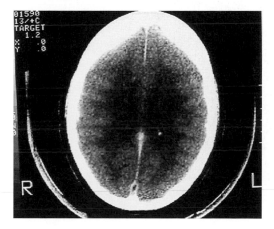

- **A.** AVM
- **B.** Low-grade astrocytoma
- **C.** Multiple sclerosis
- **D.** Normal CT
- **E.** Sagittal sinus thrombosis

70.

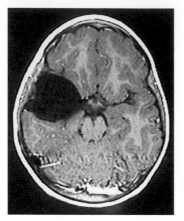

    A. Astrocytoma
    B. Arachnoid cyst
    C. Abscess
    D. Metastatic tumor

71. A patient with low back pain only and the accompanying radiograph should undergo (a)

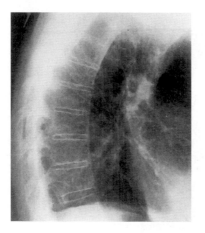

    A. CT-guided biopsy
    B. Metastatic workup
    C. Multilevel decompressive laminectomy
    D. Radiation therapy
    E. Serum antigen testing

72.

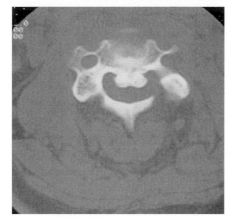

- **A.** Calcified disk herniation
- **B.** Epidural hematoma
- **C.** Meningioma
- **D.** Metastatic tumor
- **E.** Ossification of the posterior longitudinal ligament

73.

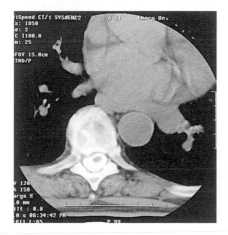

- **A.** Disk herniation
- **B.** Diskitis
- **C.** Ependymoma
- **D.** Meningioma
- **E.** Metastatic tumor

74.

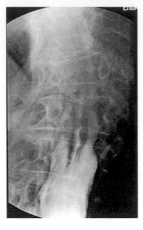

    A. Astrocytoma
    B. Diastematomyelia
    C. Ependymoma
    D. Lipoma
    E. Meningioma

75.

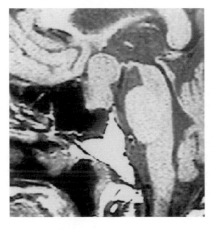

    A. Craniopharyngioma
    B. Chordoma
    C. Pituitary adenoma
    D. Rathke's cleft cyst

76.

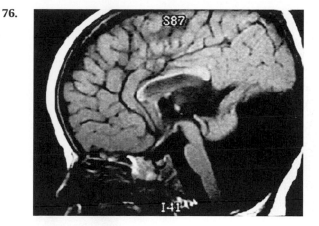

- **A.** Arachnoid cyst
- **B.** Dandy-Walker malformation
- **C.** Epidermoid cyst
- **D.** Porencephaly
- **E.** Vein of Galen aneurysm

77.

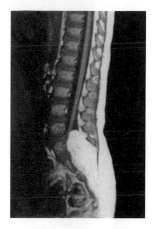

- **A.** Arachnoid cyst
- **B.** Ependymoma
- **C.** Lipomyelomeningocele
- **D.** Meningioma
- **E.** Neurenteric cyst

78. The patient whose myelogram is shown probably

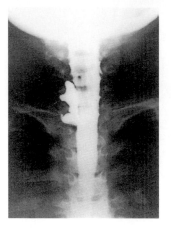

A. Has developmental cysts
B. Has multiple café-au-lait lesions
C. Is asymptomatic
D. Was recently diagnosed with lung cancer
E. Was thrown from a motorcycle

79.

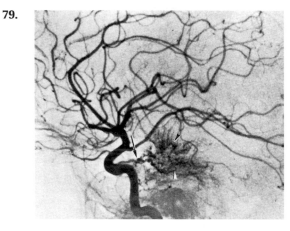

A. AVM
B. Carotid occlusion
C. Dural AVM
D. Meningioma
E. Moyamoya disease

80.

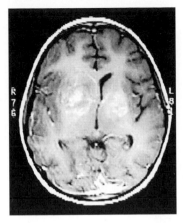

A. Glioblastoma
B. Lymphoma
C. Fahr's disease
D. Herpes simplex virus

81.

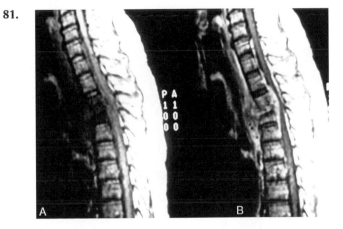

A. Disk herniation
B. Epidural abscess
C. Meningioma
D. Metastatic disease
E. Radiation change

82. The lesion shown is associated with

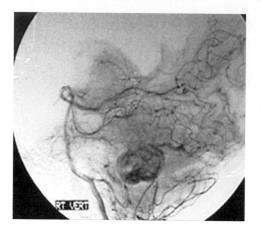

   A. Ehlers-Danlos disease
   B. Endocarditis
   C. Fibromuscular dysplasia
   D. Radiation therapy
   E. Renal cysts

83.

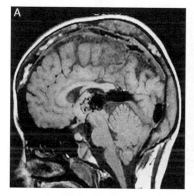 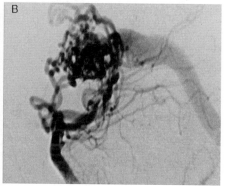

   A. Dural AVM
   B. Moyamoya disease
   C. Sagittal sinus thrombosis
   D. Subdural hematoma
   E. Vein of Galen malformation

84.

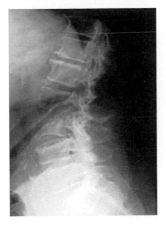

A. Chordoma
B. Diskitis
C. Metastatic disease
D. Neurofibroma
E. Normal lumbosacral radiograph

85.

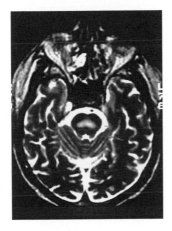

A. Human immunodeficiency virus (HIV)
B. Glioma
C. Rapid correction of hyponatremia
D. Methotrexate toxicity

86. The etiology of the process shown is

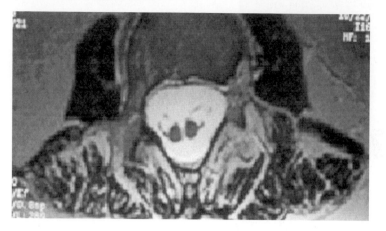

 A. Developmental
 B. Iatrogenic
 C. Infectious
 D. Neoplastic
 E. Traumatic

87.

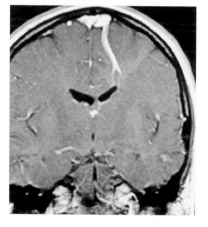

 A. AVM
 B. Fusiform aneurysm
 C. Misplaced shunt catheter
 D. Schizencephaly
 E. Venous malformation

88. This 8-year-old boy who presented with headaches, nausea, and vomiting is most likely to have a(n)

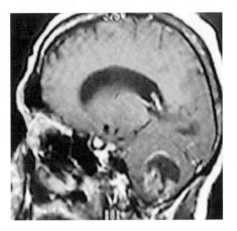

A. Astrocytoma
B. Dandy-Walker cyst
C. Hemangioblastoma
D. Medulloblastoma
E. Metastatic tumor

89.

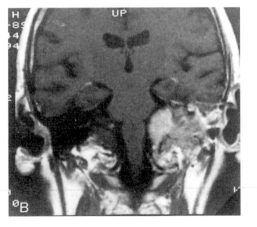

A. Acoustic neuroma
B. Chordoma
C. Giant-cell tumor
D. Glomus jugulare
E. Meningioma

319

90.

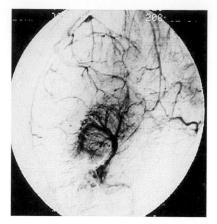

    A. No intervening normal brain
    B. Usually multiple
    C. Often associated with cavernous malformation
    D. Frequently hemorrhage

⇨ For questions **91** to **99**, identify the anatomical structures. Each response may be used once, more than once, or not at all.

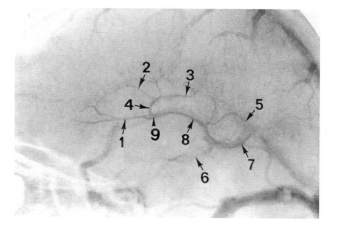

    A. Anterior caudate vein
    B. Atrial vein
    C. Basal vein of Rosenthal
    D. Internal cerebral vein
    E. Septal vein
    F. Terminal vein
    G. Thalamostriate vein
    H. Vein of Galen
    I. Venous angle

91. Structure 1

92. Structure 2

93. Structure 3

94. Structure 4

95. Structure 5

96. Structure 6

97. Structure 7

98. Structure 8

99. Structure 9

100.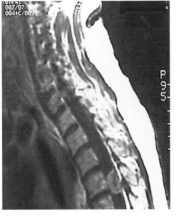

    A. Hemangioblastoma
    B. Lymphoma
    C. Meningioma
    D. Myxopapillary ependymoma
    E. Schwannoma

101. The axial postcontrast MRI shown was obtained in a patient with

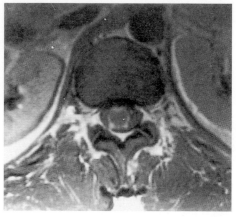

From Yoch DH. Magnetic Resonance Imaging of CNS Disease: A Teaching File, 2nd ed. St. Louis, MO: C.V. Mosby, Inc., 2002. Used with permission from Elsevier Ltd., Oxford, UK.

A. Acquired immunodeficiency syndrome (AIDS)
B. Chiari malformation
C. Disk disease
D. Neurofibromatosis
E. Severe spinal cord trauma

102.

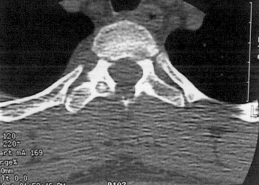

A. Giant-cell tumor
B. Osteoblastoma
C. Aneurysmal bone cyst
D. Osteoid osteoma

103. This postcontrast T1-weighted MRI illustrates

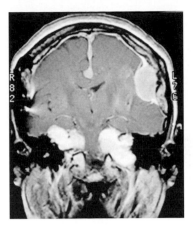

    A. Abscesses
    B. Gliomatosis cerebri
    C. Metastatic disease
    D. Multiple infarcts
    E. Neurofibromatosis type 2

104. This postcontrast T1-weighted MRI illustrates a(n)

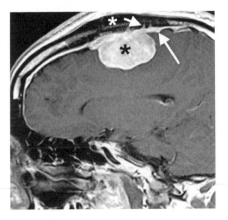

    A. Aneurysm
    B. Colloid cyst
    C. GBM
    D. Meningioma
    E. Metastasis

105.

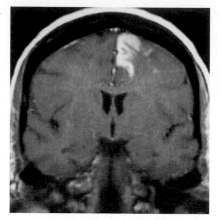

From Yoch DH. Magnetic Resonance Imaging of CNS Disease: A Teaching File, 2nd ed. St. Louis, MO: C.V. Mosby, Inc., 2002. Used with permission from Elsevier Ltd., Oxford, UK.

A. Abscess
B. Artifact
C. Hemangioblastoma
D. Infarct
E. Metastasis

106.

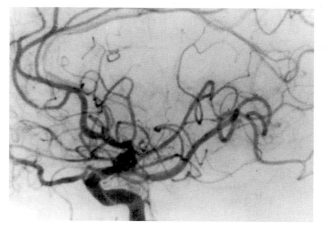

A. Aneurysm
B. AVM
C. Infarct
D. Normal angiogram
E. Persistent trigeminal artery

107. Which statement is true regarding the fracture seen here?

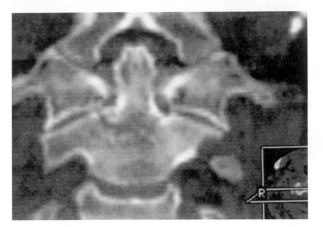

A. Type II fracture
B. Usually requires surgery
C. Requires traction
D. Treated with external orthosis

108.

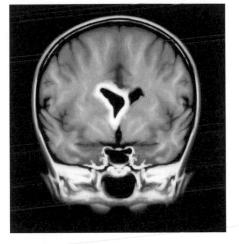

A. Abscess
B. Lymphoma
C. Multiple sclerosis
D. Periventricular leukomalacia
E. Tuberous sclerosis

109.

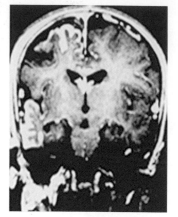

    A. Acute infarction
    B. Chronic subdural hematoma
    C. Epidermoid cyst
    D. Intracranial hypotension
    E. Sturge-Weber syndrome

▷ For questions **110** to **114**, match each of the following magnetic resonance (MR) spectroscopy peaks with the best answer.
    A. Has two peaks; involved in storage of membranous phosphoinositides
    B. Involved in maintenance of energy systems and often used as a reference
    C. Predecessor of brain lipids and participates in coenzyme A interactions
    D. Structural component of cell membranes
    E. Typical doublet located around 1.32 ppm

110. *N*-acetylaspartate (NAA)

111. Choline

112. Creatine

113. Myo-inositol (MI)

114. Lactate

115. Which of the following MR spectroscopy findings are consistent with glioblastoma?
    A. Increased NAA, increased choline, increased lactate
    B. Increased NAA, reduced choline, increased lactate
    C. Increased NAA, reduced choline, reduced lactate
    D. Reduced NAA, increased choline, increased lactate
    E. Reduced NAA, reduced choline, reduced lactate

116. The image seen here is an example of

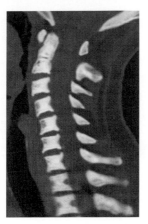

    A. Ankylosing spondylitis
    B. Diffuse idiopathic skeletal hyperostosis
    C. No pathologic process is present
    D. Osteoporosis
    E. Vertebral osteopetrosis

117. The structure seen here most likely represents

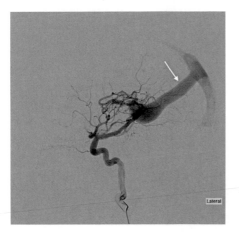

    A. Atrial vein
    B. Internal cerebral vein
    C. Median prosencephalic vein
    D. Straight sinus
    E. Vein of Galen

118. The images seen here are consistent with which of the following?

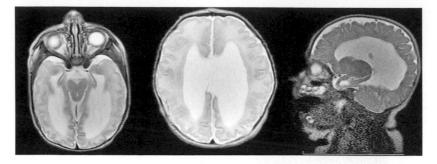

- **A.** Agenesis of the corpus callosum
- **B.** Colpocephaly
- **C.** Septo-optic dysplasia
- **D.** All of the above
- **E.** None of the above

119. The following image is most consistent with

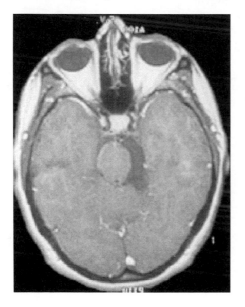

- **A.** Arachnoid cyst
- **B.** Epidermoid
- **C.** Lipoma
- **D.** Low-grade glioma
- **E.** Meningioma

120. Which of the following MRI sequences is the most sensitive for blood products?
  A.   Diffusion-weighted images
  B.   Fast spin echo
  C.   Fluid-attenuated inversion recovery
  D.   Gradient echo
  E.   MR spectroscopy

121. Which of the following is (are) true of the lesion seen here?

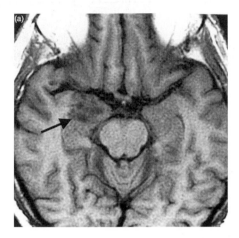

  A.   Associated with cortical dysplasia
  B.   Contains abnormal neurons and abnormal oligodendrocytes and astrocytes
  C.   Typically presents with seizures
  D.   A and C only
  E.   All of the above

6B Neuroradiology— Answer Key

1.	E	27.	A
2.	C	28.	C
3.	A	29.	B
4.	E	30.	A
5.	D	31.	A
6.	E	32.	C
7.	E	33.	B
8.	B	34.	B
9.	A	35.	B
10.	D	36.	D
11.	E	37.	A
12.	B	38.	C
13.	F	39.	B
14.	C	40.	C
15.	A	41.	E
16.	A	42.	A
17.	D	43.	C
18.	F	44.	A
19.	E	45.	A
20.	D	46.	D
21.	B	47.	D
22.	C	48.	D
23.	C	49.	C
24.	A	50.	A
25.	D	51.	D
26.	B	52.	F

53.	E	88.	A
54.	B	89.	D
55.	C	90.	C
56.	A	91.	E
57.	A	92.	A
58.	A	93.	F
59.	E	94.	G
60.	C	95.	B
61.	B	96.	C
62.	C	97.	H
63.	B	98.	D
64.	A	99.	I
65.	A	100.	C
66.	B	101.	A
67.	B	102.	D
68.	C	103.	E
69.	E	104.	D
70.	B	105.	D
71.	E	106.	C
72.	E	107.	D
73.	A	108.	B
74.	B	109.	E
75.	C	110.	C
76.	B	111.	D
77.	C	112.	B
78.	E	113.	A
79.	D	114.	E
80.	B	115.	D
81.	B	116.	E
82.	E	117.	C
83.	E	118.	D
84.	B	119.	B
85.	C	120.	D
86.	A	121.	D
87.	E		

6C Neuroradiology—Answers and Explanations

1. E –   All of the above

Risk factors for clinically evident neurologic complications in the first 24 hours after cerebral angiography include **age over 70 years (I)**, **duration of angiogram > 90 minutes (II)**, **history of TIA or stroke (III)**, and **history of systemic hypertension (IV)**. Other risk factors include patients with more than 50 to 70% stenosis of the cerebral vessels, patients whose angiograms require a higher volume of contrast, and patients referred for subarachnoid hemorrhage or who are immediately postoperative.[1]

2. C –   Hematoma

Significant **hematoma (C)** formation occurs at a rate of ~6.9 to 10.7%. **Angina (A)**, **allergic reaction (B)**, and **myocardial infarction (MI [D])** all occur with an incidence of less than 1 to 2%. Pseudoaneurysms are rare, occurring 0.05 to 0.55% of the time.[1]

3. A –   I, II, and III (tentorial artery, inferior hypophysial artery, and dorsal meningeal artery)

The meningohypophyseal trunk, the largest and most proximal branch of the cavernous carotid artery, typically has three branches: the **tentorial artery (of Bernasconi and Cassinari [I])**, the **dorsal meningeal artery (III)**, and the **inferior hypophyseal artery (the inferolateral trunk [II])**. The **superior hypophyseal artery (IV)** is a branch of the supraclinoid carotid artery.[2]

4. E –   Primitive trigeminal artery
5. D –   Primitive otic artery

332

6. E – Primitive trigeminal artery

The **primitive trigeminal artery (E)** is the most common persistent fetal anastomosis (except for the fetal posterior communicating artery, which is not an answer choice). The **primitive trigeminal artery (E)** connects the cavernous internal carotid artery (ICA) to the basilar artery. The **primitive otic artery (D)** is rare and connects the petrous ICA to the basilar artery via the internal auditory meatus. The **primitive hypoglossal artery (C)** is the second most common persistent fetal circulation, connecting the cervical ICA to the basilar artery via the hypoglossal canal. The **proatlantal intersegmental artey (B)** connects the external carotid artery (ECA) or cervical ICA with the vertebral artery, coursing between the arch of C1 and the occiput.[3,4]

7. E – Vein of Galen

The precentral cerebellar vein is a midline vessel that courses medially over the brachium pontis, parallels the roof of the fourth ventricle, and curves upward behind the inferior colliculus and precentral lobule of the vermis to drain into the **vein of Galen (E).**[2]

8. B – Anterior choroidal artery medially

Anterior temporal lobe masses characteristically displace the **anterior choroidal artery medially (B).**[2]

9. A – Isointense on T1, isointense to hyperintense on T2
10. D – Isointense on T1, hypointense on T2
11. E – Hyperintense on T1, hypointense on T2
12. B – Hyperintense on T1 and T2
13. F – Hypointense on T1, hyperintense on T2
14. C – Hypointense on T1 and T2

Blood products can be staged by their appearance on magnetic resonance imaging (MRI). Hyperacute blood contains oxyhemoglobin and is **isointense on T1 and hyperintense on T2 (A)**. Acute blood (1–3 days) contains deoxyhemoglobin and is **isointense on T1 and hypointense on T2 (D)**. The early subacute phase is associated with intracellular methemoglobin and appears **hyperintense on T1 and hypointense on T2 (E)**. The late subacute phase is associated with extracellular methemoglobin and appears **hyperintense on both T1 and T2 weighted images (B)**. The chronic phase contains hemosiderin around the periphery and appears **hypointense on both T1 and T2 (C)**. Nonparamagnetic heme pigments appear **hypointense on T1 and hyperintense on T2 (F).**[4,5]

15. A – Caroticotympanic artery
16. A – Caroticotympanic artery
17. D – Mandibulovidian artery
18. F – Tentorial artery
19. E – McConnell's capsular vessels
20. D – Mandibulovidian artery
21. B – Inferior hypophysial artery
22. C – Inferolateral trunk

23. C –   Inferolateral trunk

The **caroticotympanic artery (A)** is a vestigial hyoid artery remnant that supplies the middle and inner ear; it can provide blood supply to vascular tumors of the middle ear (i.e., glomus tympanicum). The meningohypophysial trunk gives rise to three vessels, the **tentorial artery (F)** of Bernasconi and Cassinari, the **inferior hypophysial artery (B)**, and the dorsal meningeal artery. The **inferolateral trunk (C)**, or the artery of the inferior cavernous sinus, is a remnant of the embryonic dorsal ophthalmic artery and provides branches to cranial nerves III, IV, V, and VI. The **mandibulovidian artery (D)** is a branch of the petrous internal carotid artery and is a common supply to juvenile angiofibromas. The medial trunk, or **McConnell's capsular vessels (E),** provides blood supply to the pituitary gland.[1,4]

24. A –   Cisternal segment, plexal point, plexal segment

The anterior choroidal artery (AChA) is best seen on the anteroposterior angiogram arising from the medial internal carotid artery. The cisternal AChA curves medially and posteriorly around the uncus. An abrupt "kink" is seen at the plexal point where the AChA enters the choroidal fissure. The plexal AChA then courses through the temporal horn.[2]

25. D –   Vertebral artery, internal mammary artery, thyrocervical trunk, costocervical trunk

Although this is the most common variation, others include the inferior thyroid artery sharing a common trunk with the vertebral artery, the vertebral artery from the thyrocervical trunk, the vertebral artery from the proximal common carotid artery, and the vertebral artery from the **subclavian artery distal to the thyrocervical trunk.**[1]

26. B –   A2 segment

The recurrent artery of Heubner (one of the medial striate arteries) takes origin from the **A2 segment (B)** 34 to 50% of the time, from the **A1 segment (A)** 17 to 45% of the time, and from the anterior communicating artery 5 to 20% of the time.[2]

27. A –   Diffuse dural enhancement

This **enhancement (A)** is thought to represent an increase in blood volume in the dura. Inferior displacement of the structures in the posterior fossa may accompany this finding in such cases of intracranial hypotension.[6]

28. C –   Multiple lesions (false)

Pleomorphic xanthoastrocytoma usually presents as a large single mass in a young patient with a long history of seizures. Typical findings include **cyst formation (B)**, **calcification (A)**, **superficial location (D)**, and **temporal lobe location (E)**.[6]

29. B – Left lateral ventricle

The propensity for the lateralization of choroid plexus papillomas to the **left lateral ventricle (B)** has not been explained. These large bulky tumors usually arise in the trigone.[6]

30. A – Fourth ventricle

Choroid plexus papillomas in the adult population are often found at the caudal aspect of the **fourth ventricle (A)** and frequently calcify.[6]

31. A – Adrenoleukodystrophy

The lesions of **adrenoleukodystrophy (A)** are usually symmetrical, begin in the parieto-occipital region, and spread anteriorly.[6]

32. C – Both
33. B – Chiari II malformation
34. B – Chiari II malformation
35. B – Chiari II malformation
36. D – Neither
37. A – Chiari I malformation

Chiari I malformations (A) consist of inferior displacement of the cerebellar tonsils through the foramen magnum. They usually present in early adulthood. In **Chiari II malformations (B)**, the caudal displacement of the hindbrain is more severe, with beaking of the tectum and medullary kinking often seen. Myelomeningoceles are virtually always present. **Chiari II malformations (B)** usually present in infancy. Chiari III malformations display the most severe displacement of posterior fossa structures and are often associated with a high cervical or occipital meningocele.[6]

38. C – Left common carotid artery origin from the right brachiocephalic trunk

The left common carotid artery usually arises from the aortic arch distal to the right brachiocephalic artery. In the bovine arch variant, the **left common carotid artery arises from the proximal right brachiocephalic artery (C)**. The presence of **bi-innominate arteries (A)** is rare. A **right aortic arch (D)** may be incidental or associated with congenital heart disease. A **right subclavian artery take-off distal to the left subclavian artery (E)** is associated with Down's syndrome.[1]

39. B – I, III (agenesis of the corpus callosum, periventricular leukomalacia)

Agenesis of the corpus callosum (I) and **periventricular leukomalacia (III)** can both result in colpocephaly. **Leigh's disease (II)** and **pantothenate kinase-associated neurodegeneration (formerly Hallervorden-Spatz disease [IV])** can both cause symmetric lesions of the globus pallidus but are not associated with colpocephaly.[6]

40. C – Disorder of neuronal migration

> The cleft of schizencephaly can be unilateral or bilateral, but it usually involves the region near the central sulcus. Patients can present with seizures or focal deficits. It is a **disorder of neuronal migration (C)**.[6]

41. E – All of the above

> Optic nerve thickening may be caused by nonneoplastic processes like **Graves' disease (IV)**, **orbital pseudotumor (II)**, optic neuritis, papilledema, and vascular malformations, or by tumors like **gliomas (III)**, **meningiomas (I)**, lymphomas, leukemia, and metastases.[6]

42. A – Cavernous hemangioma

> **Cavernous hemangiomas (A)** of the orbit are usually well-demarcated, vascular, intraconal lesions with smooth or lobulated borders.[7]

43. C – Both

> The **ethmoidal arteries (C)** are branches of the ophthalmic artery. They supply a portion of the anterior cranial fossa and the mucosa of the nasal septum. During embolization of the internal maxillary artery, dangerous potential anastomoses from the sphenopalatine branches of the internal maxillary artery to branches of the ophthalmic artery may be present.[1]

44. A – A rim of enhancement in the recurrent disk, diffuse enhancement in the fibrosis

> Scar tissue contains vascular granulation tissue that enhances more diffusely than a residual or recurrent disk.[6]

45. A – I, II, and III (corpus callosum, gray-white junction, and rostral brainstem)

> Lesions in diffuse axonal injury are commonly found in the corpus callosum, gray-white junction, and rostral brainstem.[8]

46. D – The high oxygen tension in the subarachnoid space prevents conversion of oxyhemoglobin to deoxyhemoglobin

> Acute subarachnoid hemorrhage is more difficult to diagnose on MRI than computed tomography (CT) because the **high oxygen tension in the subarachnoid space prevents the conversion of oxyhemoglobin to deoxyhemoglobin (D)**. Hyperacute-appearing blood containing oxyhemoglobin appears isointense on T1 and hyperintense on T2, similar to cerebrospinal fluid (CSF) signal. Susceptibility weighted images, such as gradient echo sequences, are quite sensitive for blood products in all stages, however.[4,8]

47. D – Its configuration is usually a thin, dense crescent.

The choroidal blush signifies the choroidal plexus of the eye **(A is false)** and is supplied by the ciliary branches of the ophthalmic artery **(C is false)**. It is characteristically seen as a thin crescent on the lateral projection **(B is false)** of the internal carotid angiogram. Its absence **(E is false)** can be an indirect sign of elevated intraorbital or intraocular pressure.[1]

48. D – *Citrobacter*

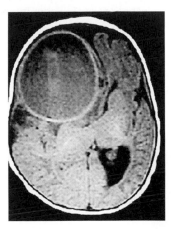

Large neonatal brain abscesses are usually caused by **Citrobacter (D)**, *Bacteroides*, *Proteus*, and various gram-negative bacilli.[4]

49. C – Fibrous dysplasia

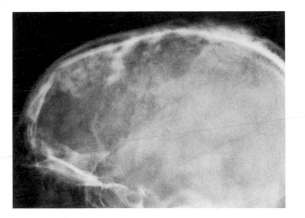

Sclerosis and thickening of the left orbit is present in this X-ray of a patient with **fibrous dysplasia (C)**.[4,9] (Courtesy of Dr. John A. Goree, Durham, NC.)

50. A – Eosinophilic granuloma

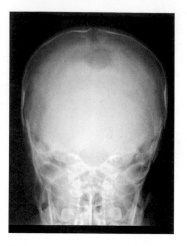

A discrete radiolucent area is seen that does not have sclerotic margins, consistent with **eosinophilic granuloma (A)**.[4,9] (Courtesy of Dr. John A. Goree, Durham, NC.)

51. D – Hemangioma

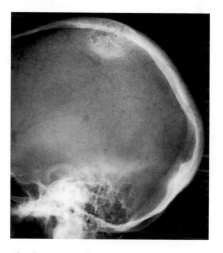

The honeycomb or sunburst pattern is characteristic of a calvarial **hemangioma (D)**.[4,10]

52. F –   Osteoma

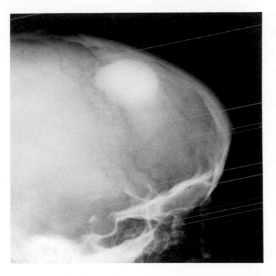

A discrete high-density lesion with smooth contours is seen, most consistent with **osteoma (F)**.[4,10]

53. E –   Multiple myeloma

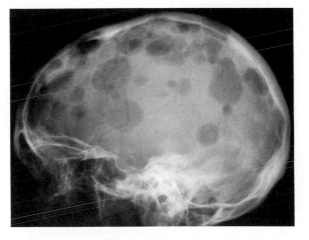

Multiple round discrete punched-out lesions are characteristic of **multiple myeloma (E)**.[4,10]

54. B – Epidermoid cyst

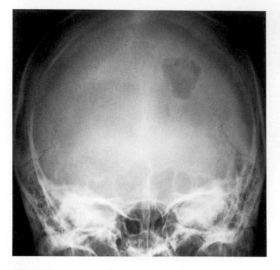

The scalloped border and sclerotic rim are characteristic of a skull **epidermoid (B)**.[4,10] (Courtesy of Dr. John A. Goree, Durham, NC.)

55. C – Cysticercosis

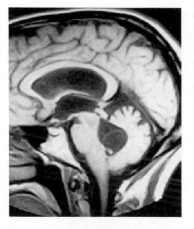

The smooth and thin-walled intraventricular cyst with a mural nodule is classic for **cysticercosis (C)**.[4]

56. A – Fetal origin of the posterior cerebral artery

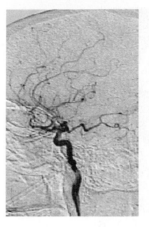

A **fetal origin of the posterior cerebral artery** (A) from the internal carotid circulation is seen in ~20% of anatomical dissections.[4]

57. A – Corpus callosum lipoma

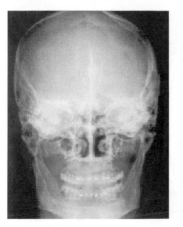

Peripheral calcification is noted in this curvilinear **lipoma of the corpus callosum (A)**.[4]

58. A – Cysticercosis

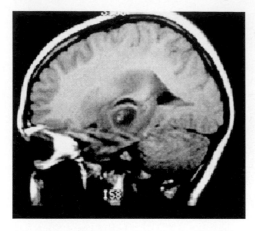

A small ring-enhancing lesion surrounded by a zone of low density is typical of **cysticercosis (A)**.[4]

59. E – Tuberous sclerosis

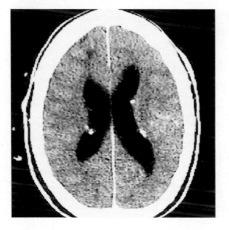

Shown are multiple calcified subependymal tubers of **tuberous sclerosis (E)**. The appearance of these hamartomatous lesions in the subependymal region is sometimes referred to as "candle guttering."[4]

60. C –   Herpes simplex virus

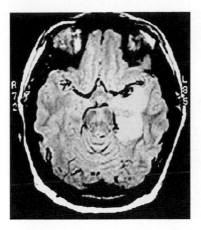

The inflammation of the mesial temporal lobe with diffuse edema is most characteristic of **herpes encephalitis (C)**. There is often associated hemorrhage.[4]

61. B –   Brainstem astrocytoma

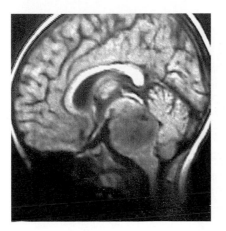

An expansile lesion of the pons is seen most consistently with **pontine glioma (brainstem astrocytoma [B])**.[4]

62. C –   Headaches

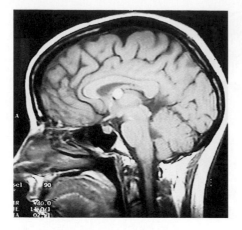

The signal intensity of colloid cysts is variable on either T1- or T2-weighted MRI. Short T1 values (hyperintense images) reflect proteinaceous material. These masses arise from the anterior roof of the third ventricle.[4]

63. B –   Cavernous hemangioma

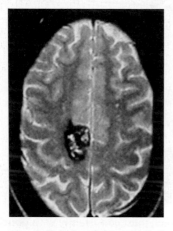

The dark halo of decreased signal is caused by iron in hemosiderin in this T2-weighted MRI. This is an almost diagnostic image of a **cavernous hemangioma (i.e., cavernous malformation [B]).**[4]

64. A – Astrocytoma

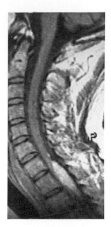

The diffuse fusiform widening of the cord with variable signal intensity is consistent with a diffuse or fibrillary **astrocytoma (A)**.[4]

65. A – Renal cell carcinoma (false)

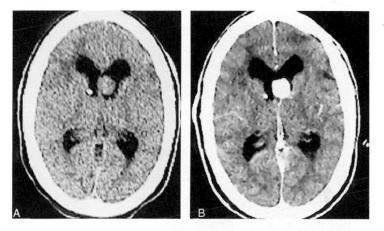

The enhancing intraventricular mass near the foramen of Monro is a subependymal giant-cell astrocytoma that is associated with tuberous sclerosis. The right ventricular calcified mass is a subependymal tuber. **Renal cell carcinoma (A)** is associated with von Hippel-Lindau syndrome, not tuberous sclerosis. The other options listed are associated with tuberous sclerosis.[4]

66. B – Ependymoma

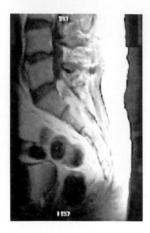

The discrete lobulated appearance of the myxopapillary **ependymoma (B)** is illustrated. These tumors originate from the conus medullaris or filum terminale.[4]

67. B – Hemangioma

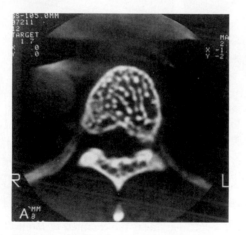

The typical polka dot, or salt-and-pepper, appearance of a **hemangioma (B)** of the vertebral body is seen.[4,8]

68. C – Heparinization

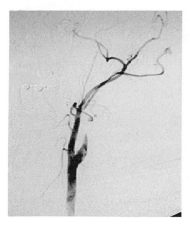

The angiogram illustrates a carotid dissection. The internal carotid gradually tapers distal to its origin: the "string sign."[4]

69. E – Sagittal sinus thrombosis

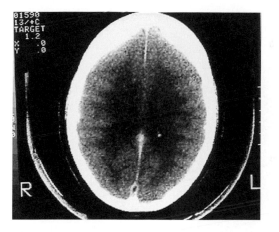

This contrast CT scan illustrates the "empty delta sign" suggestive of **sagittal sinus thrombosis (E)**. The triangle develops because of enhancement of vascular channels around the occluded sinus.[11]

70. B –   Arachnoid cyst

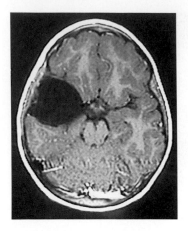

> This low-intensity extra-axial mass without surrounding edema is consistent with an **arachnoid cyst (B)**. The most common location is the middle fossa.[4]

71. E –   Serum antigen testing

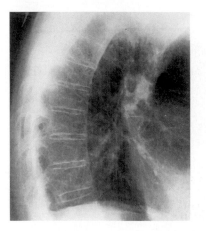

> The radiograph shows the classic "bamboo spine" configuration of ankylosing spondylitis. Although HLA-B27 testing is indicated, the results should be interpreted with caution. Although 90% of patients with clinical ankylosing spondylitis are HLA-B27 positive, < 2% of HLA-B27 patients eventually develop ankylosing spondylitis.[8]

72. E – Ossification of the posterior longitudinal ligament

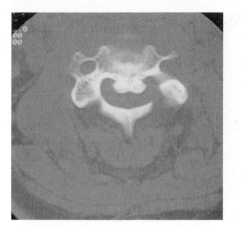

Ossification of the posterior longitudinal ligament (E) is a common cause of cervical myelopathy in patients of Asian descent. Fibrosis and hyperplasia develop initially, followed by calcification. The ossification may be diffuse or localized and may involve the dura.[4]

73. A – Disk herniation

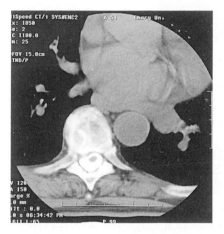

This postmyelogram CT illustrates a right-sided, partially calcified **herniated disk (A)**.

74. B – Diastematomyelia

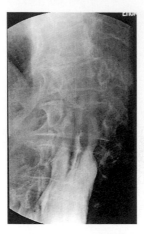

The **split cord malformation (diastematomyelia [B])** and cartilaginous septum can be seen. Patients may present with signs of a tethered cord or kyphoscoliosis.[8]

75. C – Pituitary adenoma

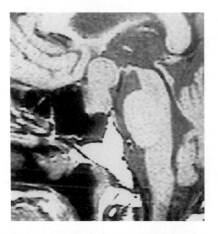

This **pituitary adenoma (C)** fills and expands the sella and also extends to the suprasellar space. **Craniopharyngiomas (A)** are more likely to be mainly suprasellar. **Rathke's cleft cysts (D)** should be cystic and are not usually this large with upward extension (though they may be). **Chordomas (B)** usually involve more bony invasion of the clivus.[4]

76. B – Dandy-Walker malformation

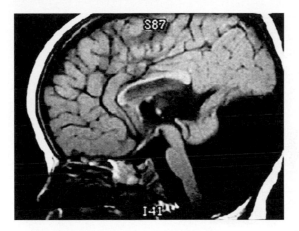

A hypoplastic vermis, high transverse sinus, and cystic dilatation of the fourth ventricle are characteristic of the **Dandy-Walker malformation (B).**[4]

77. C – Lipomyelomeningocele

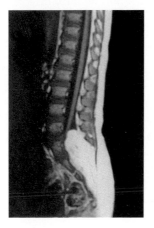

A subcutaneous lipoma that extends into the low-lying tethered spinal cord is seen.[4]

78. E –   Was thrown from a motorcycle

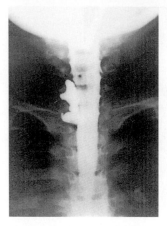

The classic appearance of pseudomeningoceles from lower cervical nerve root avulsion is seen in this myelogram.[8]

79. D –   Meningioma

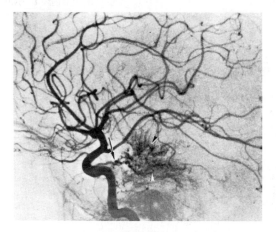

This lateral phase angiogram shows the tumor blush of a **meningioma (D)**, with a prominent contribution from the tentorial artery.[4]

80. B – Lymphoma

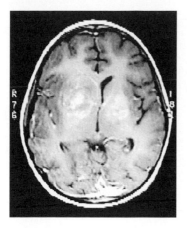

Bilateral periventricular enhancing masses are most consistent with **lymphoma (B)**. They usually enhance quite brightly. **Fahr's disease (C)** is idiopathic basal ganglia calcification and should be low-intensity on MRI. **Herpes simplex virus (HSV [D])** infection usually involves the temporal lobes. **Glioblastoma (A)** may be multicentric, but this picture is most likely a lymphoma.[4]

81. B – Epidural abscess

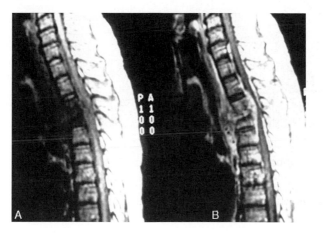

An **epidural infection (B)** is iso- or hypointense to the cord on T1-weighted MRI and hyperintense on T2-weighted and proton density unenhanced MRIs. With contrast, the solid portion of the abscess or the periphery of a liquid collection enhances.[4]

82. E – Renal cysts

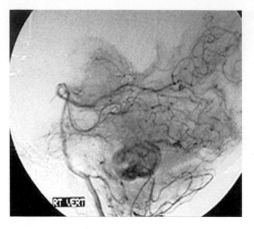

Cerebellar hemangioblastomas (tumor blush is seen in this arterial phase) are associated with **renal cysts (E)** and pancreatic cysts.[4]

83. E – Vein of Galen malformation

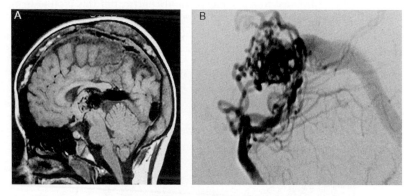

Lateral basilar artery angiogram shows early filling of the vein of Galen. **Vein of Galen malformations (E)** usually present with high-output cardiac failure in the neonate. They also may present with hydrocephalus in the infant, or subarachnoid hemorrhage, epilepsy, or mental retardation in the older child (or adult).[4]

84. B –   Diskitis

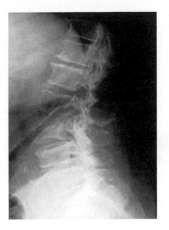

Erosion of the inferior anterior L2 end plate is noted. Plain film abnormalities in **diskitis (B)** may not become evident for weeks. They include irregularities of the end plate, loss of disk space height, and bony sclerosis.[4]

85. C –   Rapid correction of hyponatremia

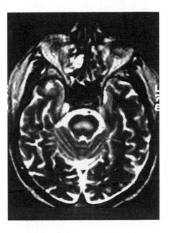

Central pontine myelinolysis is associated with the **rapid correction of hyponatremia (C)** and usually occurs in malnourished or alcoholic patients.[4]

86. A –   Developmental

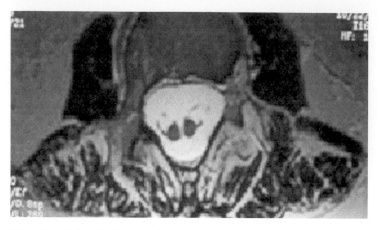

| This T2-weighted axial MRI shows the split cord of diastematomyelia, a **developmental (A)** condition. [4]

87. E –   Venous malformation

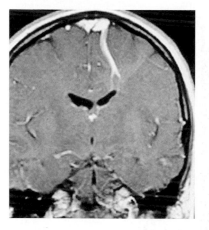

| A linear or curvilinear structure with a nidus from which emanates numerous small veins is the typical MRI appearance of a **venous angioma (E)** (i.e., developmental venous anomaly). The angiographic appearance is that of a caput medusae.[4]

88. A – Astrocytoma

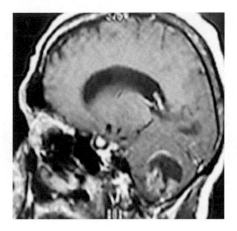

The brightly enhancing mural nodule in a large cyst is the typical appearance of the juvenile pilocytic **astrocytoma (A)** in this age group. A cerebellar **hemangioblastoma (C)**, which would be more common in an adult, may also have this appearance on MRI.[4]

89. D – Glomus jugulare

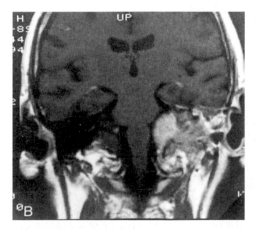

The heterogeneous "salt-and-pepper" appearance of the **glomus jugulare (D)** tumor is appreciated. These relatively rare tumors arise from rests of paraganglionic tissue along the jugular bulb. Glomus tympanicum tumors occur in the middle ear.[8]

90. C – Often associated with cavernous malformation

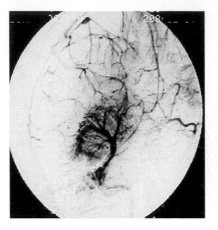

Venous malformations (developmental venous anomalies) consist of a large draining cortical vein receiving a collection of medullary veins (caput medusae). There usually is intervening normal brain **(A is false)**, unlike with arteriovenous malformations (AVMs) and capillary telangiectasias. They are **usually single (B is false)**, unlike capillary telangiectasias. They **rarely hemorrhage (D is false)** and are **often found in association with cavernous malformations (C).**[4]

91. E – Septal vein

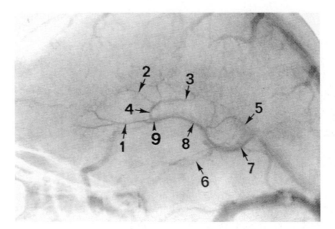

92. A – Anterior caudate vein
93. F – Terminal vein
94. G – Thalamostriate vein
95. B – Atrial vein
96. C – Basal vein of Rosenthal

97. H – Vein of Galen
98. D – Internal cerebral vein
99. I – Venous angle

⏐ For questions 91 to 99, see references 2 and 4.

100. C – Meningioma

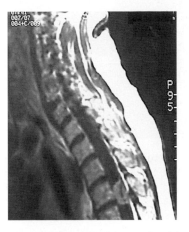

⏐ This sagittal MRI shows a dural-based mass most consistent with **meningi-**
⏐ **oma (C)**. Large **schwannomas (E)** usually show more heterogeneous contrast
⏐ enhancement.[4]

101. A – Acquired immunodeficiency syndrome (AIDS)

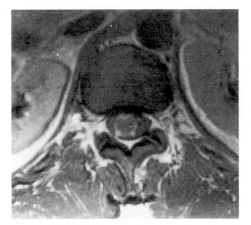

From Yoch DH. Magnetic Resonance Imaging of
CNS Disease: A Teaching File, 2nd ed. St. Louis, MO:
C.V. Mosby, Inc., 2002. Used with permission from
Elsevier Ltd., Oxford, UK.

⏐ Cytomegalovirus (CMV) is a frequent cause of polyradiculitis and myelitis in
⏐ patients with **acquired immunodeficiency syndrome (AIDS [A])**. The pial
⏐ enhancement seen is characteristic of this condition.[6]

102. D – Osteoid osteoma

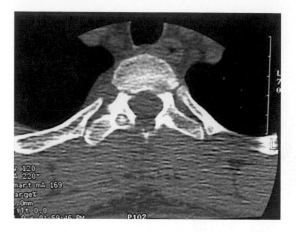

The lytic lesion with surrounding sclerosis and a central nidus is classic for **osteoid osteoma (D).** These usually present with pain that resolves with aspirin.[4]

103. E – Neurofibromatosis type 2

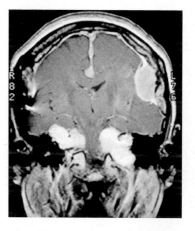

The bilateral acoustic neuromas and multiple meningiomas are consistent with **neurofibromatosis type 2 (E).**[4]

104. D – Meningioma

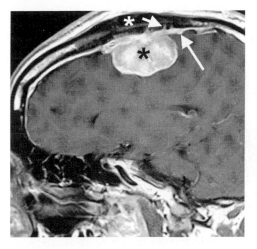

| A parafalcine **meningioma (D)** is shown.[6]

105. D – Infarct

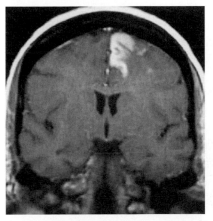

From Yoch DH. Magnetic Resonance Imaging of CNS Disease: A Teaching File, 2nd ed. St. Louis, MO: C.V. Mosby, Inc., 2002. Used with permission from Elsevier Ltd., Oxford, UK.

A gyriform pattern of contrast enhancement in the distribution of the left anterior cerebral artery (ACA) is suggestive of subacute infarction.[6]

106. C – Infarct

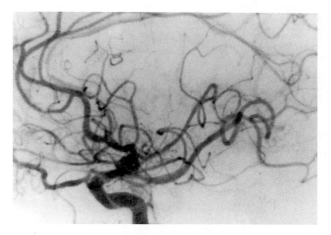

The central sulcus artery (branch of the middle cerebral artery) is not filling on this lateral ICA injection angiogram. These findings are consistent with ischemic infarction.[2]

107. D – Treated with external orthosis

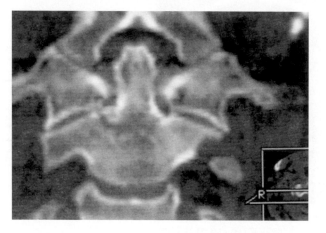

Type III odontoid fractures usually **heal well with an external orthosis (D)** (e.g., halo, Somi, Minerva). **Type II fractures (A)** will more often require surgical stabilization, especially if there are more than 6 mm of displacement.[4]

108. B – Lymphoma

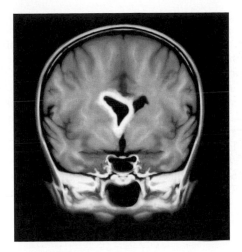

Periventricular involvement by primary central nervous system **lymphomas (B)** is common.[6]

109. E – Sturge-Weber syndrome

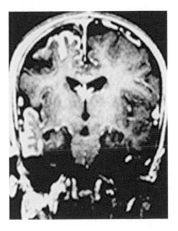

The layer of enhancement covering the hypoplastic right hemisphere represents the meningeal angioma on this postcontrast coronal MRI.[4]

110. C – Predecessor of brain lipids and participates in coenzyme A interactions
111. D – Structural component of cell membranes
112. B – Involved in maintenance of energy systems and often used as a reference
113. A – Has two peaks; involved in storage of membranous phosphoinositides

114. E – Typical doublet located around 1.32 ppm

N-acetylaspartate (NAA) is typically the most visible peak and occurs at 2 ppm. The NAA peak contains a combination of macromolecules containing *N*-acetyl groups. NAA is thought to function as a **predecessor of brain lipids and participate in coenzyme A interactions (C)**. The choline peak occurs at 3.21 ppm and is a **structural component of cell membranes (D)**. Choline in healthy membranes may not be detected in the choline peak, but the choline peak increases in situations where membranes are being destroyed (malignant tumors and degenerative disease). The creatine peak occurs at 3.03 ppm and is involved in the **maintenance of energy systems (B)**. The creatine peak is thought to be relatively stable, so it is often used as a reference. Myo-inositol (MI) has peaks at 3.56 and 4.06 ppm and is a reflection of **the storage of membranous phosphoinositides, second messengers of cell membranes (A)**. MI is located primarily in glial cells. The **lactate doublet occurs at 1.32 ppm (E)**.[12]

115. D – Reduced NAA, increased choline, increased lactate

For astrocytomas (in general), an increased choline peak, reduction of the NAA peak, and appearance of a lactate peak are typical. In cases of glioblastoma, a full reduction of the NAA peak and a sharp increase in the lactate peak often occur, which correlate with the presence of necrosis. Choice **D** is the correct answer.[12]

116. E – Vertebral osteopetrosis

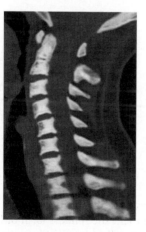

This sagittal CT scan shows an example of **vertebral osteopetrosis (E)**, a process characterized by deficient osteoclastic reabsorption leading to increased bone mineral density. Diffuse sclerosis and cortical thickening are seen here. The other choices are incorrect.[13]

117. C – Median prosencephalic vein

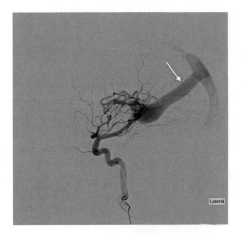

This lateral angiogram shows an example of a vein of Galen malformation, a type of arteriovenous fistula that usually presents during childhood. The *arrow* is pointing to a persistent **median prosencephalic vein (C)**, the preservation of which may be the underlying mechanism of the fistula. The *arrow* is pointed at a location too distal for the structure to represent an **atrial vein (A)**, the **internal cerebral vein (B)**, or the **vein of Galen (E)**. The **straight sinus (D)** would be at the level of the tentorium; this structure is clearly above the tentorium.[12]

118. D – All of the above

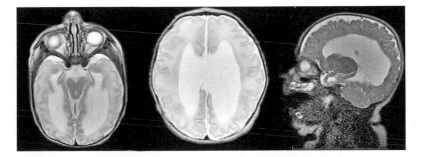

The MRI images shown here demonstrate **septo-optic dysplasia (C)**. This condition is considered by some to represent the mildest form of holoprosencephaly. There is absence of the septum pellucidum and hypoplasia of the optic nerves. The absence of the septum pellucidum gives the box-shaped configuration to the ventricles **(colpocephaly [B])**. This patient also has **agenesis of the corpus callosum (A)**, contributing to the parallel configuration of the ventricles. The correct answer is **D, all of the above**.[13]

119. B – Epidermoid

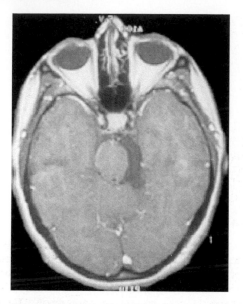

This postcontrast T1-weighted MRI image shows an example of a cerebello-pontine angle **epidermoid cyst (B)**. An **arachnoid cyst (A)** would also appear hypointense on T1; however, this location is more typical for an epidermoid lesion. A **lipoma (C)** would appear hyperintense on T1. A **low-grade glioma (D)** would be intra-axial, not extra-axial. A **meningioma (E)** would most likely show homogenous enhancement on this postcontrast image.[4]

120. D – Gradient echo

Gradient echo sequences (D) are sensitive to the magnetic field created by the iron in hemoglobin, and are therefore the most sensitive sequence for the detection of blood products of the choices listed. **Diffusion-weighted images (A)** are useful in the diagnosis of acute stroke. **Fast spin echo (B)** sequences generate traditional T1- and T2-weighted images. **Fluid-attenuated inversion recovery sequences (C)** eliminate CSF signal and are useful for lesions adjacent to the ventricular system. **MRI spectroscopy (E)** is less sensitive than gradient echo for the detection of blood products. [4]

121. D – A and C only

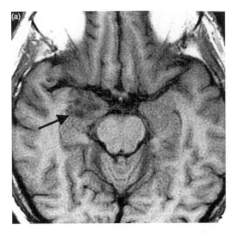

The lesion seen in this axial MRI is an example of a dysembryoplastic neuro-epithelial tumor (DNET). These lesions usually **present with seizures (C)** and are **associated with cortical dysplasia (A)**. The lesion contains abnormal oligodendrocytes and astrocytes, but normal neurons **(B is false)**. Ganglioglioma, not DNET, **contains both abnormal neurons and glial cells (B)**. **D** is the correct answer.[4,13]

References

1. Morris P. Practical Neuroangiography. Baltimore, MD: Williams & Wilkins; 1997
2. Osborn AG. Diagnostic Cerebral Angiography. Philadelphia, PA: Lippincott Williams & Wilkins; 1998
3. Apuzzo MLJ. Brain Surgery. Complication Avoidance and Management. New York: Churchill Livingstone; 1993
4. Citow JS, Macdonald RL, Refai D, eds. Comprehensive Neurosurgery Board Review. New York: Thieme Medical Publishers; 2009
5. American College of Radiology Neuroradiology Learning File. Osborne AG, Smirniotopoulos JG, eds. Videodisc Version 1.0. Mishkin, MM.
6. Yock DH Jr. Magnetic Resonance Imaging of CNS Disease: A Teaching File, 2nd ed. St. Louis, MO: Mosby; 2002
7. Winn HR, ed-in-chief. Neurological Surgery, 5th ed. Philadelphia, PA: W.B. Saunders; 2003
8. Tindall GT, Cooper PR, Barrow DL, eds. The Practice of Neurosurgery. Baltimore, MD: Williams & Wilkins; 1995
9. Burger PC, Scheithauer BW, Vogel FS, eds. Surgical Pathology of the Nervous System and Its Coverings, 4th ed. New York: Churchill Livingstone; 2002
10. Burger PC, Scheithauer BW, Vogel FS. Surgical Pathology of the Nervous System and Its Coverings, 3rd ed. New York: Churchill Livingstone; 1991
11. McKhann II GM, Kitchen ND, Manju H. Questions and Answers Color Review of Clinical Neurology and Neurosurgery. New York: Thieme Medical Publishers; 2003
12. Kornienko VN, Pronin IN. Diagnostic Neuroradiology. Moscow: Springer; 2009
13. Borden NM, Forseen SE. Pattern Recognition Neuroradiology. New York: Cambridge University Press; 2011

7A Clinical Skills/ Critical Care—Questions

➡ For questions **1** to **6**, match the anesthetic agent with the description. Each response may be used once, more than once, or not at all.

    A. Enflurane
    B. Etomidate
    C. Halothane
    D. Isoflurane
    E. Ketamine
    F. Thiopental

1. Increases cerebral blood flow (CBF) and cerebral metabolic rate of oxygen consumption ($CRMO_2$)

2. Of the volatile anesthetics, it increases CBF the least.

3. Induces seizure discharges

4. Dissociative anesthetic

5. Decreases CBF and $CRMO_2$ and produces cardiovascular depression

6. Decreases CBF and $CRMO_2$ and suppresses adrenocortical response to stress

7. Which antiemetic medication lowers seizure threshold?
    A. Phenergan
    B. Droperidol
    C. Tigan
    D. Zofran
    E. Reglan

8. The most appropriate drug to administer to a stable patient with a narrow complex supraventricular tachycardia (no serious signs or symptoms) after vagal stimulation is
    A. Adenosine
    B. Digoxin
    C. Procainamide
    D. Quinidine
    E. Verapamil

9. Each is true of fat embolism *except*
   A. Cerebral manifestations frequently occur in the absence of pulmonary manifestations.
   B. Increased serum lipase occurs in up to half of all patients.
   C. Petechia over the shoulders and chest is a classic finding.
   D. Symptoms typically occur 12 to 48 hours after trauma.
   E. Tachycardia and tachypnea are characteristic.

10. Gamma irradiation of blood helps prevent
    A. Graft-versus-host disease
    B. Hemolytic transfusion reactions
    C. Hepatitis B transmission
    D. Nonhemolytic transfusion reactions
    E. Transfusion siderosis

11. Citrate toxicity from massive transfusions results from the
    A. Binding of free ionized Ca^{2+}
    B. Decrease of 2,3-diphosphoglyceric acid (DPG) levels
    C. Inactivation of factors 5 and 8
    D. Interaction with platelets, rendering them dysfunctional
    E. Precipitation of autoimmune hemolytic anemia

⇨ For questions **12** to **14**, match the description with the disease.
    A. Cushing's disease
    B. Ectopic adrenocorticotropic hormone (ACTH) production
    C. Both
    D. Neither

12. Cortisol is suppressed with low-dose dexamethasone.

13. Cortisol is suppressed with high-dose dexamethasone.

14. Increase in urinary 17-hydroxycorticosteroids after a metyrapone test

15. Which of the following scenarios reflects an iron deficiency anemia?
    A. Decreased mean corpuscular volume (MCV) and decreased total iron binding capacity (TIBC)
    B. Decreased MCV and increased TIBC
    C. Decreased MCV and normal TIBC
    D. Increased MCV and decreased TIBC
    E. Increased MCV and increased TIBC

16. Prolongation of bleeding time usually occurs in
    I. von Willebrand's disease
    II. Use of nonsteroidal anti-inflammatory agents
    III. Uremia
    IV Factor VII deficiency
    A. I, II, III
    B. I, III
    C. II, IV
    D. IV
    E. All of the above

17. Drugs that antagonize the anticoagulant effect of warfarin (Coumadin) include
    I.   Cholestyramine
    II.   Phenobarbital
    III. Rifampin
    IV   Cimetidine
    A.   I, II, III
    B.   I, III
    C.   II, IV
    D.   IV
    E.   All of the above

18. Side effects of thiazide diuretics include
    I.   Insulin resistance
    II.   Hyponatremia
    III. Hypokalemia
    IV.   Flushing
    A.   I, II, III
    B.   I, III
    C.   II, IV
    D.   IV
    E.   All of the above

19. Plasma levels of phenytoin (Dilantin) are increased by all of the following *except*
    A.   Carbamazepine
    B.   Cimetidine
    C.   Coumadin
    D.   Isoniazid
    E.   Sulfonamides

20. The most common electrocardiogram (EKG) finding(s) in patients with pulmonary emboli is
    A.   A peaked T wave
    B.   An S1-Q3-T3 pattern
    C.   Rightward shift of the QRS axis
    D.   Sinus tachycardia (ST) and T wave changes
    E.   Bradycardia

21. Which of the following disorders leads to hypernatremia?
    A.   Addison's disease
    B.   Hyperaldosteronism
    C.   Hypothyroidism
    D.   Renal failure
    E.   Syndrome of inappropriate antidiuretic hormone (SIADH)

22. The most common acid–base disturbance in mild to moderately injured patients without severe renal, circulatory, or pulmonary decompensation is
    A.   Respiratory acidosis and metabolic alkalosis
    B.   Respiratory alkalosis and metabolic acidosis
    C.   Respiratory or metabolic acidosis
    D.   Respiratory or metabolic alkalosis

23. The reabsorption of Na$^+$ ions in the thin ascending Henle's loop
    A. Is by active transport
    B. Is by a Na$^+$–K$^+$ exchange pump
    C. Passively follows the active transport of Cl$^-$ ions
    D. Passively follows the active transport of water molecules

⇨ For questions **24** to **27**, match the antiplatelet agent with the description. Each response may be used once, more than once, or not at all.
    A. Abciximab (ReoPro)
    B. Aspirin
    C. Clopidogrel (Plavix)
    D. Eptifibatide (Integrilin)
    E. Ticlopidine (Ticlid)

24. Of the two prodrugs that block the Gi-coupled platelet adenosine diphosphate (ADP) receptor, it has a slightly more favorable toxicity profile.

25. Is the Fab fragment of a monoclonal antibody directed against the IIb/IIIa receptor

26. Is a cyclic peptide inhibitor of the arginine-glycine-aspartate (RGD) binding site on the glycoprotein IIb/IIIa

27. Blocks production of thromboxane A2

28. Which laboratory finding in disseminated intravascular coagulation (DIC) correlates most closely with bleeding?
    A. Decreased fibrinogen
    B. Increased fibrin degradation products
    C. Increased prothrombin time (PT)
    D. Increased partial thromboplastin time (PTT)
    E. Increased thrombin time (TT)

29. The definition of oxygen saturation is the
    A. Amount of oxygen dissolved in plasma
    B. Fractional concentration of inspired oxygen
    C. Partial pressure of oxygen in the blood
    D. Percentage of hemoglobin that is bound to oxygen
    E. Ratio of unbound to bound hemoglobin

30. Metabolic responses to trauma include each of the following *except*
    A. Hypoglycemia
    B. Increased rate of lipolysis
    C. Increased Na$^+$ reabsorption
    D. Increased water reabsorption
    E. Metabolic alkalosis

31. A normal PT, a prolonged PTT, and a bleeding disorder would result from a deficiency of factor
    A. II
    B. V
    C. VIII
    D. X
    E. XII

⇨ For questions **32** to **37**, match the coagulation factor with the description. Each response may be used once, more than once, or not at all.

    A.   Factor II
    B.   Factor VII
    C.   Factor VIII
    D.   Factor IX
    E.   Factor X

32. Shortest half-life

33. Reflects the extrinsic pathway

34. Deficient or abnormal in hemophilia A (classic)

35. Deficient in hemophilia B (Christmas disease)

36. All except this factor are vitamin K–dependent factors.

37. Deficiency of factor II or this factor results in prolonged PT and PTT.

⇨ For questions **38** to **45**, match the combination of laboratory values with the hematologic diagnosis. Each response may be used once, more than once, or not at all.

    A.   Abnormal PT, PTT, and bleeding time
    B.   Abnormal PT, normal PTT and bleeding time
    C.   Normal PT, PTT, and bleeding time
    D.   Normal PT, abnormal PTT and bleeding time
    E.   Hypercoagulable state
    F.   Normal PT, abnormal PTT, normal bleeding time

38. Antithrombin III deficiency

39. DIC

40. von Willebrand's disease

41. Dysfibrinogenemia

42. Malnutrition

43. Factor VII deficiency

44. Factor XIII deficiency

45. Factor VIII deficiency

⇨ For questions **46** to **52**, match the acid–base disturbance with the description or diagnosis. Each response may be used once, more than once, or not at all.

    A.   Increased anion gap metabolic acidosis
    B.   Non-anion gap metabolic acidosis
    C.   Metabolic alkalosis
    D.   Respiratory acidosis
    E.   Respiratory alkalosis

46. Often occurs with hypokalemia

47. Addison's disease

48. Salicylate overdose (early stage)

49. Myasthenia gravis

50. Ethylene glycol overdose

51. Cushing's disease

52. Primary aldosteronism

53. The formula for mean arterial pressure is (DBP, diastolic blood pressure; SBP, systolic blood pressure)
- **A.** (DBP + SBP)/2
- **B.** DBP + (SBP − DBP)/2
- **C.** DBP/2 + SBP/3
- **D.** DBP + (SBP − DBP)/3
- **E.** DBP/2 + (SBP − DBP)/3

⇨ For questions **54** to **60**, match the description with the syndrome.
- **A.** Multiple endocrine neoplasia (MEN) type I (Werner's syndrome)
- **B.** MEN type IIA (Sipple's syndrome)
- **C.** Both
- **D.** Neither

54. Parathyroid hyperplasia or adenoma

55. Pancreatic islet cell hyperplasia, adenoma, or carcinoma

56. Pituitary hyperplasia or adenoma

57. Pheochromocytomas are common.

58. Medullary thyroid carcinomas are common.

59. Mucosal and gastrointestinal neuromas

60. Marfanoid features

61. Characteristics of primary hyperaldosteronism include each of the following *except*
- **A.** Edema
- **B.** Hypokalemia
- **C.** Increased diastolic blood pressure
- **D.** Metabolic alkalosis
- **E.** Suppression of plasma renin activity

62. Adequacy of pulmonary ventilation is assessed by
- **A.** FiO_2
- **B.** Oxygen saturation
- **C.** $PaCO_2$
- **D.** Partial pressure of O_2 in blood
- **E.** Tidal volume

⟹ For questions **63** to **68**, match the abnormality in the EKG with the diagnosis. Each response may be used once, more than once, or not at all.

    A. Atrial fibrillation
    B. J-point elevation
    C. Peaked T wave
    D. Prolonged QT interval
    E. U wave

63. Hypocalcemia

64. Hypokalemia

65. Hyperkalemia

66. Hypothermia

67. Hyperthyroidism

68. Quinidine toxicity

69. Which of the following is *false* of malignant hyperthermia?
    A. Calcium is released from the muscle cell's sarcoplasmic reticulum.
    B. End-tidal pCO_2 increases
    C. It is precipitated by the use of inhalational anesthetics.
    D. Treatment is with dantrolene.
    E. Use of succinylcholine can help prevent it.

70. Of the following, the best choice for *Clostridium difficile* enterocolitis is
    A. Clindamycin orally
    B. Metronidazole (Flagyl) orally
    C. Penicillin G orally
    D. Penicillin VK intravenously
    E. Vancomycin intravenously

⟹ For questions **71** to **73**, match the description with the process.

    A. Cardiac tamponade
    B. Tension pneumothorax
    C. Both
    D. Neither

71. Pulsus paradoxus

72. Increased venous pressure

73. Increased pulse pressure

74. Meningitis occurring within 72 hours after a basilar skull fracture is most commonly secondary to
    A. *Haemophilus influenzae*
    B. *Neisseria meningitidis*
    C. *Staphylococcus aureus*
    D. *Staphylococcus epidermidis*
    E. *Streptococcus pneumoniae*

75. Postoperative shunt infections are most commonly caused by
    A. Coagulase-negative staphylococci
    B. *H. influenzae*
    C. *Pseudomonas* species
    D. *S. aureus*
    E. *S. pneumoniae*

76. The most likely cause of a fever occurring in the first 24 hours after surgery is
    A. Atelectasis/postoperative inflammation
    B. Deep vein thrombosis
    C. Pneumonia
    D. Urinary tract infection
    E. Wound infection

⟹ For questions **77** to **81**, match the description with the drug.
    A. Dobutamine
    B. Dopamine
    C. Both
    D. Neither

77. A positive inotropic agent

78. Has very little effect on α-adrenergic receptors

79. Is the drug of choice in septic shock

80. Has no effect on β2 receptors

81. Has a dose-related effect

82. Of the following, the most common cause of neonatal meningitis is
    A. *H. influenzae*
    B. *Listeria* species
    C. *N. meningitidis*
    D. Staphylococci
    E. Group B streptococci

83. Each of the following is true of nitroprusside *except*
    A. Cyanide accumulation may lead to metabolic acidosis
    B. The cyanide is reduced to thiocyanate in the liver
    C. The half-life of thiocyanate is 3 to 4 days
    D. Thiocyanate is excreted in the gastrointestinal (GI) tract
    E. With prolonged administration, accumulation of thiocyanate may cause an acute toxic psychosis

84. Isoproterenol
    A. Acts almost exclusively on α-receptors
    B. Decreases SBP
    C. Increases DBP
    D. Increases peripheral vascular resistance (PVR)
    E. Relaxes smooth muscle

85. Splenectomy for hereditary spherocytosis
    A. Corrects the anemia
    B. Corrects the defects in red blood cells
    C. Has no effect on red blood cell survival
    D. Should not be preceded by vaccination
    E. Should be performed before age 3

⇨ For questions **86** to **92**, match the time period after creation of a wound with the event occurring during wound healing. Each response may be used once, more than once, or not at all.
    A. 12 hours
    B. 5 days
    C. 17 days
    D. 42 days
    E. 2 years

86. Epithelial migration occurs.

87. Increase in tensile strength occurs at least up to this point.

88. Wound contraction begins.

89. Maximum amount of total collagen occurs at this time.

90. Visible collagen synthesis begins.

91. Significant gain in tensile strength begins at this time.

92. The rapid increase in collagen content slows considerably at this point.

93. Each of the following is consistent with the Zollinger-Ellison syndrome *except* a(n)
    A. Decrease in serum gastrin with secretin injection
    B. Duodenal ulcer
    C. Duodenal wall gastrinoma
    D. Pancreatic gastrinoma
    E. Increased serum gastrin level

⇨ For questions **94** to **99**, match the description with the disease.
    A. Type I (distal) renal tubular acidosis (RTA)
    B. Type II (proximal) RTA
    C. Both
    D. Neither

94. Non-anion gap acidosis

95. Hyperkalemia

96. Nephrocalcinosis commonly occurs.

97. Urine pH > 5.5

98. Defect in reabsorption of bicarbonate

99. Hypokalemia

100. The percentage of extracellular fluid represented by plasma volume is approximately
   A.   5%
   B.   15%
   C.   20%
   D.   40%
   E.   60%

101. Each of the following occurs in venous air embolism *except* a(n)
   A.   Decrease in cardiac output
   B.   Increase in end-tidal pCO_2
   C.   Increase in pulmonary artery pressure
   D.   Increase in pulmonary vascular resistance
   E.   Ventilation-perfusion mismatch

102. The most sensitive noninvasive monitor of venous air embolism is
   A.   Auscultation of the chest with a stethoscope
   B.   End-tidal pCO_2
   C.   End-tidal pN_2
   D.   Precordial Doppler
   E.   Pulmonary artery catheterization

103. Which EKG change in the anterior leads is the most characteristic finding in sub-endocardial ischemia?
   A.   Hyperacute T wave
   B.   Q wave
   C.   ST depression
   D.   ST elevation
   E.   T wave inversion

104. Which set of laboratory values is most consistent with hypothyroidism of hypothalamic or pituitary origin?
   A.   Decreased thyroid-stimulating hormone (TSH) and decreased free thyroxine (T4)
   B.   Decreased TSH and increased free T4
   C.   Decreased TSH and normal free T4
   D.   Increased TSH and decreased free T4
   E.   Increased TSH and increased free T4

105. Of the following treatment options for hyperkalemia, which one *does not* alter serum potassium?
   A.   Calcium
   B.   Cation-exchange resins
   C.   Hemodialysis
   D.   Insulin
   E.   Sodium bicarbonate

For questions **106** to **111**, match the acid–base disturbance with the arterial blood gas result. Each response may be used once, more than once, or not at all.

    A.   Respiratory acidosis
    B.   Respiratory acidosis and metabolic acidosis
    C.   Metabolic acidosis
    D.   Metabolic acidosis and compensatory respiratory alkalosis
    E.   Respiratory alkalosis
    F.   Respiratory alkalosis and compensatory metabolic acidosis
    G.   Uninterpretable

106. $pH = 7.5$, $pCO_2 = 30$, $HCO_3 = 19$

107. $pH = 7.3$, $pCO_2 = 52$, $HCO_3 = 29$

108. $pH = 7.35$, $pCO_2 = 17$, $HCO_3 = 9$

109. $pH = 7.55$, $pCO_2 = 32$, $HCO_3 = 12$

110. $pH = 7.22$, $pCO_2 = 55$, $HCO_3 = 22$

111. $pH = 7.25$, $pCO_2 = 28$, $HCO_3 = 12$

112. If Qs and Qt are pulmonary shunt and total blood flow, respectively, and Cc, Ca, and Cv are the oxygen contents of end-capillary, arterial, and mixed venous blood, respectively, then the shunt fraction $Qs/Qt =$

    A. $Cc/(Cc - Cv)$
    B. $(Ca - Cv)/Cv$
    C. $(Cv - Ca)/Cc$
    D. $(Cc - Ca)/(Cc - Cv)$
    E. $(Ca + Cv)/(Ca + Cc + Cv)$

113. Atropine toxicity produces each of the following *except*

    A.   Blurred vision
    B.   Decreased intestinal peristalsis
    C.   Dry mouth
    D.   Increased pulse
    E.   Increased sweating

114. Each of the following is true of hyperosmolar coma *except*

    A.   Free fatty acid concentration is lower than in ketoacidosis
    B.   Glucose concentration is higher than in ketoacidosis
    C.   It is more common in type 1 diabetes mellitus than in type 2 diabetes mellitus
    D.   Mortality is more than 50%
    E.   Volume depletion is usually severe

For questions **115** to **119**, match the autonomic drug with the description. Each response may be used once, more than once, or not at all.

    A.   Clonidine
    B.   Isoproterenol
    C.   Phenoxybenzamine
    D.   Phentolamine
    E.   Prazosin

115. β agonist

116. Pure α1 antagonist

117. Noncompetitive α antagonist

118. Competitive, nonselective α antagonist

119. Central α2 agonist

120. The most appropriate cholinergic agent to be used in urinary retention is
- **A.** Acetylcholine
- **B.** Bethanechol
- **C.** Carbachol
- **D.** Choline
- **E.** Methacholine

121. Which of the following is false of polycythemia vera?
- **A.** Budd-Chiari syndrome is common.
- **B.** Hyperuricemia can complicate the disorder.
- **C.** It is the most common of the myeloproliferative disorders.
- **D.** Massive splenomegaly is usually the presenting sign.
- **E.** The use of alkylating agents should be avoided.

122. The serum osmolarity of a patient with a sodium level of 130 meq/L, K of 4.0 meq/L, glucose of 126 mg/dL, and blood urea nitrogen (BUN) of 28 mg/dL is
- **A.** 276
- **B.** 285
- **C.** 296
- **D.** 304
- **E.** 310

123. Each of the following is a result of the use of positive end-expiratory pressure (PEEP) in the ventilated patient *except*
- **A.** Decreased cerebral perfusion pressure
- **B.** Decreased physiologic dead space
- **C.** Decreased work of breathing
- **D.** Improved lung compliance
- **E.** Predisposition to barotraumas

124. The oxyhemoglobin dissociation curve is shifted to the right (decreased oxygen affinity) by
- I. Acidosis
- II. Decreased 2,3-diphosphoglyceric acid (2,3-DPG)
- III. Fever
- IV Banked blood
- **A.** I, II, III
- **B.** I, III
- **C.** II, IV
- **D.** IV
- **E.** All of the above

125. Gastrointestinal carcinoid tumors are most frequently found in the
   A. Appendix
   B. Colon
   C. Ileum
   D. Rectum
   E. Stomach

126. Alkalinization of the urine promotes excretion of
   I. Salicylates
   II. Tricyclic antidepressants
   III. Phenobarbital
   IV. Amphetamines
   A. I, II, III
   B. I, III
   C. II, IV
   D. IV
   E. All of the above

⇨ For questions **127** and **128**, match the description with the substance.
   A. Cryoprecipitate
   B. Fresh frozen plasma
   C. Both
   D. Neither

127. Reliably effective in von Willebrand's disease

128. Used in the treatment of hemophilia B

129. The free water deficit in a dehydrated 70-kg man with an Na^+ of 160 is
   A. 2 L
   B. 4 L
   C. 6 L
   D. 7 L
   E. 8 L

⇨ For questions **130** to **134**, match the autonomic drug with the description. Each response may be used once, more than once, or not at all.
   A. Amrinone
   B. Dopamine
   C. Epinephrine
   D. Neo-Synephrine
   E. Norepinephrine

130. Pure α agonist

131. Does not interact with α or β receptors

132. Effects vary significantly with dose administered.

133. Primarily an α agonist with mild β1 activity

134. Balanced α and β agonist properties

135. Thallium intoxication causes each of the following *except*
A. Cardiac dysfunction
B. GI disturbance
C. Hirsutism
D. Lower extremity joint pain
E. Peripheral neuropathy

136. Which of the following symptoms is *least* characteristic of acute intermittent porphyria?
A. Abdominal pain
B. Hypotension
C. Polyneuropathy
D. Psychosis
E. Tachycardia

137. A patient on his third hospital day in the neuro intensive care unit abruptly develops bradycardia, hyperlipidemia, and rhabdomyolysis while on the ventilator. The most appropriate next step is
A. Acquire cardiology consultation
B. Discontinue the offending agent
C. Initiate broad-spectrum antibiotics
D. Insulin administration
E. Renal dialysis

138. Which of the following descriptions best describes Cheyne-Stokes respiration?
A. Breathing is irregularly interrupted, and each breath varies in rate and depth
B. Few rapid deep breaths alternate with apneic cycles (2–3 second pause in full inspiration) in short cycles
C. Increase in rate and depth of respiration leading to respiratory alkalosis
D. Waxing and waning hyperpnea regularly alternates with shorter apneic periods
E. None of the above

139. Cushing's reflex refers to
A. Increased heart rate in response to increased intracranial pressure
B. Increased systolic arterial pressure in response to increased intracranial pressure
C. Parasympathetic outflow in response to increased intracranial pressure
D. All of the above
E. None of the above

Clinical Skills/
Critical Care—Answer Key

1.	E	27.	B
2.	D	28.	A
3.	A	29.	D
4.	E	30.	A
5.	F	31.	C
6.	B	32.	B
7.	A	33.	B
8.	A	34.	C
9.	A	35.	D
10.	A	36.	C
11.	A	37.	E
12.	D	38.	E
13.	A	39.	A
14.	A	40.	D
15.	B	41.	A
16.	A	42.	B
17.	A	43.	B
18.	A	44.	C
19.	A	45.	F
20.	D	46.	C
21.	B	47.	B
22.	D	48.	E
23.	C	49.	D
24.	C	50.	A
25.	A	51.	C
26.	D	52.	C

53.	D	92.	D
54.	C	93.	A
55.	A	94.	C
56.	A	95.	D
57.	B	96.	A
58.	B	97.	A
59.	D	98.	B
60.	D	99.	C
61.	A	100.	C
62.	C	101.	B
63.	D	102.	D
64.	E	103.	C
65.	C	104.	A
66.	B	105.	A
67.	A	106.	E
68.	D	107.	A
69.	E	108.	D
70.	B	109.	F
71.	A	110.	B
72.	C	111.	C
73.	D	112.	D
74.	E	113.	E
75.	A	114.	C
76.	A	115.	B
77.	C	116.	E
78.	A	117.	C
79.	D	118.	D
80.	D	119.	A
81.	B	120.	B
82.	E	121.	D
83.	D	122.	B
84.	E	123.	B
85.	A	124.	B
86.	A	125.	A
87.	E	126.	A
88.	B	127.	A
89.	D	128.	D
90.	B	129.	C
91.	B	130.	D

131. A
132. B
133. E
134. C
135. C

136. B
137. B
138. D
139. B

7C Clinical Skills/Critical Care— Answers and Explanations

1. E –   Ketamine
2. D –   Isoflurane
3. A –   Enflurane
4. E –   Ketamine
5. F –   Thiopental
6. B –   Etomidate

Isoflurane (D), enflurane (A), and halothane (C) are all inhalational (volatile) anesthetics. All inhalational anesthetics reduce the metabolic rate of the brain, but also increase cerebral blood flow (CBF), which may lead to increases in intracranial pressure (ICP). At low doses all halogenated anesthetics have a similar effect on cerebral blood flow, but at higher doses enflurane and isoflurane increase CBF less than halothane. A combination of nitrous oxide and halothane increases CBF more than halothane alone. Of the volatile anesthetics listed, isoflurane (D) increases cerebral blood flow the least. Enflurane (A), at high doses, has cerebral irritant effects that can lead to spike-and-wave electroencephalogram (EEG) patterns. Etomidate (B) is a carboxylated imidazole that is sometimes used for induction of anesthesia—its use is associated with adrenal suppression, even after a single dose. Ketamine (E) is a dissociative anesthetic that increases cerebral blood flow, cerebral oxygen consumption, and ICP. Thiopental (F) is a short-acting barbiturate that is used for induction of general anesthesia—it rapidly crosses the blood–brain barrier and causes reductions in both $CMRO_2$ and CBF; the reduction in $CMRO_2$ is greater than the reduction in CBF, however. Thiopental (F) is associated with a myocardial depressant effect and increased venous pooling, which may lead to decreased blood pressure, stroke volume, and cardiac output.[1,2]

7. A –   Phenergan

Phenergan (A), a phenothiazine antiemetic, has been shown to lower the seizure threshold.[3]

8. A –   Adenosine

> **Adenosine (A)** at an initial dose of 6 mg over 1 to 3 seconds, followed by a repeat of 12 mg in 1 to 2 minutes as needed, is the initial drug of choice. If lidocaine is ineffective, procainamide at a dose of 20 to 30 mg/min for a maximum of 17 mg/kg is given.[4,5]

9. A –   Cerebral manifestations frequently occur in the absence of pulmonary manifestations (false)

> Fat embolism syndrome may occur after long bone fractures or soft tissue injury and burns. The syndrome is characterized by **pulmonary insufficiency (E)**, neurologic symptoms, anemia, and thrombocytopenia. Onset of symptoms typically occurs within the first **1–2 days following trauma (D)**. A **petechial rash (C)** in nondependent areas is present in up to 50% of cases. Neurologic involvement does not develop in the absence of pulmonary abnormalities unless there is the rare event of a paradoxical embolus through a patent foramen ovale **(A is false)**.[6,7]

10. A –   Graft-versus-host disease

> Graft-versus-host disease may occur when blood donor lymphocytes attack the normal tissues of the transfusion recipient (particularly in immunocompromised patients). Transfusion-associated graft-versus-host disease may result if viable lymphocytes in blood are not irradiated.[8]

11. A –   Binding of free ionized Ca^{2+}

> Anticoagulants such as heparin, citrate, and EDTA **bind calcium (A)**. Banked blood contains the anticoagulant citrate. Massive transfusions can lead to acute hypocalcemia in the critically ill patient.[5,6]

12. D –   Neither
13. A –   Cushing's disease
14. A –   Cushing's disease

> Cushing's syndrome is the condition of overt glucocorticoid exposure regardless of the etiology. **Cushing's disease (A)** is Cushing's syndrome caused by an ACTH-producing pituitary adenoma. The dexamethasone suppression test is used to differentiate Cushing's syndrome of various etiologies. Generally, ACTH production and cortisol secretion are not suppressed by low- or high-dose dexamethasone if the source of ACTH is an **ectopic ACTH-producing tumor (B)**. In **Cushing's disease (A)**, however (ACTH-producing pituitary adenoma), the high-dose dexamethasone suppression test is expected to suppress ACTH and cortisol secretion. The metyrapone test is a test of ACTH reserve and simulates 11-hydroxylase deficiency. Administration of metyrapone inhibits cortisol synthesis, increasing ACTH secretion and increasing adrenal production, and thus urinary excretion, of 17-hydroxycorticosteroids. An ACTH-producing pituitary adenoma is expected to respond to the metyrapone test, while an **ectopic ACTH-producing tumor (B)** is not.[9,10]

15. B – Decreased MCV and increased TIBC

Chronic iron deficiency results in a microcytic hypochromic anemia characterized by low mean corpuscular volume (MCV) values and decreased serum hemoglobin. The most common cause of a hypochromic, microcytic anemia is iron deficiency anemia, in which the serum iron concentration is decreased and total iron binding capacity (TIBC) is increased. A normal or decreased TIBC is not consistent with iron deficiency anemia **(A, C)**. An increased MCV is consistent with a macrocytic anemia as may be seen in B_{12} or folate deficiency **(D, E)**, but not iron deficiency anemia.[8,11]

16. A – I, II, III (von Willebrand's disease, nonsteroidal anti-inflammatory agents, and uremia)

An abnormal bleeding time in a patient with a normal platelet count suggests qualitative platelet dysfunction or abnormal platelet-vessel wall interactions. Possible causes for an increased bleeding time include the **use of aspirin or NSAIDs (II)**, **uremic platelet dysfunction (III)**, and **von Willebrand's disease (I)**. Although patients with von Willebrand's disease usually have an abnormal bleeding time, the bleeding time may occasionally be normal due to cyclical variations in the von Willebrand factor. **Factor VII deficiency (IV)** causes prolongation of the prothrombin time (PT), but elevations of the partial thromboplastin time (PTT) and bleeding time are not characteristic.[8,11]

17. A – I, II, III (cholestyramine, phenobarbital, rifampin)

Several drugs can antagonize the effects of warfarin through a variety of mechanisms such as reduced absorption of warfarin in the GI tract caused by **cholestyramine (I)**; increased clearance of warfarin via induction of hepatic enzymes (CYP2C9) by **barbiturates (phenobarbital [II])**, carbamazepine, or **rifampin (III)**; and by ingestion of large amounts of vitamin K. **Cimetidine (IV)** promotes the effects of warfarin via inhibition of CYP2C9, decreasing the metabolism of warfarin. Other drugs that inhibit CYP2C9 are amiodarone, azole antifungals, clopidogrel, cotrimoxazole, disulfiram, fluoxetine, isoniazid, metronidazole, sulfinpyrazone, tolcapone, and zafirlukast.[8,12]

18. A – I, II, III (insulin resistance, hyponatremia, and hypokalemia)

Metabolic side effects of thiazide diuretics include **hyponatremia (I)** and **hypokalemia (III)** from renal loss, hyperuricemia from uric acid retention, **carbohydrate intolerance (I)**, and hyperlipidemia. Niacin is associated with **flushing (IV)**.[8,12]

19. A – Carbamazepine

Any drug metabolized by CYP2C9 or CYP2C10 can increase the plasma concentration of phenytoin by decreasing its metabolism. These drugs include, but are not limited to, **cimetidine (B)**, **warfarin (C)**, **isoniazid (D)**, and **sulfonamides (E)**. **Carbamazepine (Tegretol [A])** decreases plasma levels of phenytoin (Dilantin) by enhancing its metabolism. Conversely, phenytoin reduces serum levels of carbamazepine.[8,12]

20. D – Sinus tachycardia and T wave changes

Nonspecific **sinus tachycardia (ST) and T wave changes (D)** occur in 66% of patients. Only one-third of patients with massive emboli have the **S1-Q3-T3 pattern (B)** of acute cor pulmonale, right bundle branch block, and **right axis deviation (C)**. The utility of EKG in suspected pulmonary embolism (PE) is in establishing or excluding other diagnoses such as acute myocardial infarction.[6,11]

21. B – Hyperaldosteronism

Aldosterone (B) stimulates sodium reabsorption in the renal collecting duct, leading to increased serum sodium concentration. **SIADH (E)** leads to hyponatremia because of inappropriate retention of free water despite low serum osmolality. **Addison's disease (A)** and **hypothyroidism (C)** are associated with SIADH. A severely compromised glomerular filtration rate, as in **renal failure (D)**, increases the fractional reabsorption of water in the renal proximal tubule, predisposing these patients to hyponatremia.[4,10]

22. D – Respiratory or metabolic alkalosis

Respiratory and metabolic alkalosis are the most common acid–base disturbances in mild to moderately injured patients without severe renal, circulatory, or pulmonary decompensation.[6]

23. C – Passively follows the active transport of Cl⁻ ions

Sodium transport by both the thin ascending and thin descending loop of Henle is almost entirely **passive and follows Cl⁻ ions (C)**. Sodium ions are actively transported in the early and distal convoluted tubule and in the thick ascending limb.[8,13]

24. C – Clopidogrel
25. A – Abciximab
26. D – Eptifibatide
27. B – Aspirin

Aspirin (B) inactivates cyclooxygenase, the enzyme that produces the precursor of thromboxane A2. **Ticlopidine (E)** and **clopidogrel (C)** are thienopyridines that inhibit $P2Y_{12}$, a G-protein-coupled receptor for adenosine diphosphate (ADP) on the platelet. They are both prodrugs requiring conversion to the active metabolite. Thrombocytopenia and leukopenia occur less commonly with clopidogrel than with ticlopidine. **Abciximab (ReoPro [A])** and **eptifibatide (Integrilin [D])** are the inhibitors of glycoprotein IIb/IIIa receptor, but the former is the Fab fragment of a humanized monoclonal antibody against the receptor, and the latter is a cyclic peptide inhibitor of the arginine-glycine-aspartate (RGD) binding site on the receptor.[12]

28. A – Decreased fibrinogen

Disseminated intravascular coagulation (DIC) is a consumptive coagulopathy characterized by widespread microvascular thrombosis, thrombocytopenia, and depletion of circulating coagulation factors. Thrombocytopenia, reduced fibrinogen levels, and **prolongation of the prothrombin time (C)** are the result of depletion, while the **elevated D-dimer (B)** is due to increased thrombolysis. While all of these abnormalities can be observed in DIC, **decreased fibrinogen (A)** correlates most closely with bleeding.[5,8]

29. D – Percentage of hemoglobin that is bound to oxygen

The oxygen saturation refers to the percentage of hemoglobin (Hb) that is bound to oxygen. In other words: Oxygen saturation = (Hb bound to oxygen / Total Hb).[5,14]

30. A – Hypoglycemia (false)

Hyperglycemia, not **hypoglycemia (A)**, is one of the metabolic responses to trauma.[6]

31. C – VIII

Deficiency of factors **II (A)**, **V (B)**, or **X (D)** causes prolonged PT and PTT. A deficiency of factor **XII (E)** causes a prolonged PTT but no clinical bleeding. Only a **factor VIII deficiency (C, hemophilia A)** would cause a prolonged PTT, normal PT, and a bleeding disorder.[8,11]

32. B – Factor VII
33. B – Factor VII
34. C – Factor VIII
35. D – Factor IX
36. C – Factor VIII
37. E – Factor X

The prothrombin time (PT) measures the integrity of the extrinsic and common pathways (factors **VII [B]**, **X [E]**, V, prothrombin, and fibrinogen). The activated partial thromboplastin time (aPTT) measures the integrity of the intrinsic and common pathways of coagulation (factors XII, XI, **IX [D]**, **VIII [C]**, **X [E]**, and V). Hemophilia A is caused by a deficiency in **factor VIII (C)**. Hemophilia B (Christmas disease) is caused by a **factor IX (D)** deficiency. The vitamin K–dependent factors are factors **II (A)**, **VII (B)**, **IX (D)**, and **X (E)**. A deficiency of **factor II (A)**, V, or **X (E)** would result in prolongation of PT and PTT. **Factor VII (B)** has the shortest half-life of the options listed.[8,11]

38. E – Hypercoagulable state
39. A – Abnormal PT, PTT, and bleeding time
40. D – Normal PT, abnormal PTT and bleeding time
41. A – Abnormal PT, PTT, and bleeding time
42. B – Abnormal PT, normal PTT and bleeding time
43. B – Abnormal PT, normal PTT and bleeding time
44. C – Normal PT, PTT, and bleeding time

45. F –   Normal PT, abnormal PTT, and normal bleeding time

> The two conditions listed that would cause **prolongation of the PT, PTT, and bleeding time (A)** are disseminated intravascular coagulation and dysfibrinogenemia. Factor VII deficiencies and nutritional factor deficiencies result in **prolongation of the PT (vitamin K–dependent factors) without prolongation of the PTT or bleeding time (B)**. Factor XIII deficiency is not detected by routine laboratory screening and is characterized by **normal PT, PTT, and bleeding times (C)**. von Willebrand's disease (vWD) is a disorder of platelet–vessel wall interaction, and the **bleeding time is therefore prolonged. The PTT is also prolonged in vWD due to a concomitant factor XIII deficiency; the PT is normal (D)**. Antithrombin III is the major physiologic inhibitor of thrombin; its deficiency leads to unregulated thrombin formation, resulting in a **hypercoagulable state (E)**. A factor VIII deficiency (hemophilia A) results in a **normal PT, abnormal PTT, and normal bleeding time (F)**.[8,11]

46. C –   Metabolic alkalosis
47. B –   Non-anion gap metabolic acidosis
48. E –   Respiratory alkalosis
49. D –   Respiratory acidosis
50. A –   Increased anion gap metabolic acidosis
51. C –   Metabolic alkalosis
52. C –   Metabolic alkalosis

> An **anion gap metabolic acidosis (A)** is caused by fixed acids such as is seen in lactic acidosis, ketoacidosis, late salicylate toxicity, methanol poisoning, and ethylene glycol poisoning. A **non-anion gap metabolic acidosis (B)** is caused by decreased bicarbonate levels with a compensatory increase in chloride ions as is seen in diarrhea, early renal insufficiency, increased chloride load, and type II renal tubular acidosis. Addison's disease is a form of primary adrenal insufficiency caused by the autoimmune-mediated destruction of the adrenal gland. Addison's disease is associated with a hyperkalemic **non-anion gap metabolic acidosis (B)** and decreased extracellular fluid volume due to decreased mineralocorticoid activity in the kidney. Conversely, in situations where there is increased mineralocorticoid activity, there is a tendency toward expansion of the extracellular fluid volume and hypokalemic **metabolic alkalosis (C)** as is seen in cases of Cushing's disease and primary aldosteronism. **Respiratory acidosis (D)** is caused by hypoventilation and carbon dioxide retention as can be seen in myasthenia gravis. **Respiratory alkalosis (E)** is the earliest abnormality and may be the only acid–base disorder in some patients with salicylate overdose. Production of a mixture of endogenous acids, from a metabolic block, may later lead to metabolic acidosis.[3,8,10]

53. D –   DBP + (SBP − DBP)/3

> The mean arterial pressure can be estimated by adding the diastolic pressure to one-third of the pulse pressure. This formula assumes that diastole makes up one-third of the cardiac cycle.[5,6]

54. C –   Both
55. A –   Multiple endocrine neoplasia (MEN) type I (Werner's syndrome)
56. A –   Multiple endocrine neoplasia (MEN) type I (Werner's syndrome)
57. B –   MEN type IIA (Sipple's syndrome)
58. B –   MEN type IIA (Sipple's syndrome)
59. D –   Neither
60. D –   Neither

> **MEN type I (Werner's syndrome [A])** can be remembered as the "PPP" syndrome because it is characterized by parathyroid, pancreatic, and pituitary tumors. **MEN type IIA (Sipple's syndrome [B])** is characterized by medullary thyroid carcinoma, pheochromocytoma, and tumors of the parathyroid glands. Rarely, pheochromocytomas may be seen in **MEN type I (A)**. MEN type IIB (also known as MEN type III) is associated with medullary thyroid carcinoma, pheochromocytoma, gastrointestinal and mucosal neuromas, and a marfanoid habitus.[8,10]

61. A –   Edema

> Hyperaldosteronism stimulates sodium reabsorption in the collecting ducts, causing renal potassium wasting and leading to a **hypokalemic (B)**, hypochloremic **metabolic alkalosis (D)**. Both primary and secondary hyperaldosteronism present with **hypertension (C)**. Primary hyperaldosteronism, or Conn's syndrome, is caused by autologous production of aldosterone either by an adrenal adenoma or adrenal hyperplasia and causes **feedback inhibition of the renin-angiotensin system (E)**. Secondary hyperaldosteronism occurs as a result of increased tone in the renin-angiotensin system, usually caused by renal vascular disease. Secondary hyperaldosteronism usually responds to angiotensin-converting enzyme (ACE) inhibitors. In the absence of associated disorders, **edema (A)** is characteristically absent.[8,10]

62. C – $PaCO_2$

> The partial pressure of arterial CO_2 is directly related to the rate of CO_2 production by the body and inversely related to the rate of alveolar ventilation. Of the choices listed, the adequacy of pulmonary ventilation is best assessed by **$PaCO_2$ (C)**.[5,8,14]

63. D –   Prolonged QT interval
64. E –   U wave
65. C –   Peaked T wave
66. B –   J-point elevation
67. A –   Atrial fibrillation
68. D –   Prolonged QT interval

> Hyperthyroidism is associated with **atrial fibrillation (A)**. Hypothermia is associated with pronounced waves at the QRS-ST interval known as **J-waves (B)** or Osborn waves. Hyperkalemia is associated with **peaked T waves (C)**. A **prolonged QT interval (D)** can be seen with hypocalcemia and quinidine toxicity. Hypokalemia is associated with **U waves (E)**.[3,5,8]

69. E – Use of succinylcholine can help prevent malignant hyperthermia (false).

> Malignant hyperthermia is an inherited disorder characterized by fever and rigidity that involves **excessive release of calcium from the sarcoplasmic reticulum (A)** of skeletal muscle precipitated by **inhalational anesthetics (C)** and **depolarizing neuromuscular blocking agents such as succinylcholine (E is false)**. Diagnosis can be made by an **early rise in end-tidal CO$_2$ (B)** followed by muscle rigidity and fever that may progress to rhabdomyolysis and renal failure. The administration of **dantrolene (D)** is critical in the treatment of this disorder.[3,5,8]

70. B – Metronidazole (Flagyl) orally

> For the treatment of *Clostridium difficile*, a 10-day course of **oral metronidazole (B)** is the preferred treatment. Intravenous metronidazole can be used in patients who cannot receive oral medications. Oral vancomycin is also effective in the treatment of this infection, but it is a second-line agent in an effort to limit vancomycin use. Oral vancomycin is the treatment of choice in pregnant or lactating females. **Intravenous vancomycin (E)** is not effective in this setting.[5,8]

71. A – Cardiac tamponade
72. C – Both
73. D – Neither

> **Cardiac tamponade (A)** occurs when pericardial fluid causes an increase in pericardial pressure and resultant decrease in ventricular filling. Physical exam in cardiac tamponade reveals jugular venous distention from increased atrial (venous) pressures, narrowing of the pulse pressure, and pulsus paradoxus (inspiratory drop in systolic pressure is > 15 mm Hg). In **tension pneumothorax (B)**, intrathoracic pressure is elevated, which impairs ventricular filling, leading to increased atrial (venous) pressure.[5,6,11]

74. E – *Streptococcus pneumoniae*

> ***Streptococcus pneumoniae* (E)** is the most common cause of meningitis in the adult population.[3,15]

75. A – Coagulase-negative staphylococci

> **Coagulase-negative staphylococci (*S. epidermidis* [A])** are the most common cause of postoperative shunt infections.[3,15]

76. A – Atelectasis/postoperative inflammation

> Fever is present in 15–40% of patients in the first postoperative day, is usually self-limited, and is attributed to **atelectasis or postoperative inflammation (A)**. Atelectasis as a cause of fever is somewhat controversial; some authors argue that it is not atelectasis itself, but instead, postoperative inflammation that is the cause of early postoperative fever. **Deep vein thrombosis (B)**, **urinary tract infection (D)**, **pneumonia (C)**, and **wound infection (E)** are less likely to cause fever on the first postoperative day.[5,15]

77. **C –** Both
78. **A –** Dobutamine
79. **D –** Neither
80. **D –** Neither
81. **B –** Dopamine

> **Dobutamine (A)** is a strong β1 receptor agonist and a weak β2 receptor agonist. β1 stimulation causes a positive chronotropic and ionotropic effect. **Dobutamine (A)** is typically used in patients with decompensated systolic heart failure who also have a normal blood pressure. **Dopamine (B)** has dose-dependent effects and, at a low dose, causes changes in renal and splanchnic blood flow as well as increased sodium excretion by the kidneys. At intermediate doses, **dopamine (B)** has a positive ionotropic and chronotropic effect via agonism of β1 receptors, although the ionotropic effect of dopamine is much less than that of dobutamine. At high doses, dopamine stimulates α receptors, causing systemic vasoconstriction and increased cardiac afterload, counteracting the increase in cardiac output. **Both (C)** dopamine and dobutamine stimulate β2 receptors, which causes some degree of peripheral vasodilatation (only at low doses for dopamine). Norepinephrine is the first-line pressor of choice in septic shock.[4,5]

82. **E –** Group B streptococci

> Gram-negative bacilli (*Escherichia coli*) and **group B streptococci (E)** are the most common causes of neonatal meningitis, followed by *Listeria* **(B)**. *Streptococcus pneumoniae* is the most common pathogen in the 4- to 12-week age range. *H. influenzae* **(A)** is most common in the 3-month to 3-year range. *N. meningitidis* **(C)** is the most common pathogen in children and young adults.[3,8]

83. **D –** Thiocyanate is excreted in the GI tract (false)

> Nitroprusside is reduced by smooth muscle, and nitrous oxide and cyanide are released. **Cyanide is reduced to thiocyanate in the liver (B)** by the action of liver rhodanese, and the **thiocyanate is then excreted in the urine (D is false)**. The **half-life of thiocyanate is ~3 days (C)** in patients with normal renal function. Prolonged administration of nitroprusside or infusions at high doses may lead to **accumulation of cyanide (causing lactic acidosis [A])** or **accumulation of thiocyanate (causing psychosis [E])**.[12]

84. **E –** Relaxes smooth muscles

> Isoproterenol is a nonselective β-receptor agonist, **acting almost exclusively on β receptors (A is false)**. It **increases (or leaves unchanged) systolic blood pressure (B is false)** and **decreases diastolic blood pressure (C is false)**, and mean arterial pressure typically falls. It also **decreases peripheral vascular resistance (D is false)** and **relaxes smooth muscle (E)**.[12]

85. A – Corrects the anemia

Splenectomy for hereditary spherocytosis leads to **normal or near normal red blood cell (RBC) survival (B is false)**, **correcting the anemia (A)**. Splenectomy does not correct the underlying defect in red cell membrane structure **(B is false)** and should be performed after age 4–5, when the risk of severe infections is lower **(E is false)**. Patients undergoing splenectomy should be given a polyvalent pneumococcal vaccine several weeks before surgery to reduce the risk of bacterial sepsis **(D is false)**.[8,11]

86. A – 12 hours
87. E – 2 years
88. B – 5 days
89. D – 42 days
90. B – 5 days
91. B – 5 days
92. D – 42 days

This question refers to the time line for wound healing associated with a surgical incision with approximated edges (healing by primary intention). In the **first 12 hours of wound healing (A)**, epithelial cells migrate to the wound edge laying down basement membrane as they travel, fusing in the midline. Within **5 days (B)** visible collagen synthesis has begun, the wound begins to gain tensile strength, and wound contraction begins. Within **6 weeks (42 days [D])**, the wound reaches its maximum amount of total collagen and collagen synthesis slows considerably. The wound may not reach its greatest tensile strength for a full **2 years (E)**.[6,7]

93. A – Decrease in serum gastrin with secretin injection (false)

Gastrinomas of the pancreas (D) or **duodenal wall (C)** cause an **increase in the serum gastrin level (E)**. **Peptic ulcer disease of the duodenum (B)** caused by gastric acid production associated with a gastrinoma is known as the Zollinger-Ellison syndrome. Intravenous secretin increases serum gastrin in patients with a gastrinoma **(A is false)**.[8,10]

94. C – Both
95. D – Neither
96. A – Type I RTA
97. A – Type I RTA
98. B – Type II RTA

99. C – Both

> **Type I (classic, or distal) renal tubular acidosis (RTA; A)** is a hypokalemic, hyperchloremic metabolic acidosis caused by a selective defect in distal acidification (inability to lower urinary pH sufficiently in the distal nephron). The urinary pH is therefore inappropriately high in **type I RTA (A)** with a urine pH > 5.5. Nephrocalcinosis and nephrolithiasis are common in **type I RTA (A)**. **Type II (proximal) RTA (B)** is a hyperchloremic, hypokalemic metabolic acidosis that is caused by a selective defect in proximal acidification—urine pH is usually acidic in periods of acidosis. **Proximal RTA (B)** is rare and usually found in patients with Fanconi's syndrome. The loss of 15% or more of filtered bicarbonate at a normal serum bicarbonate level is pathognomonic of **RTA type II (B)**. Hyperkalemia is found in **RTA type IV**. Nephrocalcinosis is rare in **RTA type II (B)**, and the urine pH is less than 5.5 in this type. **Both (C)** RTA type I and type II result in non-anion gap metabolic acidosis.[8,11]

100. C – 20%

> For the average adult male, total body water (TBW) makes up approximately **60% (E)** of body weight. Intracellular fluid makes up **60% (E)** of the TBW and extracellular fluid makes up **40% (D)** of the TBW. Extracellular fluid is comprised of interstitial fluid (75%), transcellular fluid (5%), and **blood plasma (20% [C])**.[13]

101. B – Increase in end-tidal pCO_2 (false)

> Small air bubbles in the circulation can obstruct vascular flow. Venous air embolism can travel to the pulmonary circulation obstructing small vessels, causing pulmonary vasoconstriction, **increased pulmonary vascular resistance (D)**, and, therefore, **increased pulmonary artery pressure (C)**. Decreased pulmonary perfusion in areas of preserved ventilation results in a **ventilation–perfusion mismatch (E)** leading to **decreased end-tidal pCO_2 (B is false)**. Air in the right atrium may lead to impaired cardiac filling, and therefore a **reduction in cardiac output (A)**.[1,7,11]

102. D – Precordial Doppler

> The most sensitive test for venous air embolism is transesophageal echocardiography. The most sensitive noninvasive monitor is the **precordial Doppler (D)**.[1]

103. C – ST depression

> Subendocardial ischemia is associated with **ST depression (C)** in the anterior leads. Transmural ischemia may lead to **ST elevation (D)** in the electrocardiogram (EKG).[8]

104. A – Decreased thyroid-stimulating hormone (TSH) and decreased free thyroxine (T4)

> Under normal conditions, thyrotropin-releasing hormone (TRH) is secreted by the hypothalamus, driving TSH production by the anterior pituitary and T4 production by the thyroid gland. Primary hypothyroidism is caused by dysfunction of the thyroid gland itself, and would result in **increased levels of TSH and TRH with low T4 levels (D)**. In cases of secondary or tertiary hypothyroidism (pituitary or hypothalamic dysfunction, respectively), there is a **reduction in T4 levels as well as a reduction in TSH levels (A)**. To distinguish between secondary and tertiary hypothyroidism, a TRH challenge must be administered, and the TSH response measured (as TRH is difficult to measure in vivo). In cases of tertiary hypothyroidism (hypothalamic dysfunction), the pituitary gland will appropriately produce TSH in response to a TRH challenge. In secondary hypothyroidism (pituitary dysfunction), the pituitary gland will not produce TSH in response to a TRH challenge test. **Choices B and E** are hyperthyroid states (increased free T4). **Choice C** is a euthyroid state (normal free T4). Note: Occasionally, in patients with hypothyroidism of pituitary or hypothalamic origin, serum TSH concentrations may be slightly increased rather than decreased if the form of TSH secreted is immunoactive but not bioactive.[8,10]

105. A – Calcium

> **Calcium gluconate (A)** infusion is useful for cardiotoxicity (antagonizes the membrane effects of potassium), but it does not reduce serum potassium concentrations. **Cation-exchange resins (B)** such as Kayexalate enhance potassium clearance across the intestinal mucosa reducing serum potassium. **Hemodialysis (C)** is effective for reducing the serum potassium concentration in patients with renal failure. The administration of **insulin (D)** and dextrose causes a transient decrease in serum potassium levels by driving potassium into muscle cells. The administration of **sodium bicarbonate (E)** also causes a transient reduction in serum potassium levels via cellular shifts.[5,8]

106. E – Respiratory alkalosis
107. A – Respiratory acidosis
108. D – Metabolic acidosis and compensatory respiratory alkalosis
109. F – Respiratory alkalosis and compensatory metabolic acidosis
110. B – Respiratory acidosis and metabolic acidosis

111. C – Metabolic acidosis

The first step in the diagnosis of acid–base disorders is determining whether the primary abnormality is an acidosis or an alkalosis, which can be determined by the pH. If the pH and pCO_2 are both abnormal, a change in the same direction indicates a primary metabolic disorder; a change in opposite directions indicates a primary respiratory disorder. If either the pH or pCO_2 is normal, there must be a mixed metabolic and respiratory disorder; if the pH is normal, the direction change in $PaCO_2$ identifies the nature of the respiratory disorder, and if the $PaCO_2$ is normal, the change in pH identifies the nature of the metabolic disorder. If there is a primary metabolic alkalosis or acidosis, the measured serum bicarbonate should be used to calculate the expected pCO_2. If the measured pCO_2 is higher than predicted by the formula, a respiratory acidosis is also present. If the measured pCO_2 is lower than predicted by the formula, a respiratory alkalosis is present. If a primary respiratory acidosis or alkalosis is present, the measured $PaCO_2$ should be used to calculate an expected pH value. If the pH is lower than expected, a metabolic acidosis is also present. If the pH is higher than expected, a metabolic alkalosis is also present. Formulas helpful in the calculation of simple acid–base disturbances are listed here.[4,5]

Acid–base disorder	1 degree abnormality	2 degree response	Expected degree of compensatory response
Metabolic acidosis	Decr. $[HCO_3]$	Decr. pCO_2	$pCO_2 = (1.5 \times [HCO_3]) + 8$
Metabolic alkalosis	Incr. $[HCO_3]$	Incr. pCO_2	$\Delta\, pCO_2 = 0.6 \times \Delta[HCO_3]$
Respiratory acidosis (Chronic)	Incr. pCO_2	Incr. $[HCO_3]$	$\Delta\, [HCO_3] = 0.4 \times \Delta\, pCO_2$
Respiratory alkalosis (Chronic)	Decr. pCO_2	Decr. $[HCO_3]$	$\Delta\, [HCO_3] = 0.50 \times \Delta\, pCO_2$

112. D – $(Cc - Ca)/(Cc - Cv)$

The shunt fraction is the portion of the cardiac output that represents the intrapulmonary shunt (Qs/Qt). The shunt fraction can be estimated from measurements of the oxygen content of arterial blood, mixed venous blood, and pulmonary capillary blood. The shunt fraction is expressed as $(Qs/Qt) = [(Cc - Ca)/(Cc - Cv)]$ **(D)**. Since pulmonary capillary oxygen tension cannot be directly measured, it is estimated with the patient on 100% O_2.[5,14]

113. E – Increased sweating (false)

High doses of atropine (> 10 mg) may cause a **rapid, thready pulse (D)**; **blurry vision (A)**; skin dryness and flushing; ataxia, hallucinations; **dry mouth (C)**; delirium; urinary retention; **decreased intestinal peristalsis (B)**; dilated pupils; and coma. Decreased sweating is a manifestation of atropine toxicity **(E is false)**.[12]

114. C – It is more common in type 1 diabetes mellitus than in type 2 diabetes mellitus (false)

> Hyperosmolar, nonketotic diabetic coma is usually a complication of type 2 diabetes mellitus **(C is false)**. The other responses regarding hyperosmolar nonketotic coma are true. The free fatty acid and glucose concentrations tend to be higher than in ketoacidosis **(A and B)**. Volume depletion is usually more severe **(E)** than in ketoacidosis, and mortality is greater than 50% **(D)**.[8]

115. B – Isoproterenol
116. E – Prazosin
117. C – Phenoxybenzamine
118. D – Phentolamine
119. A – Clonidine

> **Clonidine (A)** is a centrally acting α2 receptor agonist that is used in the treatment of hypertension. **Isoproterenol (B)** is a nonselective β agonist. **Phenoxybenzamine (C)** is an irreversible α agonist that is somewhat selective for α1 receptors. **Phentolamine (D)** is a competitive nonselective antagonist at α1 and α2 receptors. **Prazosin (E)** is a highly selective α1 agonist.[2,8]

120. B – Bethanechol

> **Bethanechol (B)** and **carbachol (C)** selectively stimulate the urinary and gastrointestinal (GI) tract. **Carbachol (C)** is less desirable for urinary retention, however, because it has greater nicotinic action at autonomic ganglia.[12]

121. D – Massive splenomegaly is usually the presenting sign.

> Polycythemia vera is a chronic myeloproliferative disorder that results in increased red cell mass. **It is the most common of the myeloproliferative disorders (C)**. More than 20% of patients present with thrombosis; there is a 10% incidence of abdominal major vessel thrombosis such as the **Budd-Chiari syndrome (A)**. The diagnosis is generally made by increased hemoglobin and hematocrit on routine CBC **(D is false)**. **Hyperuricemia may complicate the disorder (B)**, and **alkylating agents are generally avoided (E)**. Although massive splenomegaly can be the presenting sign, the disorder is usually first recognized by a high hematocrit **(D is false)**.[8,11]

122. B – 285

> Serum osmolarity can be calculated from the formula
>
> $$\text{Serum osmolarity} = 2(\text{Na} + \text{K}) + \text{Glucose}/18 + \text{BUN}/2.8$$
> $$= 2(130 + 4) + 126/18 + 28/2.8$$
> $$= 2(134) + 7 + 10 = 285,$$
>
> where BUN = blood urea nitrogen.[13]

123. B – Decreased physiologic dead space (false)

> Positive end-expiratory pressure (PEEP) **increases physiologic dead space (B is false)** by raising intra-alveolar pressure and lung perfusion, thereby impairing CO_2 elimination.[5]

124. B – I, III (acidosis and fever)

The oxyhemoglobin dissociation curve is shifted to the right by **acidosis (I)**, **fever (III)**, **increased 2,3-diphosphoglyceric acid (DPG [II is false])**, and hypoxemia, and to the left by alkalosis, hypothermia, **banked blood (IV)**, and **decreased 2,3-DPG (II)**.[4,13]

125. A – Appendix

Forty-six percent of carcinoid tumors of the GI tract are located in the **appendix (A)**, the most common site for GI carcinoids. The **ileum (28% [C])** and the **rectum (17% [D])** are less frequently involved.[6,7]

126. A – I, II, III (salicylates, tricyclic antidepressants, and phenobarbital)

The excretion of weak acids is facilitated by alkalinization of the urine and serum. Compounds such as **phenobarbital (III)**, **salicylates (I)**, chlorpropamide, **tricyclic antidepressants (II)**, 2,4-dichlorophenoxyacetic acid, diflunisal, fluoride, and methotrexate are weak acids. **Amphetamines (IV)** are weak bases, the excretion of which is enhanced by acidification of the urine.[12,16]

127. A – Cryoprecipitate
128. D – Neither

von Willebrand's disease is an autosomal dominant condition of altered hemostasis resulting from a deficiency of von Willebrand factor (vWF). vWF, under normal conditions, aids in platelet–platelet and platelet–subendothelial interactions and stabilizes factor VIII. Treatment goals include replacing vWF and factor VIII, which is best accomplished with the administration of **cryoprecipitate (A)**. Hemophilia B is caused by a deficiency of factor IX that causes inadequate generation of thrombin by the coagulation cascade. Historically, **fresh frozen plasma (FFP [B])** was the treatment of choice for factor replacement in hemophilia. The use of FFP, however, has been supplanted by the use of recombinant factor IX, with a reduced risk of bloodborne diseases and transfusion reactions.[11]

129. C – 6 L

Free water deficit can be calculated from the formula:

Free water deficit (L) = [(Na − 140)/140] × body weight (kg) × 0.6
$$= [(160 - 140)/140] \times 70 \times 0.6$$
$$= 20 / 2 \times 0.6 = 6 \text{ L}$$

130. D – Neo-Synephrine (phenylephrine)
131. A – Amrinone (inamrinone)
132. B – Dopamine
133. E – Norepinephrine

134. C – Epinephrine

Amrinone (A) and milrinone are phosphodiesterase inhibitors that prevent the degradation of cAMP, resulting in positive cardiac inotropy and vascular smooth muscle contraction. **Dopamine (B)** has dose-dependent pharmacologic and hemodynamic effects. At intermediate doses, dopamine increases cardiac output via stimulation of cardiac β receptors; at higher doses, peripheral vasoconstriction occurs, which may cause undesirable increases in afterload in patients with a tenuous cardiac status. **Epinephrine (C)** stimulates both α and β adrenergic receptors. **Neo-Synephrine (phenylephrine [D])** is a pure α1 receptor agonist. **Norepinephrine (E)** has similar activity as compared with epinephrine at α and β1 receptors, but has relatively little action at β2 receptors.[8,12,16]

135. C – Hirsutism (false)

Thallium intoxication is characterized by **cardiac dysfunction (A)**, **gastrointestinal disturbance (B)**, **alopecia (C is false)**, **lower limb joint pain (D)**, and **peripheral neuropathy (E)**. Thallium poisoning causes alopecia, not **hirsutism (C)**.[3,17]

136. B – Hypotension (false)

Acute intermittent porphyria is characterized by colicky **abdominal pain (A)**, **psychosis (D)**, **(a predominantly motor) polyneuropathy (C)**, and **tachycardia (E)**. Hypertension, not **hypotension (B)**, typically occurs during an attack.[18]

137. B – Discontinue the offending agent

The triad of bradycardia, hyperlipidemia, and rhabdomyolysis is consistent with a propofol infusion syndrome in this ventilated neuro intensive care patient. This disorder involves the abrupt onset of heart failure, bradycardia, lactic acidosis, hyperlipidemia, and rhabdomyolysis. It typically occurs in the setting of high-dose, prolonged propofol infusions. The most appropriate next step after making the diagnosis is to **discontinue the offending agent (B)**. A **cardiology consult (A)** may be necessary if external pacing is needed, but the propofol needs to be discontinued. **Renal dialysis (E)** may become necessary depending on the severity of the rhabdomyolysis but is not the next best step. **Antibiotic therapy (C)** would be appropriate for sepsis, but not for the propofol infusion syndrome. **Insulin administration (D)** is unlikely to be helpful.[5]

138. D – Waxing and waning hyperpnea regularly alternates with shorter apneic periods

> Cheyne-Stokes respiration is characterized by **waxing and waning hyperpnea regularly alternating with shorter apneic periods (D)** and is thought to be related to isolation of the brainstem respiratory centers from the cerebrum rendering them more sensitive to carbon dioxide. Central neurogenic hyperventilation is an **increase in rate and depth of respiration leading to respiratory alkalosis (C)** associated with lesions of the lower midbrain and upper pontine tegmentum. Apneustic breathing is caused by either basilar artery occlusion or low pontine lesions and is characterized by a **few rapid deep breaths alternating with apneic cycles (2–3 second pause in full inspiration [B])**. With Biot breathing, or ataxic breathing, **breathing is irregularly interrupted and each breath varies in rate and depth (A)**; Biot breathing is associated with lesions of the dorsomedial medulla.[18]

139. B – Increased systolic arterial pressure in response to increased intracranial pressure

> Cushing was the first neurosurgeon to recognize that increases in intracranial pressure (ICP) compromise cerebral blood flow. Cushing's reflex refers to the **rise in systemic arterial pressure (B)** due to **increased sympathetic activity (C is false)** in response to rises in ICP. As the systemic arterial pressure rises, **bradycardia may also occur (A is false)**. The triad of hypertension, bradycardia, and abnormal breathing is known as Cushing's triad.[13,19]

References

1. Barash PG, Cullen BF, Stoelting RK, eds. Clinical Anesthesia, 4th ed. Philadelphia, PA: Lippincott Williams & Wilkins; 2001
2. Katzung BG, ed. Basic and Clinical Pharmacology, 9th ed. New York: McGraw-Hill; 2004
3. Citow JS, Macdonald RL, Refai D, eds. Comprehensive Neurosurgery Board Review. New York: Thieme Medical Publishers; 2009
4. Gomella LG, ed. Clinician's Pocket Reference, 9th ed. New York: McGraw-Hill; 2002
5. Marino P. The ICU Book. Philadelphia, PA: Lippincott, Williams, and Wilkins; 2007
6. Schwartz SI, ed. Principles of Surgery, 7th ed. New York: McGraw-Hill; 1999
7. Kumar VK, Abbas AK, Fausto N, eds. Robbins and Cotran: Pathologic Basis of Disease, 7th ed. Philadelphia, PA: Elsevier; 2005
8. Braunwald E, Fauci AS, et al, eds. Harrison's Principle's of Internal Medicine, 15th ed. New York: McGraw-Hill; 2001
9. Winn HR, ed-in-chief. Neurological Surgery, 5th ed. Philadelphia, PA: W.B. Saunders; 2003
10. Kacsoh B. Endocrine Physiology. New York: McGraw-Hill; 2000
11. Goldman L, Ausiello D, eds. Cecil Textbook of Medicine, 22nd ed. Philadelphia, PA: Saunders; 2004
12. Brunton LL, Lazo JS, Parker KL, eds. Goodman & Gilman's the Pharmacological Basis of Therapeutics, 11th ed. New York: McGraw-Hill; 2006
13. Boron WF, Boulparp EL, eds. Medical Physiology. A Cellular and Molecular Approach. Philadelphia, PA: Elsevier; 2005
14. West JB. Respiratory Physiology: The Essentials, 6th ed. Baltimore, MD: Williams & Wilkins; 2000

15. Apuzzo MLJ. Brain Surgery. Complication Avoidance and Management. New York: Churchill Livingstone; 1993
16. Marini JJ, Wheeler AP. Critical Care Medicine-the Essentials. Baltimore, MD: Williams & Wilkins; 1989
17. Nelson JS, Mena H, Parisi JE, Schochet SS, eds. Principles and Practice of Neuropathology, 2nd ed. New York: Oxford University Press; 2003
18. Ropper AH, Brown RH. Principles of Neurology, 8th ed. New York: McGraw-Hill; 2005
19. Quinones-Hinojosa A, ed. Schmidek & Sweet Operative Neurosurgical Techniques, 6th ed. Philadelphia, PA: Elsevier; 2012

Index

A

A1 segment. *See* anterior cerebral artery
α2βγδ, 169, 189
abciximab (ReoPro), 371, 388
abducens nerve, 21, 50, 50*f*
    Dorello's canal and, 125, 126, 156
    superior orbital fissure and, 125, 126, 156
abducens nucleus, discrete unilateral lesion of, 129, 160
abductor pollicis longus, 3, 31
    posterior interosseous nerve and, 128, 159
abnormal optokinetic response, 56, 85
absence seizures, 72, 102
α-bungarotoxin, 178, 198, 199
abuse, of child, 14, 42
acetylcholine quanta, defect in release of, Eaton-Lambert syndrome and, 65, 93
acetylcholine (ACh) receptor
    receptor, 169, 189
    release of, from neuromuscular junction, 170, 191
ACh. *See* acetylcholine receptor
achromatopsia, 76, 106
acid maltase deficiency, 67, 86
acoustic neuroma, 15, 44, 237, 282
    high-frequency loss and, 70, 99
    middle fossa and, 3, 30
    suboccipital transmeatal approach to, 11, 39
acquired immunodeficiency syndrome (AIDS), 322, 359
    dementia and, 215, 260
acromegaly, carpal tunnel syndrome and, 63, 92
ACTH. *See* adrenocorticotropic hormone
action potential
    events occurring during, 172, 192
    velocity of, 172, 192
acute hyperextension, central cord syndrome and, 66, 95
acute mononeuropathy, diabetes complications and, 66, 95
acute multiple sclerosis, cerebrospinal fluid and, 57
acute subarachnoid hemorrhage, 299, 336
acute type II odontoid fracture, posterior C1-2 instrumented fusion, 24, 53
adductor brevis, obturator nerve and, 132, 164
adductor magnus, sciatic nerve and, 124, 154, 155

adductor pollicis, ulnar nerve and, 113, 143
adenosine, 368, 386
Aδ fibers, 176, 196
Adie's syndrome, characteristics of, 59
adrenocorticotropic hormone (ACTH), 72, 102
    pro-opiomelanocortin and, 171, 191
adrenoleukodystrophy, 214, 259
adults, choroid plexus papillomas in, 297, 335
adult somnambulism, 67, 96
α-fetoprotein, in endodermal sinus tumors, 212, 256
agenesis of corpus callosum, 328, 365
agraphia, alexia without, 61, 90
AICA. *See* anteroinferior cerebellar artery
AIDS. *See* acquired immunodeficiency syndrome
alar ligaments, 133, 165
alar plate, 130, 162
Alexander's disease, 214, 231, 259, 276
alexia, without agraphia, 61, 90
alpha, 56, 86
ALS. *See* amyotrophic lateral sclerosis
Alzheimer's disease, 74, 103
Alzheimer's type II astrocytes, hepatic failure and, 210, 254
amantadine, 65, 95
α-melanocyte-stimulating hormone (MSH), pro-opiomelanocortin and, 171, 191
υ-aminobutyric acid (GABA), deficiency of, 61, 91
AMPA. *See* quisqualate/α-amino-3-hydroxy-5-methyl-4-isoxazoleproprionic acid receptor only
amrinone (inamrinone), 380, 399, 400
amygdala, 119, 149
    anterior choroidal artery and, 112, 142
    stria terminalis and, 120, 149
    telencephalon and, 121, 150
amyloid angiopathy, 215, 241, 260, 286
amyloidosis, carpal tunnel syndrome and, 63, 92
amyotrophic lateral sclerosis (ALS), 61, 75, 91, 105, 211, 234, 255, 279
anaplastic astrocytoma, 238, 283
aneurysms
    anterior communicating artery, diabetes insipidus and, 4, 32
    bacterial arterial (mycotic), subacute bacterial endocarditis and, 14, 43
    bacterial intracranial, 14, 43